New Aspects of the Renin Angiotensin System in Cardiovascular and Renal Diseases

Edited By

Dulce Elena Casarini
Department of Medicine - Nephrology Division
Escola Paulista de Medicina
Universidade Federal de São Paulo
Brazil

Danielle Yuri Arita
Department of Medicine – Nephrology Division
Escola Paulista de Medicina
Universidade Federal de São Paulo
Brazil

Tatiana Sousa Cunha
Department of Science and Technology
Escola Paulista de Medicina
Universidade Federal de São Paulo
Brazil

Juliana Almada Colucci
Department of Medicine – Nephrology Division
Escola Paulista de Medicina
Universidade Federal de São Paulo
Brazil

advertisements or ideas contained in the Work.

Limitation of Liability:

In no event will Bentham Science Publishers, its staff, editors and/or authors, be liable for any damages, including, without limitation, special, incidental and/or consequential damages and/or damages for lost data and/or profits arising out of (whether directly or indirectly) the use or inability to use the Work. The entire liability of Bentham Science Publishers shall be limited to the amount actually paid by you for the Work.

General:

1. Any dispute or claim arising out of or in connection with this License Agreement or the Work (including non-contractual disputes or claims) will be governed by and construed in accordance with the laws of the U.A.E. as applied in the Emirate of Dubai. Each party agrees that the courts of the Emirate of Dubai shall have exclusive jurisdiction to settle any dispute or claim arising out of or in connection with this License Agreement or the Work (including non-contractual disputes or claims).
2. Your rights under this License Agreement will automatically terminate without notice and without the need for a court order if at any point you breach any terms of this License Agreement. In no event will any delay or failure by Bentham Science Publishers in enforcing your compliance with this License Agreement constitute a waiver of any of its rights.
3. You acknowledge that you have read this License Agreement, and agree to be bound by its terms and conditions. To the extent that any other terms and conditions presented on any website of Bentham Science Publishers conflict with, or are inconsistent with, the terms and conditions set out in this License Agreement, you acknowledge that the terms and conditions set out in this License Agreement shall prevail.

Bentham Science Publishers Ltd.
Executive Suite Y - 2
PO Box 7917, Saif Zone
Sharjah, U.A.E.
Email: subscriptions@benthamscience.org

BENTHAM
SCIENCE

CONTENTS

FOREWORD

Research on the pleiotropic actions and consequences of the renin angiotensin system (RAS) and its many effector components remains fascinating and interesting because new surprises continue to emerge and provide fodder for further analysis and new experimental directions. The older paradigm was so straightforward and simple focusing primarily on the circulating RAS and a single effector peptide, angiotensin II [Ang II]. However, we now know that the system is much more complex exhibiting multiple actions of various active components *via* different receptors and utilizing various important enzymatic pathways. In this exciting new e-book by Dr. Casarini and her colleagues, a number of important new concepts are presented which further demonstrate the complexity of the RAS system and the many effector components. As pointed out in the first few chapters, evidence obtained during the previous one or two decades has led to an expanded view of the RAS serving paracrine, intracrine, and endocrine functions. Our attention is also directed to the findings that many other angiotensin peptides also exert bioactive roles.

Several of the subsequent chapters then delve into the intricacies of the local tissue RAS activities focusing on the paracrine and intracrine functions of Ang II in the heart and kidneys as well as other angiotensin peptides including Ang 1-7. The more recently discovered components of the tissue RAS, including ACE2 and the prorenin receptor, are also integrated into the overall interactions that occur at the tissue and cellular level and also within the intratubular network in the kidneys. Our attention is then directed to a consideration of the complex enzymatic pathways that are responsible for the generation of the various angiotensin peptides. The roles of tonin, ACE and ACE2 and ACE polymorphisms are examined.

Additional chapters discuss the novel developments related to the ACE2/Mas axis and how it influences formation and action of Ang 1-7, and our evolving concepts regarding the renin-prorenin receptor and their possible roles in regulating the local formation and activities of Ang 1-7 and the prorenin receptor. Completing the book, the remaining chapters deal with RAS related pathophysiology and the roles of immunity and inflammation activated by Ang II, the interactions with the nitric oxide system and catecholamines, and how emotional stress and exercise may alter the activity of the RAS. Finally, a consideration of how the activity of the RAS is modulated in animal models of hypertension and diabetes provides further insights on pathophysiological contributions of the RAS in disease states.

In this e-book, Dr. Casarini and her associates have provided us with an outstanding array of topics which are covered in-depth and will be of tremendous value not only to investigators directly involved in studies of the RAS but also to all colleagues who are interested in obtaining a comprehensive appreciation of the current state of knowledge regarding the regulation and roles of the many components of the "modern" RAS.

L. Gabriel Navar
Department of Physiology
Center of Biomedical Research
Excellence in Hypertension and Renal Biology
Tulane University School of Medicine
USA

PREFACE

The idea of publishing a book on the new aspects of the renin-angiotensin system (RAS) in cardiovascular and renal diseases has been developed during the past few years. The need for a book that describes the new approaches of the RAS in the development of cardiovascular and renal diseases and the trend of future research became apparent. The book describes the important role of systemic and local RAS in the development of heart and kidney diseases and its relationship with the immune system, stress and exercise; as well as provides data on the biochemical and pathological changes in these diseases.

Understanding the mechanisms of participation of this system in cardiovascular and intrarenal modulation can lead us to better understand the pathogenesis of diseases such as diabetes, hypertension and chronic renal failure. Even knowing the therapeutic interventions for these diseases, there are many challenges in integrating traditional medical literature and increased information of new technologies that facilitate the comprehension of the molecular and cellular mechanisms.

We have been very fortunate to enlist a group of renowned experts in RAS research for this book, and very grateful to the dedication and contribution of our authors. We hope that book will be useful for researchers working in the field of the RAS.

Danielle Yuri Arita
Tatiana Sousa Cunha
Juliana Almada Colucci
Dulce Elena Casarini
Federal University of São Paulo
São Paulo, Brazil

List of Contributors

A.H. Jan Danser	Division of Pharmacology and Vascular Medicine, Department of Internal Medicine, Erasmus MC, Rotterdam, The Netherlands
Alexandre Costa Pereira	Laboratory of Genetic and Molecular Cardiology, Heart Institute, University of Sao Paulo, Sao Paulo, Brazil
Alexis A. Gonzalez	Instituto de Química, Pontificia Universidad Católica de Valparaíso, Chile. Department of Physiology, Tulane University, School of Medicine, New Orleans, LA, USA
Allyson C. Marshall	The Hypertension & Vascular Disease Center, Department of Physiology & Pharmacology, Wake Forest University School of Medicine, Winston-Salem, North Carolina, USA
Amanda Aparecida Ribeiro	Nephrology Division, Department of Medicine, Escola Paulista de Medicina, Universidade Federal de São Paulo, Sao Paulo, Brazil
Anderson José Ferreira	Departments of Morphology, Biological Sciences Institute, Federal University of Minas Gerais, Belo Horizonte, Minas Gerais, Brazil
Andrea Sanches	Department of Physiological Sciences, Piracicaba Dental School, University of Campinas, Brazil
Andréia Cristina Febba Gomes	Nephrology Division, Department of Medicine, Escola Paulista de Medicina, Universidade Federal de São Paulo, Sao Paulo, Brazil
Bryan A. Wilson	The Hypertension & Vascular Disease Center, Department of Physiology & Pharmacology, Wake Forest University School of Medicine, Winston-Salem, North Carolina, USA
Bruno Sevá Pessôa	Nephrology Division, Department of Medicine, Escola Paulista de Medicina, Universidade Federal de São Paulo, Sao Paulo, Brazil
Candice M. Thomas	Division of Molecular Cardiology, Department of Medicine, Texas A&M Health Science Center, College of Medicine; Scott & White; Central Texas Veterans Health Care System, Temple, Texas, USA
Danielle Sanches Aragão	Nephrology Division, Department of Medicine, Escola Paulista de Medicina, Universidade Federal de São Paulo, Sao Paulo, Brazil
Danielle Yuri Arita	Nephrology Division, Department of Medicine, Escola Paulista de Medicina, Universidade Federal de São Paulo, Sao Paulo, Brazil
Debra I. Diz	The Hypertension & Vascular Disease Center, Department of Physiology & Pharmacology, Wake Forest University School of Medicine, Winston-Salem, North Carolina, USA
Dulce Elena Casarini	Nephrology Division, Department of Medicine, Escola Paulista de Medicina, Universidade Federal de São Paulo, Sao Paulo, Brazil

Ebaa Azayadneh	The Hypertension & Vascular Disease Center, Department of Physiology & Pharmacology, Wake Forest University School of Medicine, Winston-Salem, North Carolina, USA
Fernanda Aparecida Ronchi	Nephrology Division, Department of Medicine, Escola Paulista de Medicina, Universidade Federal de São Paulo, Sao Paulo, Brazil
Fernanda Barrinha Fernandes	Nephrology Division, Department of Medicine, Escola Paulista de Medicina, Universidade Federal de São Paulo, Sao Paulo, Brazil
Fernanda Klein Marcondes	Department of Physiological Sciences, Escola de Odontologia de Piracicaba, University of Campinas, Brazil
Fernanda Rezende	University of Mogi das Cruzes, Sao Paulo, Brazil
Flavia F. Jung	Washington Hospital, Washington DC, USA
Hossam A. Shaltout	The Hypertension & Vascular Disease Center, Department of Physiology & Pharmacology, Wake Forest University School of Medicine, Winston-Salem, North Carolina, USA
Ingrid Kazue Mizuno Watanabe	Nephrology Division, Department of Medicine, Escola Paulista de Medicina, Universidade Federal de São Paulo, Sao Paulo, Brazil
Isabela Bezerra Loyola	Nephrology Division, Department of Medicine, Escola Paulista de Medicina, Universidade Federal de São Paulo, Sao Paulo, Brazil
Ivana Cynthia Moraes Silva	University of Sao Paulo, Medical School, Heart Institute, Hypertension Unit, Sao Paulo, Brazil
James C. Rose	The Hypertension & Vascular Disease Center, Department of Physiology & Pharmacology, Wake Forest University School of Medicine, Winston-Salem, North Carolina, USA
Janaína Barcellos Ferreira	University of Sao Paulo Medical School, Heart Institute, Hypertension Unit, Sao Paulo, Brazil
Jorge Luiz Pesquero	Department of Physiology and Biophysics, Biological Sciences Institute, Federal University of Minas Gerais, Minas Gerais, Brazil
José Eduardo Krieger	Laboratory of Genetic and Molecular Cardiology, Heart Institute, University of Sao Paulo, Sao Paulo, Brazil
José Geraldo Mill	Department of Physiological Sciences, Federal University of Espírito Santo, Vitória, Espírito Santo, Brazil
Juliana Almada Colucci	Nephrology Division, Department of Medicine, Escola Paulista de Medicina, Universidade Federal de São Paulo, Sao Paulo, Brazil
Juliana Dinéia Perez Brandão	Nephrology Division, Department of Medicine, Escola Paulista de Medicina, Universidade Federal de São Paulo, Sao Paulo, Brazil
Kátia Bilhar Scapini	University of Sao Paulo, Medical School, Heart Institute, Hypertension Unit, Sao Paulo, Brazil

Kátia De Angelis	Nove de Julho University, Sao Paulo, Brazil
Kenneth M. Baker	Division of Molecular Cardiology, Department of Medicine, Texas A&M Health Science Center, College of Medicine; Scott & White; Central Texas Veterans Health Care System, Temple, Texas, USA
Kleiton Augusto dos Santos	Nephrology Division, Department of Medicine, Escola Paulista de Medicina, Universidade Federal de São Paulo, Sao Paulo, Brazil
L. Gabriel Navar	Department of Physiology and Tulane Hypertension and Renal Center, Tulane University, School of Medicine, New Orleans, LA, USA
Larissa Emi Matsumoto	Nephrology Division, Department of Medicine, Escola Paulista de Medicina, Universidade Federal de São Paulo, Sao Paulo, Brazil
Larissa Miranda Pereira	Division of Molecular Cardiology, Department of Medicine, Texas A&M Health Science Center, College of Medicine; Scott & White; Central Texas Veterans Health Care System, Temple, Texas, USA. Nephrology Division, Department of Medicine, Universidade Federal de São Paulo, Sao Paulo, Brazil
Lília Firoozmand	Science and Technology Institute, Universidade Federal de São Paulo, São José dos Campos, Brazil
Lilian dos Santos	Nephrology Division, Department of Medicine, Escola Paulista de Medicina, Universidade Federal de São Paulo, Sao Paulo, Brazil
Lilian Saemi Arita	Nephrology Division, Department of Medicine, Escola Paulista de Medicina, Universidade Federal de São Paulo, Sao Paulo, Brazil
Lisete C. Michelini	Department of Physiology, Institute of Biomedical Science, University of São Paulo, Sao Paulo, Brazil
Ludimila Forechi	Department of Physiological Sciences, Federal University of Espírito Santo, Vitória, Brazil
Lys Angela Favaroni Mendes Salgado Ribeiro	Nephrology Division, Department of Medicine, Escola Paulista de Medicina, Universidade Federal de São Paulo, Sao Paulo, Brazil
Marcelo Perim Baldo	Department of Physiological Sciences, Federal University of Espírito Santo, Vitória, Espírito Santo, Brazil
Maria Cláudia Costa Irigoyen	University of Sao Paulo Medical School, Heart Institute, Hypertension Unit, Sao Paulo, Brazil
Maria José Costa Sampaio Moura	Life Sciences Center, Pontifical Catholic University of Campinas, Brazil
Marie Doki Nogueira	Nephrology Division, Department of Medicine, Escola Paulista de Medicina, Universidade Federal de São Paulo, Sao Paulo, Brazil

Mark C. Chappell	The Hypertension & Vascular Disease Center, Department of Physiology & Pharmacology, Wake Forest University School of Medicine, Winston-Salem, North Carolina, USA
Mercia de Paula Lima	Department of Physiology and Biophysics, Biological Sciences Institute, Federal University of Minas Gerais, Brazil
Minolfa C. Prieto	Department of Physiology and Tulane Hypertension and Renal Center, Tulane University, School of Medicine, New Orleans, LA, USA
Nádia de Sousa da Cunha Bertoncello	Science and Technology Institute, Universidade Federal de São Paulo, São José dos Campos, Brazil
Nestor Schor	Nephrology Division, Department of Medicine, Escola Paulista de Medicina Universidade Federal de São Paulo, Sao Paulo, Brazil
Qian Chen Yong	Division of Molecular Cardiology, Department of Medicine, Texas A&M Health Science Center, College of Medicine; Scott & White; Central Texas Veterans Health Care System, Temple, Texas, USA
Rafaela Costa	Department of Physiological Sciences, Escola de Odontologia de Piracicaba, University of Campinas, Brazil
Rajesh Kumar	Division of Molecular Cardiology, Department of Medicine, Texas A&M Health Science Center, College of Medicine; Scott & White; Central Texas Veterans Health Care System, Temple, Texas, USA
Rebeca Caldeira Machado	Department of Physiological Sciences, Federal University of Espírito Santo, Vitória, Espírito Santo, Brazil
Roberto Mesquita Soler	Department of Urology, Escola Paulista de Medicina, Federal University of São Paulo, São Paulo, Brazil
Robson Augusto Souza dos Santos	Department of Physiology and Biophysics, Biological Sciences Institute, Federal University of Minas Gerais, Belo Horizonte, MG, Brazil
Rodolfo Mattar Rosa	Nephrology Division, Department of Medicine, Escola Paulista de Medicina, Universidade Federal de São Paulo, Sao Paulo, Brazil
Rodrigo Araújo Fraga-Silva	Institute of Bioengineering, Ecole Polytechnique Fédérale de Lausanne, Lausanne, Switzerland
Rodrigo Yokota	Nephrology Division, Department of Medicine, Escola Paulista de Medicina, Universidade Federal de São Paulo, Sao Paulo, Brazil
Rosana Inácio dos Reis	Department of Biochemistry, Biomembrane Structure Unity, University of Oxford, England, United Kingdom
Roseli Peres Moreira	Nephrology Division, Department of Medicine, Escola Paulista de Medicina, Universidade Federal de São Paulo, Sao Paulo, Brazil
Sebastião Donato Silva Jr	Department of Physiology, Institute of Biomedical Science, University of São Paulo, São Paulo, Brazil

Silvia Lacchinni	Department of Anatomy, Institute of Biomedical Science, University of Sao Paulo, Sao Paulo, Brazil
Tatiana Sousa Cunha	Science and Technology Institute, Universidade Federal de São Paulo, São José dos Campos, Brazil
Valéria Alves Fernades	Departmentof Physiology and Biophysics, Universidade Federal de São Paulo, Brazil
Vander José das Neves	School of Physical Education and Sports, University of Sao Paulo, São Paulo, Brazil
Vanessa Oliveira	Nephrology Division, Department of Medicine, Escola Paulista de Medicina, Universidade Federal de São Paulo, Sao Paulo, Brazil
Wen Chen	Division of Molecular Cardiology, Department of Medicine, Texas A&M Health Science Center, College of Medicine; Scott & White; Central Texas Veterans Health Care System, Temple, Texas, USA
Zaira Palomino Jara	Nephrology Division, Department of Medicine, Escola Paulista de Medicina, Universidade Federal de São Paulo, Sao Paulo, Brazil

New Aspects of the Renin Angiotensin System in Cardiovascular and Renal Diseases

New Aspects of the Renin Angiotensin System in Cardiovascular and Renal Diseases

Editors: Dulce Elena Casarini, Danielle Yuri Arita, Tatiana Sousa Cunha & Juliana Almada Colucci

ISBN (eBook): 978-1-68108-313-1

ISBN (Print): 978-1-68108-314-8

First published in 2016.

CHAPTER 1

Renin Angiotensin System: Old System with New Different Components

Danielle Yuri Arita[1], **Rosana Inácio dos Reis**[2], **Bruno Sevá Pessôa**[1] and **Dulce Elena Casarini**[1,*]

[1] *Nephrology Division, Medicine Department, Escola Paulista de Medicina, Universidade Federal de Sao Paulo, São Paulo, Brazil*

[2] *Department of Biochemistry, Biomembrane Structure Unity, University of Oxford, England, United Kingdom*

Abstract: Recently, the continuing and increasing interest in the renin angiotensin system (RAS) after discovery of new peptides and enzymes, has been stimulating us to review the new concepts described in the literature. The classical RAS is a system in which renin acts on angiotensinogen (Agt) to form angiotensin I (Ang I) that is cleaved to the active peptide angiotensin II (Ang II) by angiotensin converting enzyme (ACE). The Ang II pharmacological actions occur after their interaction with Ang II type 1 and type 2 receptors (AT1R; AT2R). In the last decade, a new concept of local tissue RAS systems has been described in different organs, and also intracellular RAS has been stated, allowing expansion of the concept of functions of this system as endocrine, paracrine, autocrine and intracrine. This first chapter provides brief overview on the history of the RAS components, circulating and tissue RAS, and outlines the physiological functions of the RAS major active substance, Ang II. Here, we also describe other bioactive angiotensins, such as Ang III, Ang IV, Ang (1-7), Ang (1-12), angiotensin A and alamandine. Moreover, we report the studies on ACE2 and chymase, enzymes identified during the last years. The recent advances in the understanding of the RAS will provide new opportunities to treat and prevent hypertension and cardiovascular diseases.

* **Corresponding author Dulce Elena Casarini:** Rua Botucatu, 740 – 2° andar, Department of Medicine/Nephrology Division, Vila Clementino – São Paulo/SP, Brazil CEP 04023-900; Phone: +55 11 5904-1687; E-mail: casarini.elena@unifesp.br.

Dulce Elena Casarini, Danielle Yuri Arita, Tatiana Sousa Cunha & Juliana Almada Colucci (Eds.)

Keywords: ACE, ACE2, Alamandine, Angiotensin A, Angiotensin converting enzyme 2, Angiotensin I-converting enzyme, Angiotensin II, Angiotensin III, Angiotensin IV, Angiotensin (1-7), Angiotensin (1-12), Chymases, Enzymes, RAS, Receptors, Renin, Renin angiotensin system.

INTRODUCTION

Recently, the continuing and increasing interest in the renin angiotensin system (RAS) has been stimulating us to review and present the discoveries concerning the system. To briefly introduce this book, we will describe the classic and new components of the RAS. More than one hundred years ago, Tirgersted and Bergman (1898) discovered the RAS by detecting a pressor effect under intravenous injection when using an alcoholic extracts of renal cortex of rabbits. They called this substance renin [1]. The characterization of renin as an enzyme was proposed by Kohlstaedt *et al.*, in 1940 [2]. At the same period, Braun-Menendez and Irvine (1940) discovered the active substance angiotensin [3] and Skeggs *et al.* (1954) described two forms of this peptide, termed as angiotensin I (Ang I) and angiotensin II (Ang II) [4]. The RAS is a complex hormonal system; it is known that there are two RAS: plasma-localized, which acts *via* blood circulation regulating cardiovascular system function, and tissue-localized, regulating specific long-term changes. Both systems are crucial for hydro-electrolyte balance and blood pressure regulation. In the literature, it has been described that RAS is presently described as an endocrine, paracrine, autocrine and intracrine, system [5]. While, the intracellular system has important role in cellular homeostasis reflecting in renal function.

The RAS modulation is focused on the activity of Ang II, as well as other products of Ang I metabolism, as Ang (1-7), which has contrary actions of Ang II. The cascade is initiated with the formation of the decapeptide Ang I by renin, an aspartyl protease secreted and released by the juxtaglomerular apparatus of the kidney, after cleavage of Leu-Val peptide bond of angiotensinogen (Agt), which is produced by organs as liver, kidney, brain, heart. Prieto *et al.* (2009) described the renin production in the collecting duct cells that are able to liberate in this portion Ang I [6]. Renin produced by kidney is a rate-limiting regulator enzyme of the circulating and tissue RAS activity.

In the circulation renin is released as prorenin that can be converted to active renin by proteolytic and non-proteolytic cleavage. Intracellular renin was described to be derived from local synthesis, but also as a result of uptake from the circulation being active in cellular compartment [7, 8].

Ang I is hydrolyzed to Ang II by angiotensin converting enzyme (ACE), a kininase classified as metallo-endopeptidase [9]. Then, Ang II binds to two specific receptors, Ang II type 1 receptor (AT1R) and Ang II type 2 receptor (AT2R), to follow up biological functions [5, 10]. ACE is expressed on the surfaces of the endothelial cells, epithelial and mesangial cells [8, 11, 12]. Besides of the pulmonary epithelial cells, ACE is also expressed in many other tissues in the organism. In the literature, two ACE forms are described in human as a product of alternative splicing, the germinal and somatic ones. Somatic ACE is expressed in the lung, kidney, intestine, placenta, pancreas, adrenal and choroid plexus. Whilst, the germinal ACE is present in testes during the spermatogenesis. Both forms of ACE are anchored to plasma membrane [13].

ACE have been described as soluble forms in circulation and in many fluids as intestinal and urine [14 - 18]. Further, ACE is able to inactivate bradykinin a vasodilator peptide from Kallikrein-Kinin System. ACE can interact with Ang II and evoke calcium and other signaling molecules in cells expressing only ACE, promoting an increase of reactive oxygen species [19, 20].

On the basis of classical RAS, the pharmacological actions of Ang II occur *via* AT1Rs resulting in cellular proliferation; vasoconstriction, cardiac contractility, increased renal tubule Na^+ reabsorption; aldosterone, vasopressin, and endothelin secretion; activation of the sympathetic nervous system (Fig. **1**).

Ang II also acts *via* AT2Rs but have opposite actions to the AT1Rs under most circumstances [21, 22].

RAAS at Present

RAS profile in the last ten-fifteen years was extended, when new different components appeared, as well as independent actions were described for tissue and circulating systems demonstrating the independence of these two compartments [23 - 26]. Actually, two counter-regulatory pathways were described, the ACE2/Ang (1-7)/Mas receptor axis, and the AT2R pathway, that opposes the actions of AT1R [7].

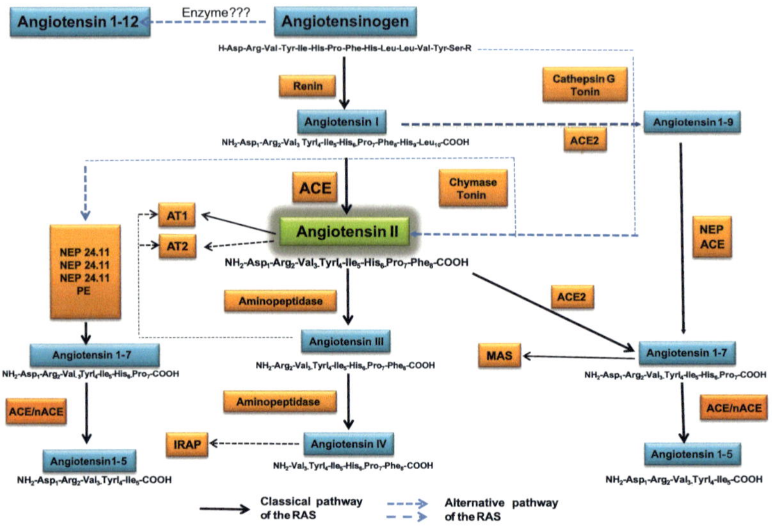

Fig. (1). View of the RAS. RPR, renin/pro renin receptor; Mas, mas oncogene receptor for Ang (1-7); AT2R, angiotensin type 2 receptor; AT1R, angiotensin type 1 receptor; IRAP, insulin-regulated aminopeptidase; Ang IV receptor AMPA, aminopeptidase A; AMPM, aminopeptidase M; ACE, angiotensin converting enzyme; ACE2, angiotensin converting enzyme 2; NEP, Neutral endopeptidase. (Drawn by Casarini, DE. 2015).

The classical elements of the circulating and local RAS are: prorenin, renin, Agt, ACE, Ang I, and Ang II. Other types of angiotensins angiotensin III (Ang III), angiotensin IV (Ang IV), Ang (1-7), receptors renin and prorenin (R/P-R), AT4 or insulin-regulated membrane aminopeptidase (IRAP), Mas and enzymes ACE 2, elastase, chymase, cathepsin G, tonin, are also involved in the RAS functions [22, 25]. In addition to Ang (1-7), other active angiotensin peptides were described in the last years: angiotensin A (Ang A) which has an N-terminal substitution of Ala1 instead of Asp1 Ala1-Ang II [27]; the Ang (1-12), an isolated peptide from rat intestine and present in different organs [28]. Although Ang I generation is abolished by renin inhibitors, they do not inhibit the generation of both Ang A and Ang (1-12), suggesting a renin-independent pathway within tissues.

This topic briefly describes the modulation and physiology of new RAS active enzymes and angiotensins.

ACE2

ACE2 is a metalloenzyme able to hydrolize Ang I to Angiotensin 1-9 (Ang 1-9), and Ang II to generate Ang (1-7) [29, 30] which was described in kidney, heart, hypothalamus, testis and aortic wall. ACE2 and Ang (1-7) play an important role in cardiovascular and renal physiology, counterbalancing the activity and actions of ACE and Ang II [31, 32]. The detection of ACE2 activity in kidney and heart increased in rats treated with ACE inhibitors evidenciated the local production of Ang (1-7) [33]. Especially in the kidney ACE2 has a protective role regulating the effects of Ang II [22].

Chymase

Chymase is an enzyme stored in secretory granules of mast cells and its activity is only detected in tissues but not in the circulation. The enzyme is inactive in normal vascular tissue; however, it can generate Ang II in damage arterial walls [34]. Cardiac chymase is important in atherosclerosis [35], type 2 diabetes [36], and heart failure [37]. Ahmad *et al.* (2014) described the presence of Ang-1-12 and chymase in the diseased cardiomyocytes of neonatal rat myocytes and human atrial appendages [38]. It was postulated that the intracellular generation of of Ang II *via* chymase pathway is independent of inhibition of Ang II formation by ACE inhibitors or AT1 receptors blockers [39].

Angiotensin III and IV

Aminopeptidases are enzymes able to cleave Ang II generating Ang III and Ang IV. Ang III has similar function as Ang II acting *via* AT1 or AT2 receptors resulting in vasoconstriction and release of aldosterone [22].

Ang III is cleaved by aminopeptidase M producing Ang IV that has effects different from those described for other angiotensins. Ang IV cause vasorelaxation in cerebral, renal, and vascular beds binding to the specific receptor named as insulin-regulated aminopeptidase (IRAP) found in specialized vesicles containing the insulin-sensitive glucose transporter GLUT4. Despite the binding with the specific receptor, this peptide can also binding the AT1 receptor [8, 40].

Angiotensin (1-7)

ACE2 is able to cleave Ang I forming Ang 1- 9, which is degraded by ACE to Ang 1- 7. ACE2 and prolil carboxipeptidase hydrolizes Ang II to Ang 1- 7. Furthermore, Neutral endopeptidases and Prolyl endopeptidases are able to hydrolize Ang I and Ang II to generate Ang 1- 7 [22]. This peptide was described as a vasodilator peptide antagonizing the pharmacological actions of Ang II mediated *via* AT1R [31, 41].

Ang (1-7) mediates vasodilating and antiproliferative actions through Mas receptor, an orphan heterotrimeric guanine nucleotide-binding protein-coupled receptor [42]. Ferraro *et al.* (2005) showed that this peptide showed in vascular endothelial and smooth muscle cells an anti-growth action to facilitate diuresis and natriuresis, and acted as an antiarrhythmic agent [43].

Moreover, Ang (1-7) potentiates the vasodilation caused by bradykinin [42, 43].

Angiotensin (1-12)

Nagata *et al.* (2006) described a dodecapeptide Ang (1-12) from the rat small intestine [44]. This peptide opens a possibility of alternative Ang II generation, more dependent on chymase than renin action in the heart. In rats, Ang (1-12) increased blood pressure, which was abrogated by the administration of ACE inhibitors and antagonists of AT1R [45, 46].

High levels of Ang (1-12) were detected in aorta, heart, and kidneys, differing from circulating levels that are lower than those of Ang I and Ang II. These differences suggested a dissociation of the physiological role of this peptide in tissues and circulation [47]. Chymase is an enzyme able to cleave Ang (1-12) in the heart. In plasma, this peptide is hydrolyzed by ACE generating Ang I. Moniwa *et al.* (2013) described the action of ACE upon Leu10- Leu11 bond of Ang (1-12) generating Ang I [28].

Although the enzyme responsible for the production of Ang (1-12) from Agt was not described in the literature, some authors suggested the enzymes kallikrein, cathepsin, and chymase as possible candidates.

Angiotensin A

Ang A was described in human plasma as a result of Ang II modification, by enzymatic decarboxylation of Asp1 generating Ala1-Ang II [48]. This peptide has affinity for both AT1Rs and AT2Rs, but higher for AT2Rs. The pressor and renal vasoconstrictor effects of Ang A were described in rats similarly as those of Ang II through AT1Rs [49].

The quantification of Ang A plasma levels is very difficult even when using nano-liquid chromatography–tandem mass spectroscopy assay [48].

Alamandine

Alamandine is the new angiotensin peptide generated from Ang A by human ACE-2 [27]. This peptide has in the N-terminal portion the substitution of Asp1 by Ala1 Ala1-Ang (1-7) (Ala^1-Arg^2-Val^3-Tyr^4,Ile^5,His^6-Pro^7). Alamandine has similar properties to Ang (1-7), but differs from Ang A, which presents vasoconstrictor actions. Moreover, Alamandine might exert its actions through MrgD receptor [50, 51]. Similarly to Ang (1-7), Alamandine induces blood pressure reduction when administered in spontaneously hypertensive rats. Studies with aortic rings from Mas deficient mice demonstrated that alamandine induced vasorelaxation [51]. The real function of circulating Alamandine in humans is uncertain, despite the increased levels in patients with end-stage renal disease, [27].

PERSPECTIVES

The discovery of Ang (1-12) and Alamandine and its receptor MrgD, expanded the concepts of the RAS. Ang (1-12) was described as an important peptide in the heart suggesting the importance of tissue RAS. The local tissue RAS assumes an important physiological and pathophysiological role, especially with the description of Ang II being able to intracellularly modulate the renal Na^+ reabsorption in proximal tubule and blood pressure. The recent advances in the understanding of the components and actions of the RAS show that this system regulates more physiological functions than previously believed. It will provide the opportunities to treat and prevent hypertension and cardiovascular diseases.

CONFLICT OF INTEREST

The authors confirm that they have no conflict of interest to declare for this publication.

ACKNOWLEDGEMENTS

We would like to thank CAPES [Coordenação de Aperfeiçoamento de Pessoal de nível Superior], CNPq [Conselho Nacional de Desenvolvimento Científico e Tecnológico] and FAPESP [Fundação de Amparo a Pesquisa do Estado de São Paulo].

REFERENCES

[1] Tigerstedt R, Bergman P. Niere und Kreislauf. Skand Arch Physiol 1898; 8(1): 223-71. [http://dx.doi.org/10.1111/j.1748-1716.1898.tb00272.x]

[2] Kohlstaedt KG, Page IH. The liberation of renin by perfusion of kidneys following reduction of pulse pressure. J Exp Med 1940; 72(2): 201-16. [http://dx.doi.org/10.1084/jem.72.2.201] [PMID: 19871017]

[3] Braun-Menendez E, Fasciolo JC, Leloir LF, Muñoz JM. The substance causing renal hypertension. J Physiol 1940; 98(3): 283-98. [http://dx.doi.org/10.1113/jphysiol.1940.sp003850] [PMID: 16995204]

[4] Skeggs LT Jr, Marsh WH, Kahn JR, Shumway NP. The existence of two forms of hypertensin. J Exp Med 1954; 99(3): 275-82. [http://dx.doi.org/10.1084/jem.99.3.275] [PMID: 13130799]

[5] Kumar R, Thomas CM, Yong QC, Chen W, Baker KM. The intracrine renin-angiotensin system. Clin Sci 2012; 123(5): 273-84. [http://dx.doi.org/10.1042/CS20120089] [PMID: 22590974]

[6] Prieto-Carrasquero MC, Botros FT, Kobori H, Navar LG. Collecting Duct Renin: A major player in Angiotensin II-dependent Hypertension. J Am Soc Hypertens 2009; 3(2): 96-104. [http://dx.doi.org/10.1016/j.jash.2008.11.003] [PMID: 20046983]

[7] Carey RM. Newly discovered components and actions of the renin-angiotensin system. Hypertension 2013; 62(5): 818-22. [http://dx.doi.org/10.1161/HYPERTENSIONAHA.113.01111] [PMID: 24082058]

[8] Herichova I, Szantoova K. Renin-angiotensin system: upgrade of recent knowledge and perspectives. Endocr Regul 2013; 47(1): 39-52.

[http://dx.doi.org/10.4149/endo_2013_01_39] [PMID: 23363256]

[9] Frühbeck G. The adipose tissue as a source of vasoactive factors. Curr Med Chem Cardiovasc Hematol Agents 2004; 2(3): 197-208.
[http://dx.doi.org/10.2174/1568016043356255] [PMID: 15320786]

[10] Bermann MA, Walsh MF, Sowers JS. Angiotensin-II Biochemistry and Physiology: Update on Angiotensin-I1 Receptor. Blockers. Cardiovasc Drug Rev 2007; 15: 75-100.
[http://dx.doi.org/10.1111/j.1527-3466.1997.tb00325.x]

[11] Camargo de Andrade MC, Di Marco GS, de Paulo Castro Teixeira V, *et al.* Expression and localization of N-domain ANG I-converting enzymes in mesangial cells in culture from spontaneously hypertensive rats. Am J Physiol Renal Physiol 2006; 290(2): F364-75.
[http://dx.doi.org/10.1152/ajprenal.00110.2005] [PMID: 16106038]

[12] Mei Wang PH, Andrade MC, Quinto BM, *et al.* N-domain angiotensin-I converting enzyme is expressed in immortalized mesangial, proximal tubule and collecting duct cells. Int J Biol Macromol 2015; 72: 380-90.
[http://dx.doi.org/10.1016/j.ijbiomac.2014.07.043] [PMID: 25193099]

[13] Wei L, Alhenc-Gelas F, Soubrier F, Michaud A, Corvol P, Clauser E. Expression and characterization of recombinant human angiotensin I-converting enzyme. Evidence for a C-terminal transmembrane anchor and for a proteolytic processing of the secreted recombinant and plasma enzymes. J Biol Chem 1991; 266(9): 5540-6.
[PMID: 1848554]

[14] Casarini DE, Alves KB, Araujo MS, Stella RC. Endopeptidase and carboxypeptidase activities in human urine which hydrolyze bradykinin. Brazilian journal of medical and biological research = Revista brasileira de pesquisas medicas e biologicas / Sociedade Brasileira de Biofisica (et al) 1992; 25(3): 219-9.
[PMID: 1341917]

[15] Casarini DE, Carmona AK, Plavnik FL, Zanella MT, Juliano L, Ribeiro AB. Calcium channel blockers as inhibitors of angiotensin I-converting enzyme. Hypertension 1995; 26(6 Pt 2): 1145-8.
[http://dx.doi.org/10.1161/01.HYP.26.6.1145] [PMID: 7498985]

[16] Deddish PA, Marcic B, Jackman HL, Wang HZ, Skidgel RA, Erdös EG. N-domain-specific substrate and C-domain inhibitors of angiotensin-converting enzyme: angiotensin-(1-7) and keto-ACE. Hypertension 1998; 31(4): 912-7.
[http://dx.doi.org/10.1161/01.HYP.31.4.912] [PMID: 9535414]

[17] Hattori MA, Del Ben GL, Carmona AK, Casarini DE. Angiotensin I-converting enzyme isoforms (high and low molecular weight) in urine of premature and full-term infants. Hypertension 2000; 35(6): 1284-90.
[http://dx.doi.org/10.1161/01.HYP.35.6.1284] [PMID: 10856278]

[18] Marques GD, Quinto BM, Plavinik FL, Krieger JE, Marson O, Casarini DE. N-domain angiotensin I-converting enzyme with 80 kDa as a possible genetic marker of hypertension. Hypertension 2003; 42(4): 693-701.
[http://dx.doi.org/10.1161/01.HYP.0000085784.18572.CB] [PMID: 12900433]

[19] Lazartigues E, Feng Y, Lavoie JL. The two fACEs of the tissue renin-angiotensin systems: implication

in cardiovascular diseases. Curr Pharm Des 2007; 13(12): 1231-45. [http://dx.doi.org/10.2174/138161207780618911] [PMID: 17504232]

[20] Guimarães PB, Alvarenga EC, Siqueira PD, *et al.* Angiotensin II binding to angiotensin I-converting enzyme triggers calcium signaling. Hypertension 2011; 57(5): 965-72. [http://dx.doi.org/10.1161/HYPERTENSIONAHA.110.167171] [PMID: 21422380]

[21] Carey RM, Siragy HM. Newly recognized components of the renin-angiotensin system: potential roles in cardiovascular and renal regulation. Endocr Rev 2003; 24(3): 261-71. [http://dx.doi.org/10.1210/er.2003-0001] [PMID: 12788798]

[22] Fyhrquist F, Saijonmaa O. Renin-angiotensin system revisited. J Intern Med 2008; 264(3): 224-36. [http://dx.doi.org/10.1111/j.1365-2796.2008.01981.x] [PMID: 18793332]

[23] Albiston AL, McDowall SG, Matsacos D, *et al.* Evidence that the angiotensin IV (AT(4)) receptor is the enzyme insulin-regulated aminopeptidase. J Biol Chem 2001; 276(52): 48623-6. [http://dx.doi.org/10.1074/jbc.C100512200] [PMID: 11707427]

[24] Danser AH. Local renin-angiotensin systems: the unanswered questions. Int J Biochem Cell Biol 2003; 35(6): 759-68. [http://dx.doi.org/10.1016/S1357-2725(02)00178-4] [PMID: 12676161]

[25] De Mello WC, Frohlich ED. Clinical perspectives and fundamental aspects of local cardiovascular and renal Renin-Angiotensin systems. Front Endocrinol (Lausanne) 2014; 5: 16. [http://dx.doi.org/10.3389/fendo.2014.00016] [PMID: 24600438]

[26] Paul M, Poyan Mehr A, Kreutz R. Physiology of local renin-angiotensin systems. Physiol Rev 2006; 86(3): 747-803. [http://dx.doi.org/10.1152/physrev.00036.2005] [PMID: 16816138]

[27] Lautner RQ, Villela DC, Fraga-Silva RA, *et al.* Discovery and characterization of alamandine: a novel component of the renin-angiotensin system. Circ Res 2013; 112(8): 1104-11. [http://dx.doi.org/10.1161/CIRCRESAHA.113.301077] [PMID: 23446738]

[28] Moniwa N, Varagic J, Simington SW, *et al.* Primacy of angiotensin converting enzyme in angiotensin-(1-12) metabolism. Am J Physiol Heart Circ Physiol 2013; 305(5): H644-50. [http://dx.doi.org/10.1152/ajpheart.00210.2013] [PMID: 23812388]

[29] Donoghue M, Hsieh F, Baronas E, *et al.* A novel angiotensin-converting enzyme-related carboxypeptidase (ACE2) converts angiotensin I to angiotensin 1-9. Circ Res 2000; 87(5): E1-9. [http://dx.doi.org/10.1161/01.RES.87.5.e1] [PMID: 10969042]

[30] Tipnis SR, Hooper NM, Hyde R, Karran E, Christie G, Turner AJ. A human homolog of angiotensin-converting enzyme. Cloning and functional expression as a captopril-insensitive carboxypeptidase. J Biol Chem 2000; 275(43): 33238-43. [http://dx.doi.org/10.1074/jbc.M002615200] [PMID: 10924499]

[31] Danilczyk U, Penninger JM. Angiotensin-converting enzyme II in the heart and the kidney. Circ Res 2006; 98(4): 463-71. [http://dx.doi.org/10.1161/01.RES.0000205761.22353.5f] [PMID: 16514079]

[32] Der Sarkissian S, Huentelman MJ, Stewart J, Katovich MJ, Raizada MK. ACE2: A novel therapeutic target for cardiovascular diseases. Prog Biophys Mol Biol 2006; 91(1-2): 163-98.

[http://dx.doi.org/10.1016/j.pbiomolbio.2005.05.011] [PMID: 16009403]

[33] Ishiyama Y, Gallagher PE, Averill DB, Tallant EA, Brosnihan KB, Ferrario CM. Upregulation of angiotensin-converting enzyme 2 after myocardial infarction by blockade of angiotensin II receptors. Hypertension 2004; 43(5): 970-6.
[http://dx.doi.org/10.1161/01.HYP.0000124667.34652.1a] [PMID: 15007027]

[34] Timmermans PB, Wong PC, Chiu AT, *et al.* Angiotensin II receptors and angiotensin II receptor antagonists. Pharmacol Rev 1993; 45(2): 205-51.
[PMID: 8372104]

[35] Ihara M, Urata H, Kinoshita A, *et al.* Increased chymase-dependent angiotensin II formation in human atherosclerotic aorta. Hypertension 1999; 33(6): 1399-405.
[http://dx.doi.org/10.1161/01.HYP.33.6.1399] [PMID: 10373223]

[36] Rafiq K, Sherajee SJ, Fan YY, *et al.* Blood glucose level and survival in streptozotocin-treated human chymase transgenic mice. Chin J Physiol 2011; 54(1): 30-5.
[http://dx.doi.org/10.4077/CJP.2011.AMM008] [PMID: 21786536]

[37] Kokkonen JO, Lindstedt KA, Kovanen PT. Role for chymase in heart failure: angiotensin II-dependent or -independent mechanisms? Circulation 2003; 107(20): 2522-4.
[http://dx.doi.org/10.1161/01.CIR.0000074786.92067.AA] [PMID: 12777313]

[38] Ahmad S, Varagic J, Groban L, *et al.* Angiotensin-(1-12): a chymase-mediated cellular angiotensin II substrate. Curr Hypertens Rep 2014; 16(5): 429.
[http://dx.doi.org/10.1007/s11906-014-0429-9] [PMID: 24633843]

[39] Ferrario CM, Ahmad S, Nagata S, *et al.* An evolving story of angiotensin-II-forming pathways in rodents and humans. Clin Sci 2014; 126(7): 461-9.
[http://dx.doi.org/10.1042/CS20130400] [PMID: 24329563]

[40] Chai SY, Fernando R, Peck G, *et al.* The angiotensin IV/AT4 receptor. Cell Mol Life Sci 2004; 61(21): 2728-37.
[http://dx.doi.org/10.1007/s00018-004-4246-1] [PMID: 15549174]

[41] Burns KD. The emerging role of angiotensin-converting enzyme-2 in the kidney. Curr Opin Nephrol Hypertens 2007; 16(2): 116-21.
[http://dx.doi.org/10.1097/MNH.0b013e3280123c0e] [PMID: 17293686]

[42] Santos RA, Ferreira AJ. Angiotensin-(1-7) and the renin-angiotensin system. Curr Opin Nephrol Hypertens 2007; 16(2): 122-8.
[http://dx.doi.org/10.1097/MNH.0b013e328031f362] [PMID: 17293687]

[43] Ferrario CM, Trask AJ, Jessup JA. Advances in biochemical and functional roles of angiotensin-converting enzyme 2 and angiotensin-(1-7) in regulation of cardiovascular function. Am J Physiol Heart Circ Physiol 2005; 289(6): H2281-90.
[http://dx.doi.org/10.1152/ajpheart.00618.2005] [PMID: 16055515]

[44] Nagata S, Kato J, Sasaki K, Minamino N, Eto T, Kitamura K. Isolation and identification of proangiotensin-12, a possible component of the renin-angiotensin system. Biochem Biophys Res Commun 2006; 350(4): 1026-31.
[http://dx.doi.org/10.1016/j.bbrc.2006.09.146] [PMID: 17045572]

[45] Cummins PM. A new addition to the renin-angiotensin peptide family: proAngiotensin-12 (PA12). Cardiovasc Res 2009; 82(1): 7-8.
[http://dx.doi.org/10.1093/cvr/cvp053] [PMID: 19211622]

[46] Kobori H, Nangaku M, Navar LG, Nishiyama A. The intrarenal renin-angiotensin system: from physiology to the pathobiology of hypertension and kidney disease. Pharmacol Rev 2007; 59(3): 251-87.
[http://dx.doi.org/10.1124/pr.59.3.3] [PMID: 17878513]

[47] Ferrario CM. New physiological concepts of the renin-angiotensin system from the investigation of precursors and products of angiotensin I metabolism. Hypertension 2010; 55(2): 445-52.
[http://dx.doi.org/10.1161/HYPERTENSIONAHA.109.145839] [PMID: 20026757]

[48] Jankowski V, Vanholder R, van der Giet M, *et al.* Mass-spectrometric identification of a novel angiotensin peptide in human plasma. Arterioscler Thromb Vasc Biol 2007; 27(2): 297-302.
[http://dx.doi.org/10.1161/01.ATV.0000253889.09765.5f] [PMID: 17138938]

[49] Yang R, Smolders I, Vanderheyden P, *et al.* Pressor and renal hemodynamic effects of the novel angiotensin A peptide are angiotensin II type 1A receptor dependent. Hypertension 2011; 57(5): 956-64.
[http://dx.doi.org/10.1161/HYPERTENSIONAHA.110.161836] [PMID: 21464395]

[50] Gembardt F, Grajewski S, Vahl M, Schultheiss HP, Walther T. Angiotensin metabolites can stimulate receptors of the Mas-related genes family. Mol Cell Biochem 2008; 319(1-2): 115-23.
[http://dx.doi.org/10.1007/s11010-008-9884-4] [PMID: 18636314]

[51] Balakumar P, Jagadeesh G. A century old renin-angiotensin system still grows with endless possibilities: AT1 receptor signaling cascades in cardiovascular physiopathology. Cell Signal 2014; 26(10): 2147-60.
[http://dx.doi.org/10.1016/j.cellsig.2014.06.011] [PMID: 25007996]

CHAPTER 2

The Important Role of Systemic and Local Renin-Angiotensin System

Danielle Sanches Aragão, Lilian Saemi Arita, Rodrigo Yokota, Lilian dos Santos, Larissa Emi Matsumoto, Marie Doki Nogueira, Fernanda Aparecida Ronchi and **Danielle Yuri Arita***

Nephrology Division, Medicine Department, Escola Paulista de Medicina, Universidade Federal de São Paulo, Sao Paulo, Brazil

Abstract: Knowledge of renin-angiotensin system (RAS) has evolved through the years from the classical endocrine system view, which explains the homeostasis and arterial blood pressure control, to a more complex system, including new components and independent local RAS acting intracellularly and within different organs. It is well-known that the circulating RAS plays a physiological and important role in blood pressure regulation through direct effects on vascular smooth muscle, aldosterone secretion and sodium, potassium and water equilibrium. The potent vasopressor peptide Angiotensin (Ang) II is the key regulator of the system and the Ang 1-7 counter-regulates Ang II actions. Components are generated in liver (angiotensinogen), kidneys [renin] and vascular endothelial cell membranes (angiotensin I -converting enzyme) and secreted to the circulation to generate systemic Ang II. Recently, the focus of interest in the RAS changed the role of tissue/local system in specific tissue. Ang II synthesis within tissues from angiotensinogen and enzymes is defined as local RAS. The activation of the circulating and/or local RAS plays a fundamental role in the pathogenesis of hypertension and chronic kidney disease. RAS blockade with angiotensin I-converting enzyme (ACE) inhibitors or Ang II receptor blockers is a major approach to treat cardiovascular and renal diseases. However, it is still unclear if a dual blockade exerts a better protection than single blockade or shows a higher risk for renal complications and hyperkalemia.

* **Corresponding author Danielle Yuri Arita:** Rua Botucatu, 740 – 2° andar, Department of Medicine/Nephrology Division Vila Clementino – Sao Paulo/SP, Brazil CEP 04023-900; Phone: +55 11 5904-1687; E-mail: arita@unifesp.br.

Dulce Elena Casarini, Danielle Yuri Arita, Tatiana Sousa Cunha & Juliana Almada Colucci (Eds.)

Keywords: ACE inhibitors, Angiotensinogen, Angiotensins, Angiotensin converting enzyme 2, Angiotensin I-converting enzyme, Angiotensin II-receptor blockers, Cardiac diseases, Cells, Chronic kidney diseases, Heart, Kidney, Local RAS, RAS blockade, Renin, Renin-angiotensin system, Systemic RAS.

CLASSICAL AND NEW VISION OF THE RAS

The renin-angiotensin system (RAS) has been studied for more than a century and the deep investigative research over the last years have well established the role of the RAS as a main component in the control of arterial blood pressure, cardiovascular, renal and adrenal function, and fluid and electrolyte homeostasis. RAS is identified as a dual vasoactive system, acting as both a circulating endocrine and a local tissue paracrine system [1 - 5].

In the classical view, the RAS is a hormone coordinated cascade of sequential enzymatic steps, which the first is the release of angiotensinogen (AGT) produced in the liver, cleaved by renin, which is released from the juxtaglomerular cells in the kidney generating angiotensin I (Ang I). This peptide is further processed by angiotensin-I converting enzyme (ACE) into angiotensin II (Ang II), the key regulator of the system. In addition, alternative enzymes generate Ang II, such as cathepsins and chymase, however it has been established that ACE is the key enzyme in the regulation of Ang II production in the cascate [1, 3, 6].

Ang II is a potent vasoconstrictor acting on different target organs, including blood vessels, kidney and heart. This peptide influences many physiological processes such as fluid and electrolyte balance, homeostasis and blood pressure. The effects of this potent peptide are mediated by two different receptors: AT1 and AT2. AT1 receptor (AT1R) is responsible for the majority action of Ang II in the heart, kidney and adrenal glands, including vasoconstriction, aldosterone and vasopressin release, sodium and water retention, cell proliferation and sympathetic facilitation. In most cases, the actions of the AT2 receptor (AT2R) counterbalance to those of the AT1R and are partly mediated by activation of kallikrein-kinin system [7].

Due to the great importance of the RAS, many studies have been conducted and important discoveries have been occurred and contributed to a new vision of this system, such as the identification of new enzymes, new peptides, novel receptors and new functions. In 2000, two distinct groups described a new ACE homologue enzyme, called ACE2, which catalyzes Ang II into the biologically active peptide, angiotensin 1-7 (Ang 1-7) and also cleaves Ang I into angiotensin 1-9 (Ang 1-9), an inactive peptide. Importantly, the metabolization of Ang II into Ang 1-7 by ACE2 is much more efficient than the conversion of Ang I into Ang 1-9 [8, 9]. Ang 1-7 generation was also demonstrated by the cleavage of Ang I by the neutral endopeptidase also called neprilysin, a cell surface zinc metalloendopeptidase involved in peptide hydrolysis at the extracellular surface of the plasma membrane [10]. In 2007, Santos *et al.* [11] described the new receptor for Ang 1-7, the Mas proto-oncogene, which is mainly expressed in many organs, such as brain, testis, kidney, heart and vessels [12]. Studies demonstrate that Ang 1-7 contributes to the control of blood pressure in the cardiovascular and renal systems *via* actions that, within the heart, kidney, and the blood vessels, opposing the actions of Ang II [11, 13].

There are other active peptides generated through the cleavage of Ang II that may have important actions in the local RAS. Among them, the angiotensin III (Ang III) is generated by the cleavage of Ang II by aminopeptidase A, which is itself converted to angiotensin IV (Ang IV) by aminopeptidase N. These peptides have affinity to AT1R and AT2R, and AT2R and IRAP (insulin-regulated aminopeptidase), respectively. The interaction of Ang IV with its receptor, AT4R, has been comprehensively reviewed and research findings about Ang III and Ang IV lead to the conclusion that theses peptides are biologically active in the brain, supporting the possibility that Ang I and Ang II are precursor molecules for these active forms [5, 14]. Despite the existence of other components of the system, Ang II is still considered as the primary effector hormone of the RAS.

Tissue Sites of Local RAS

Nowadays, the existence of local or tissue-based RAS and angiotensin production at tissue sites is firmly established, being described as a key player in the pathophysiology of cardiovascular and renal diseases [5, 15, 16]. In the tissue RAS, Ang II is generated from components that are mainly of local origin. In some tissues, the enzymes responsible for producing Ang II from AGT may be different from the circulating RAS, like cathepsin D and chymase [6].

The synthesis of most of RAS components has been detected in the heart, being 75% of cardiac Ang II is synthesized locally [17]. RAS components are also found in the kidney and distinguished amounts of Ang II can be formed in the tissue sites [15]. Besides the presence of local RAS in the heart and kidneys, components of the system were described in other tissues like liver, pancreas, adrenal glands, brain, blood vessels, and adipose tissue, acting as a autocrine and/or paracrine system [5].

The local RAS exerts different actions in several organs. In some organs, the tissue system operates independently of the circulating one, however, at the kidney and heart, local and systemic RAS act in cooperation. In fact, the RAS is now considered much more than an autocrine regulatory system involved in fluid and salt hemodynamic. The presence of tissue-based RAS has conducted to the finding of new roles for angiotensins as paracrine and autocrine or even intacrine systems [4, 5]. Growing interest has led on the possibility that the local production of Ang II may be more important than circulating Ang II in tissue sites of local RAS such as the control of cardiovascular and renal function.

The Intracellular RAS

Evidences suggest the existence of an intracellular (intacrine) RAS (iRAS) may be present through different theoretical pathways [3 - 5].

1) The first, a transient iRAS, which the components formed intracellularly are transferred *via* secretory vesicles to the cell surface. Renin, angiotensinogen and ACE providing from intravesicular generation of Ang II are transported by these secretory vesicles. Intracellularly formed Ang II would be used *in situ* and/or secreted [18]; 2) The second, a non-secreted constitutive system, which is formed by a differently spliced non-secreted renin isoform; a membrane bound ACE and Ang receptors mainly localized in the mitochondria and nucleus [19 - 21]. 3) The third, a hybrid system described as the interaction between the secreted and constitutive iRASs. The roles of the intracellular RASs are distinct, which are located in different compartments subcellularly and are controlled separately from the autocrine/paracrine RAS [22]. All components must be confined within the

same cell to have a functional and independently operated intracellular system [23]. Studies suggest that intracellular RAS may have a predominant role in some cell types and pathological conditions [24].

Renin is a secretory glycoprotein produced, stored and released by the kidney. The intracellular isoforms can also be found in the heart, brain and adrenal glands. Renin can be expressed by secreted (pro)renin and a non-secreted intracellular renin. This type of renin is produced exclusively for use within the cell as it lacks the signal peptide that allows it to be secreted and is constitutively active. Renin has been detected inside the cell in the cytosol, nucleus and mitochondria. It has been described a possibility of an association between AT1R in the nuclei and intracellular renin regulation, suggesting that the components of the iRAS are located in different compartments inside the cell. The cytosolic renin protein exerts functions different and even opposite to those of secretory renin. The iRenin is driven into mitochondria *via* an ATP-dependent mechanism and the membrane potential of the organelle, showing an important role in mitochondrial bioenergetics. Whereas secretory renin increases necrotic death rates of cardiac cells, the cytosolic renin isoform even protects cells from necrotic death. Renin overexpression in mitochondria leads to enhanced cell apoptosis. However, it remains unknown if this form of renin has specific actions inside the cell [21, 25, 26].

Recent evidences support the concept about production of AGT locally in central and peripheral tissues, in contradiction to the previous concept about the exclusivity production of AGT by the liver. The AGT messenger ribonucleic acid (mRNA) has been found in several organs, such as heart, kidney, pancreas, adrenal gland, uterus, ovary, brain pituitary, endothelial cells and adipocytes, [3, 27]. AGT is situated into nuclei and cytoplasm [28] and, as renin and ACE, intracellular AGT seems to be synthesized in a non-glycosylated form by post-translational alteration and is not released. Studies showed that high glucose conditions resulted an accumulation of AGT intracellularly, whereas extracellular AGT concentration remained relatively unchanged [20, 29, 30].

ACE is found in a membrane-bound and in a soluble secreted form that are involved in the generation of intracellular Ang II. This enzyme has also been localized into nuclei and cytoplasm of renal, smooth muscle and endothelial cells [31, 32]. Large quantities of ACE has been found in the endoplasmic reticulum as well [33]. It has been shown differential regulation of extracellular and intracellular ACE. Furthermore, ACE inhibitors (ACEI), that are effective in blocking the production of Ang II by the extracellular form of the enzyme, these drugs have failed to inhibit intracellular ACE [20], probably due to the lack of intracellular uptake of ACEI. The aminopeptidases, APA and APN, are also found intracellularly in high amounts in plasma membranes of renal proximal tubule cells and in the brain [34, 35].

It has been described the presence of nonsecreted Ang I in different tissues including cardiac myofibroblasts and pancreatic cells, similar to the non-secreted intracellular renin, and it is involved in tissue repair and organogenesis [36, 37]. The existence of a complete and independently regulated iRAS has been shown through rising levels of intracellular renin that leads to the enhancement of intracellular Ang levels, consequently activating the intracardiac RAS associated with heart damage [23]. Ang II can be produced within secretory vesicles from AGT, renin, and ACE. Thus, Ang II can be formed and retained intracellularly from iAGT [18, 38]. Ang II are located in different cell types as cardiac myocytes, hepatoma cells, renal juxtaglomerular cells, renal proximal tubule cells, vascular smooth muscle cells and several types of brain cells [39]. It has been reported that cardiac myocytes, fibroblasts, vascular smooth muscle cells, renal proximal tubule cells synthesize Ang II intracellularly [5, 40, 41]. ATRs (types 1 and 2) are also abundant intracellularly demonstrated in many cell types [22]. Newer components were included to the RAS receptor family such as the renin/(pro)renin receptor, the AT4R and Ang 1–7 receptor in renal cells [23]. Stimulation of intracellular RAS can lead to overexpression of angiotensin receptors in the mitochondria, nucleus or plasma membranes. Different conditions, such as high glucose, can promote the enhancement of formation and migration of intracellular Ang II to the nucleus. This peptide modulates the expression of AGT and renin, generating a feedback loop [29].

The Circulating and Local RAS in Cardiovascular and Renal Homeostasis

The activity of the circulating RAS is stated mainly by renin and substantial alteration in circulating renin levels can occur rapidly, leading to changes in Ang I formation. Major stimulators of intrarenal renin released are low sodium chloride concentrations, low renal arterial pressure and epinephrine/norepinephrine. Main inhibitors of renin secretion in the kidney are Ang II, potassium and atrial natriuretic peptide.

Circulating Ang II and peptides including Ang 1-7, Ang III and Ang IV have significant biological activity through interactions with specific transmembrane receptor. Studies demonstrate that Ang 1-7 contributes to the control of blood pressure in cardiovascular and renal systems *via* actions that, within the heart, kidney, and the blood vessels, opposed the Ang II activity [11, 13]. Ang 1-7 binding to Mas receptor leads to protective actions such as vasodilatation and nitric oxide (NO) production. On the other hand, Ang III and Ang IV activities are lower than those of Ang II [14].

In the Heart

Originally, renin and its mRNA were described in the heart in 1987 [42] as well as other components of RAS required for Ang II biosynthesis in the cardiac tissue. These components are distributed in cardiomyocytes and fibroblasts, in the endothelium and vascular smooth cells of coronary arteries and vessels, evidencing a local cardiac RAS and, consequently, Ang II formation [5, 16].

Renin has been detected in cardiac atria, ventricles, and primary cultures of neonatal and adult rat ventricular myocytes. Renin mRNA levels in neonatal and adult cardiac myocytes and neonatal isolated fibroblasts are <1% of the levels reported for kidney. In human, renin mRNA has been found in the atrium and right ventricle, and renin immunostaining has been detected in the endothelium and vascular smooth muscle of coronary arteries and veins, as well as in capillaries of the myocardium [43].

Firstly, it was proposed that the cardiac (pro)renin was captured from the circulation and it was taken into the heart. This uptake means diffusion through the interstitial space and/or interaction with (pro)renin specific receptors [44]. In addition, subsequent studies confirmed the presence of three (pro)renin-binding proteins called ((P)RnBPs) that bind to (pro)renin in the tissues, acting as a (pro)renin carriers: 1) An intracellular (P)RnBP that reduces the Ang I generated by renin, being similar to the enzyme N-acyl-D-glucosamine 2-epimerase [45]; 2) The mannose 6-phosphate insulin-like growth factor II (M6P/IGFII) that not only interacts and internalizes proteins like (pro)renin with high affinity, but also stimulates prohormones intracellularly (including prorenin) [46]; 3) A high affinity receptor originally described in human mesangial cells and which gene encodes for a 350-amino acid protein, differing from any known proteins. The receptor-bound renin exhibited enhanced catalytic activity as compared to soluble form. It is able to activate prorenin as well [47, 48].

AGT is expressed in atrial muscle and neuronal fibers of conduction system and low levels in the ventricle [49]. Although it is more readily detectable than renin, cardiac mRNA of AGT is found in a lesser amount in heart than in liver, the major source of AGT production [27]. Studies using radiolabeled Ang I- and Ang II-infused indicate that most of both cardiac Ang I and Ang II are synthesized locally, and most of the Ang II is mainly originated using *in situ* synthesized Ang I [50]. And despite the synthesis of AGT exists in the cardiac tissue, we must consider that this peptide is also captured from the circulation. In other words, even though there is a local production of Ang I and Ang II, this synthesis is not dependent on production of local renin and AGT [4]. The AGT and its mRNA may have their levels enhanced in the heart by the actions of glucocorticoids, estrogen and thyroid hormones [51].

ACE is found in coronary endothelial cells and cardiac fibroblast, in larger quantities in atrium than ventricles, in all four valves, coronary vessels, aorta, pulmonary arteries, endocardium and epicardium [52].

ACE2, which cleaves Ang II into Ang 1-7 and may exert a protective effect on cardiac function and in the heart, is located in the membrane of cardiac myocytes [8]. In the heart, the conversion of Ang I to Ang II is mediated by chymase and, in human myocardial extracts, the conversion of chymase can reach over 80%, while the ACE is not greater than 11%. This suggests that chymase is an important pathway in cardiac tissue [53]. However, this issue still remains controversial because there is evidence that ACEI are extremely effective for treating heart disease [54], and in experimental conditions, these same inhibitors can block the formation of Ang II in intact cardiac veins [55]. Furthermore, as previously mentioned, endothelial cells of the vascular system can also mediate the formation of Ang II by capturing renin from circulation [56]. In cardiac fibroblasts, synthesis of Ang II occurs only in secretory pathways mediated by action of renin and ACE, stimulated by high glucose and isoprenaline [57].

Fibroblasts and cardiomyocytes express both AT1R and AT2R. However, fibroblasts recruit AT2R only in pathological conditions. While the activation of the AT1R results in stimulation of hypertrophy and proliferation of cardiac cells, the AT2R promotes the reverse effect [58 - 60].

In summary, a complete intracellular system for Ang II synthesis and actions, including signaling mechanisms and cellular effects, has been described in the heart [58, 61].

In the Kidney

Mesangial cells have all components of the RAS including renin, AGT, AT1R, somatic ACE and N-domain ACE, ACE2 and angiotensins, showing the existence of an intrarenal RAS which seems to be regulated independently of the conventional RAS present in the bloodstream [30, 31]. All RAS components were also detected in epithelial cells of the proximal tubule [62], glomerular endothelial cells [63] and collecting duct cells [64]. ACE N-domain is located in the nucleus of mesangial cells in primary culture and seems to be responsible for transcription of new genes [31]. Vidotti *et al.* [30] demonstrated the secretion of (pro)renin by mesangial cells in basal conditions, but in the presence of high concentrations of glucose occur a decrease of this secretion. After 72 hours incubation with high glucose medium, only the messenger RNA for angiotensinogen and ACE were high in mesangial cells. This indicates that high glucose concentrations induce increased generation of Ang II in these cells resulting in higher intracellular renin activity mediated by three different factors: time-dependent stimulation of transcription of the gene of (pro)renin, decreased secretion of (pro)renin and increased conversion of (pro)renin to active renin *via* cathepsin B.

Renin can also be found in proximal tubule which suggests to be endocytosed from the filtrate and stored in subapical vesicles [65], and minor renin concentrations have been determined in the tubule fluid [66]. However, substantial intratubular levels of Ang I (10- fold greater than in plasma) appear to be formed locally [67].

ACE is abundantly expressed in proximal brush border membrane and it may provide the proximity of enzyme-substrate interaction necessary for generating intratubular Ang II. Nevertheless, alternative ACE-independent pathways appear to exist. Ang II levels in proximal tubule were approximately 100-fold higher than those in plasma, showing that the proximal tubule produces and secretes Ang II at levels greater than can be accounted by glomerular filtration [68]. ACE2 may counterbalance classical RAS effects in part by metabolizing Ang II to the heptapeptide, Ang 1–7, which activates the receptor Mas, thus antagonizing the effects of local Ang II. For this reason, the role of ACE2 has received importance for recent studies [69].

Renal proximal tubule cells grown in high glucose medium showed elevated intracellular Ang II levels that were associated with increased N-acetyl-β-glucosaminidase secretion and p22*phox* protein levels. Treatment with ARBs normalized those levels, suggesting the involvement of intracellular Ang II in mediating the high-glucose effects [70]. Despite abundant evidence for the expression and function of RAS components in the proximal nephron, their precise localization is not well known with regard to the dualism between local biosynthesis and endocytotic uptake/intracellular processing [71].

Role of the RAS in Cardiac and Chronic Kidney Diseases

Disorders of RAS importantly contribute to the pathophysiology of heart and kidney diseases with subsequent complications such as myocardial infarction, chronic heart failure and end-stage renal disease. The discovery of the local RAS has revolutionized the thinking about the role of this system in cardiovascular and renal diseases [15, 16, 67].

The physiological function of the classical RAS is to maintain vascular tone through direct on vascular smooth muscle cells (VSCM) and salt and water homeostasis through aldosterone secretion [72]. Lately, the growing interest in the RAS changed the role of tissue/local RAS in specific tissue. Ang II is the major active product of the system, as mentioned before and acts directly on contraction VSCM, enhances myocardial contractility, increases sympathetic nervous system activity, stimulates thirst and salt appetite, stimulates release of catecholamines from adrenal gland and sympathetic nerve endings. Locally produced, Ang II has pathophysiological functions in cardiovascular diseases including hypertension, atherosclerosis, and heart failure, which are associated with endothelial dysfunction, vascular hyperactivity, and structural remodeling. Increased Ang II levels are also related to inflammation, apoptosis, cells growth, mitogenesis, migration and differentiation, regulation of gene expression of bioactive substances, and active multiples intracellular signaling pathways, all processes which might lead for tissue damage [67].

The local RAS has been demonstrated to have a role in hypertrophy, inflammation, fibrosis, thrombosis and oxidative stress, independent of systemic Ang II [24]. Increased levels of local Ang II are found in the heart under pathological conditions such as myocardial dysfunction, diabetes and infarction. Moreover, direct effects of this local peptide on tissue have been associated with the mechanism of end-organ damage, resulting in kidney and heart failure [24, 67].

In CKD, pathogenic mechanisms, independent from onset injury, leads to glomerular filtration changes, proteinuria, fibrosis and progressive renal function loss. Inappropriate RAS activation has been described as the largest contributor event to glomerular hypertension. Ang II is the key component in these glomerular hemodynamic alterations, determinative to progressive renal injury [67, 73]. Certainly, angiotensin-dependent mechanisms are commonly involved in glomerular capillary hypertension, which is caused by augmented systemic blood pressure and afferent arterioles vasoconstriction. Furthermore, the key peptide promotes progressive renal injury directly through several mechanisms such as immune activation, increased extracellular matrix deposition and induction of growth factor release [74].

Increased blood pressure is a physiological prevent contributor to the affection of the renal microcirculation. The pressure coming from the systemic circulation to the glomerular capillary is reduced, while glomerular hydrostatic pressure remains relative stable despite changes in blood pressure. When the auto-control response fail, it enhances hydrostatic pressure of the glomerulus, proteinuria and hyperfiltration [75].

Intrarenal RAS activity has many pathophysiological functions besides in blood pressure regulation but also in production of glomerulosclerosis and renal cell growth that contributes to the development of renal fibrosis [67, 73]. Glomerular diseases are divided into two main categories: glomerulosclerosis and glomerulonephritis due to many conditions with variety genetic and environmental factors. Although glomerulosclerosis and glomerulonephritis present distinct causes, they can both conduct to renal failure [76]. Activation of the AT1R pathway triggers pro-inflammatory mediators generation, cell proliferation and extracellular matrix synthesis that contribute to kidney injury and progress chronic kidney disease [77, 78]. It is well known that intrarenal RAS activation is major mediator of progressive renal injury in glomerulonephritis [79]. Intrarenal Ang II is augmented in chronic glomerulonephritis, promoting changes in intraglomerular pressure, increase glomerular hypertrophy, and augmented extracellular matrix deposition. Chronic glomerulonephritis is frequently characterized by progression to end-stage renal disease [79, 80].

Blocking the Systemic and Local RAS

As mentioned above, Ang II is responsible for several complications in cardiac and chronic kidney disease. Given a significant function of Ang II in provoking and maintaining glomerular hypertension and proteinuria and its harmful effects, the protection of the kidney by Ang II inhibition has been extensively studied [81, 82]. If the RAS is over active, blood pressure will be too high. Besides enhancing blood pressure by several actions, such as vasoconstriction and sodium and fluid retention, Ang II is also involved in development of atherosclerosis and contributes cardiovascular remodeling through induction of hypertrophy and fibrosis in heart [57]. Furthermore, *via* AT1R, Ang II acts as a potent activator of vascular NADPH oxidase promoting oxidative stress in the vascular wall [83]. Alternative proteases, such as chymase, kallikrein and cathepsin G, are responsible for ACE-independent Ang II production [6]. On the other hand, AT2R activation causes vasodilation and contrary actions of AT1R, such as anti-fibrotic and anti-inflammatory effects.

Several studies have been accomplished to compare the treatment with ACEI and ARB in hypertensive cardiovascular diseases, mainly renal function [84 - 86]. ACEI and ARB are effective in the treatment of hypertension and associated end-organ damage. Nevertheless, many evidences have shown that renal or cardiac failure commonly advances, even treating with RAS inhibitors. These considerations show incomplete RAS blockade and accentuate the requirement for more aggressive intervention, such as increasing dose or combination therapy [22].

Most hypotensive drugs are designed to block the RAS at different points in the pathway. RAS blockade with ACEIs or ARBs is important in the treatment of essential hypertension, [87], and heart and kidney diseases [88 - 93]. These drugs reduce cardiovascular morbidity and mortality in patients with heart failure or left ventricular dysfunction, and after myocardial infarction [94]. RAS inhibition also slows up the onset of renal insufficiency in individuals with chronic proteinuric nephropathy of diabetic or non-diabetic source [89, 95].

Besides antihypertensive effect, Ang II inhibition acts locally in the vasculature [96] and the kidney, decreasing intraglomerular pressure, improving glomerular barrier size selectivity, and reducing proteinuria [97]. Studies with ACEIs and ARBs have shown that the renoprotective benefit of these drugs is due to the antiproteinuric effect [98, 99], since the proteins cross the glomerular membrane, contributing to the ongoing renal fibrosis [100]. Both types of drugs limit the effects of Ang II. However, their mechanisms of action differ from each other.

Treatment with ACEIs *e.g.* lisinopril, ramipril, trandolapril, enalapril, lisinopril, fosinopril, perindopril, quinapril and captopril decreases plasma and local Ang II by inhibiting ACE and leading to increased levels of Ang I [101]. However, ACEIs do not fully prevent Ang II formation because other enzymes in alternative pathways, such as chymase and cathepsin G, are capable of generating Ang II [102]. ACEIs also promote the accumulation of peptides, such as bradykinin (BK) [103] and Ang 1–7 [104]. Consequently, it stimulates the release of NO, prostacyclin and other vasodilatory substances [103] through B2 receptor, inducing vasodilation and natriuresis. Nevertheless, the excessive local levels of of BK and/or substance P has also been associated to uncomfortable or serious adverse events in ACEIs-treated patients ACEIs such as coughing and angioneurotic edema [105].

ARBs (*e.g.*, valsartan, losartan, candesartan, telmisartan, olmesartan, and irbesartan) block the AT1R, inhibiting the vasoconstrictor and proliferative effects of Ang II [102], also caused by alternative pathways not blocked by ACEIs. After ARB administration The increase in plasma Ang II levels is related with the augmentation in renin release from juxtaglomerular cells [106]. This blockade also stimulates the AT2R, activating a vasodilatory and natriuretic cascade including BK, NO and cyclic GMP [107, 108]. However, ARBs blocking AT1R prevent the uptake of Ang II and the stimulation of intrarenal AGT decreasing intrarenal production of Ang II [109, 110]. It was reported that Ang II were enhanced in kidney of Ang II-infused hypertensive rats and this augmentation was prevented by ARBs [111, 112].

Indeed, renal and systemic Ang II generation is caused by increases in plasma renin levels and long-term enhance in renin formation after treatment with ACEIs and ARBs. Thereby, the use of direct renin inhibitors (DRIs) (*e.g.* aliskiren, enalkiren, remikiren, and zankiren) which specifically block the renin-angiotensinogen reaction — the first and rate-limiting step in the RAS - is to improve the therapy of hypertension [113]. Aliskiren has demonstrated antihypertensive and renoprotective efficacy lowering intrarenal Ang I and Ang II in transgenic rats for human renin and AGT [114 - 116]. Several clinical studies have been conducted to analyze the safety, tolerability and efficacy of aliskiren for long-term treatment [115, 117].

Therefore, although ACEIs and ARBs raise plasma renin levels, they promote the production of different angiotensin peptides in plasma [118]. ARBs enhance all angiotensin peptides, including Ang II and III and Ang 1–7 and ACEIs stimulate Ang I and Ang 1–7 and decrease Ang II and III generation. DRIs completely inhibit all angiotensin peptides formation [119, 120].

Optimizing RAS Blockade

In the treatment with ACEI, the conversion of Ang I to Ang II is blocked, leading to increase of Ang I. With chronic use of ACEIs, the levels of Ang II are restored nearly to baseline levels due alternative pathways where Ang I is converted by Ang II [121]. Consequently, local Ang II production presumably continues despite blockade of the RAS systemically by ACE inhibition [122]. Furthermore, ACEI therapy promotes the up-regulation of the AT1R, which are responsible for the development of some cardiovascular events such as vascular and cardiac hypertrophy, inflammatory process, fibrosis and apoptosis [123].

Specific and full blockade of the AT1R may also avoid all deleterious effects of systemic or local [124]. Nevertheless, Ang II levels increase considerably, resulting in an "overstimulation" of non-AT1R, including the AT2R, which has uncertain effects and, under certain experimental conditions, mediate deleterious effects on the cardiovascular system [121, 125]. Also, it has been reported that AT2Rs localized in adult kidney are responsible for a variety of events associated to renal disease [121]. In addition, the efficacy of ARBs may be further compromised with long-term use, because increased Ang II may compete with and displace ARBs from AT1R [126].

DRIs blocks renin activity, however this inhibition by itself is not effective since renin levels further enhances and the generation Ang I from angiotensinogen *via* non-renin pathways continues [125]. Furthermore, high plasma renin activity has also been related with the target organ damage, including kidney dysfunction and left ventricular hypertrophy in the heart [125, 127].

For all these compensatory responses, the "single blockade" results in a partial and temporary suppression of the RAS [128], since these drugs have different mechanisms of action for blocking the system, each one interfering in one specific step of the cascade [129]. RAS inhibition at two different points by using ACEI and ARBs has various clinical and pathophysiological advantages and disadvantages [122, 124].

Many studies with various degrees of congestive heart failure, such as the Randomized Evaluation of Strategies for Left Ventricular Dysfunction

(RESOLVD), Valsartan Heart Failure Trial (Val-HeFT) and Candesartan in Heart Failure Assessment of Reduction in Mortality (CHARM-ADDED) trials, have reported that dual blockade of the RAS inhibition, using ACEI and ARB, significantly decreases the morbidity in some patients compared with monotherapy. In the other hand, the Ongoing Telmisartan Alone and in combination with Ramipril Global Endpoint Trial (ONTARGET) and Valsartan in Acute Myocardial Infarction Trial (VALIANT) trials showed that dual RAS blockade did not further reduce events. [123, 129 - 131]. Moreover, the combination therapy augmented significantly the proportion of discontinuation due to hypotensive symptoms, syncope, decreased kidney function and hyperkalemia [121, 129 - 133].

The dual blockade has been most frequently used to prevent kidney disease [134]. Studies of meta-analysis demonstrate that ACEI combined with ARB significantly decreases proteinuria in both diabetic and nondiabetic patients [135].

In The Candesartan and Lisinopril in Microalbuminuria CALM study showed that the combined therapy presented better results in systolic blood pressure and albumin-creatinine than monotherapy, however serum creatinine and potassium concentration were slightly increased after combined treatment. Nevertheless, the CALM II study, using a high dose of ACEI, showed similar results in systolic blood pressure and albumin excretion rates compared to dual blockade [131, 136, 137].

In The Irbesartan in the Management of Proteinuric Patients at High Risk for Vascular Events (IMPROVE), despite the slightly reduction in blood pressure, the results showed no further improvement on urinary albumin excretion in individuals with microalbuminuria. However, patients presenting high rates of albumin excretion rates had a trend toward improve with dual blockade [128, 133]. On the other hand, the Valsartan in Combination With Lisinopril *Versus* the Respective High Dose Monotherapies in Hypertensive Patients With Microalbuminuria (VALERIA) trial reported that the dual therapy presented better results in reducing microalbuminuria despite that adverse events, such as hypotension, were slightly higher [131].

There are several studies that have investigated the dual blockade using ACEI in and ARB, some showed satisfactory results and some showed the opposite. Thereby, there are not enough data concerning the safety and efficacy of combination therapy [138]. The ideal dose for an ACEI or ARB as monotherapy or in combined therapy for an effective and total inhibition of the RAS is still uncertain.

More recently, the use of Direct Renin Inhibitors (DRIs) has been used as a new strategy to treatment of hypertension. Since the renin participates in the first and rate-limiting step in the production of Ang II, it has been postulated that DRIs, in combination with ECAI or with ARBs, may provide more complete RAS blockade and additional benefits [139].

The Aliskiren in the Evaluation of Proteinuria in Diabetes (AVOID) trial showed that the aliskiren associated with losartan reduced urinary albumin to creatinine ratio by 20% more than monotherapy with losartan, showing an organ protective properties of the treatments [123, 132, 140]. In the Aliskiren Left Ventricular Assessment of Hypertrophy (ALLAY) study, patients showed reduction in left ventricular mass with treatment with aliskiren and losartan, indicating that dual therapy using DRI may help slow or reverse cardiac end-organ damage [132]. Nevertheless, although several trials showed the effectiveness and safety of aliskiren as either monotherapy or in addition with other antihypertensive drugs have shown interesting results in the treatment of hypertension, higher side effects were expressed in patients receiving the renin inhibitor associated with ACEI or ARB in the Aliskiren Trial in Type 2 Diabetes Using Cardio-Renal Endpoints (ALTITUDE) trial, such as non-fatal stroke, renal complications, hyperkalemia, and hypotension [141]. Furthermore, the recent trial Six Months Efficacy and Safety of Aliskiren Therapy on Top of Standard Therapy, on Morbidity and Mortality in Patients with Acute Decompensated Heart Failure (ASTRONAUT) showed no improvement in the morbidity and mortality in patients with cardiovascular complications [142].

Taken together, given that the single agents can achieve only partial and not durable suppression of the RAS, it has been hypothesized that combination therapy would be more effective than either agent alone [121, 128, 129].

Numerous observational studies have suggested the use of a dual blockade of the RAS to benefit from a better cardiorenal protection since it could provide more effective inhibition of the RAS and has been considered a major approach to treat hypertension, cardiovascular and renal diseases [125, 143]. However, recent randomized controlled studies showed a higher risk for renal complications and hyperkalemia [133]; and benefits of RAS blockade must be weighed against its possible adverse effects particularly in elderly patients. Thus, the knowledge of the new RAS components are not entirely clear and are stimulating further research to elucidate the increasing complexity of this system. The new discoveries could leads to an understanding about RAS acting as a permissive contributor for the remodeling of the cardiovascular and renal systems in normal and pathophysiological conditions.

CONFLICT OF INTEREST

The authors confirm that they have no conflict of interest to declare for this publication.

ACKNOWLEDGEMENTS

The authors thank CAPES (Coordenação de Aperfeiçoamento de Pessoal de nível Superior), CNPq (Conselho Nacional de Desenvolvimento Científico e Tecnológico) and FAPESP (Fundação de Amparo a Pesquisa do Estado de São Paulo) for research grants and fellowships.

REFERENCES

[1] Skeggs LT, Dorer FE, Levine M, Lentz KE, Kahn JR. The biochemistry of the renin-angiotensin system. Adv Exp Med Biol 1980; 130: 1-27. [http://dx.doi.org/10.1007/978-1-4615-9173-3_1] [PMID: 6250339]

[2] Herichova I, Szantoova K. Renin-angiotensin system: upgrade of recent knowledge and perspectives. Endocr Regul 2013; 47(1): 39-52. [http://dx.doi.org/10.4149/endo_2013_01_39] [PMID: 23363256]

[3] Campbell DJ. Circulating and tissue angiotensin systems. J Clin Invest 1987; 79(1): 1-6. [http://dx.doi.org/10.1172/JCI112768] [PMID: 3025255]

[4] Paul M, Poyan Mehr A, Kreutz R. Physiology of local renin-angiotensin systems. Physiol Rev 2006; 86(3): 747-803. [http://dx.doi.org/10.1152/physrev.00036.2005] [PMID: 16816138]

[5] Kumar R, Thomas CM, Yong QC, Chen W, Baker KM. The intracrine renin-angiotensin system. Clin Sci 2012; 123(5): 273-84.
[http://dx.doi.org/10.1042/CS20120089] [PMID: 22590974]

[6] Kumar R, Boim MA. Diversity of pathways for intracellular angiotensin II synthesis. Curr Opin Nephrol Hypertens 2009; 18(1): 33-9.
[http://dx.doi.org/10.1097/MNH.0b013e32831a9e20] [PMID: 19077687]

[7] Kaschina E, Unger T. Angiotensin AT1/AT2 receptors: regulation, signalling and function. Blood Press 2003; 12(2): 70-88.
[http://dx.doi.org/10.1080/08037050310001057] [PMID: 12797627]

[8] Tipnis SR, Hooper NM, Hyde R, Karran E, Christie G, Turner AJ. A human homolog of angiotensin-converting enzyme. Cloning and functional expression as a captopril-insensitive carboxypeptidase. J Biol Chem 2000; 275(43): 33238-43.
[http://dx.doi.org/10.1074/jbc.M002615200] [PMID: 10924499]

[9] Vickers C, Hales P, Kaushik V, *et al.* Hydrolysis of biological peptides by human angiotensin-converting enzyme-related carboxypeptidase. J Biol Chem 2002; 277(17): 14838-43.
[http://dx.doi.org/10.1074/jbc.M200581200] [PMID: 11815627]

[10] Turner AJ, Isaac RE, Coates D. The neprilysin (NEP) family of zinc metalloendopeptidases: genomics and function. Bioessays: News and Reviews in Molecular. Cellular and Developmental Biology 2001; 23(3): 261-9.

[11] Santos RA, Ferreira AJ. Angiotensin-(1-7) and the renin-angiotensin system. Curr Opin Nephrol Hypertens 2007; 16(2): 122-8.
[http://dx.doi.org/10.1097/MNH.0b013e328031f362] [PMID: 17293687]

[12] Metzger R, Bader M, Ludwig T, Berberich C, Bunnemann B, Ganten D. Expression of the mouse and rat mas proto-oncogene in the brain and peripheral tissues. FEBS Lett 1995; 357(1): 27-32.
[http://dx.doi.org/10.1016/0014-5793(94)01292-9] [PMID: 8001672]

[13] Chappell MC. Emerging evidence for a functional angiotensin-converting enzyme 2-angiotensin-(1-7)-MAS receptor axis: more than regulation of blood pressure? Hypertension 2007; 50(4): 596-9.
[http://dx.doi.org/10.1161/HYPERTENSIONAHA.106.076216] [PMID: 17785634]

[14] Bosnyak S, Jones ES, Christopoulos A, Aguilar MI, Thomas WG, Widdop RE. Relative affinity of angiotensin peptides and novel ligands at AT1 and AT2 receptors. Clin Sci 2011; 121(7): 297-303.
[http://dx.doi.org/10.1042/CS20110036] [PMID: 21542804]

[15] Zhuo JL, Li XC. New insights and perspectives on intrarenal renin-angiotensin system: focus on intracrine/intracellular angiotensin II. Peptides 2011; 32(7): 1551-65.
[http://dx.doi.org/10.1016/j.peptides.2011.05.012] [PMID: 21699940]

[16] De Mello WC, Frohlich ED. On the local cardiac renin angiotensin system. Basic and clinical implications. Peptides 2011; 32(8): 1774-9.
[http://dx.doi.org/10.1016/j.peptides.2011.06.018] [PMID: 21729730]

[17] Danser AH, van Kats JP, Admiraal PJ, *et al.* Cardiac renin and angiotensins. Uptake from plasma *versus in situ* synthesis. Hypertension 1994; 24(1): 37-48.
[http://dx.doi.org/10.1161/01.HYP.24.1.37] [PMID: 8021006]

[18] Inagami T, Nakamaru M, Pandey KN, *et al.* Intracellular action of renin, angiotensin production and release. J Hypertens Suppl 1986; 4(4): S11-6.
[PMID: 3021940]

[19] Casarini DE, Boim MA, Stella RC, Krieger-Azzolini MH, Krieger JE, Schor N. Angiotensin I-converting enzyme activity in tubular fluid along the rat nephron. Am J Physiol 1997; 272(3 Pt 2): F405-9.
[PMID: 9087685]

[20] Cristovam PC, Arnoni CP, de Andrade MC, *et al.* ACE-dependent and chymase-dependent angiotensin II generation in normal and glucose-stimulated human mesangial cells. Exp Biol Med (Maywood) 2008; 233(8): 1035-43.
[http://dx.doi.org/10.3181/0708-RM-229] [PMID: 18480420]

[21] Clausmeyer S, Stürzebecher R, Peters J. An alternative transcript of the rat renin gene can result in a truncated prorenin that is transported into adrenal mitochondria. Circ Res 1999; 84(3): 337-44.
[http://dx.doi.org/10.1161/01.RES.84.3.337] [PMID: 10024308]

[22] Kumar R, Singh VP, Baker KM. The intracellular renin-angiotensin system: a new paradigm. Trends Endocrinol Metab 2007; 18(5): 208-14.
[http://dx.doi.org/10.1016/j.tem.2007.05.001] [PMID: 17509892]

[23] Abadir PM, Walston JD, Carey RM. Subcellular characteristics of functional intracellular renin-angiotensin systems. Peptides 2012; 38(2): 437-45.
[http://dx.doi.org/10.1016/j.peptides.2012.09.016] [PMID: 23032352]

[24] Singh VP, Le B, Khode R, Baker KM, Kumar R. Intracellular angiotensin II production in diabetic rats is correlated with cardiomyocyte apoptosis, oxidative stress, and cardiac fibrosis. Diabetes 2008; 57(12): 3297-306.
[http://dx.doi.org/10.2337/db08-0805] [PMID: 18829990]

[25] Wanka H, Kessler N, Ellmer J, *et al.* Cytosolic renin is targeted to mitochondria and induces apoptosis in H9c2 rat cardiomyoblasts. J Cell Mol Med 2009; 13(9A): 2926-37.
[http://dx.doi.org/10.1111/j.1582-4934.2008.00448.x] [PMID: 18671756]

[26] Eggena P, Zhu JH, Clegg K, Barrett JD. Nuclear angiotensin receptors induce transcription of renin and angiotensinogen mRNA. Hypertension 1993; 22(4): 496-501.
[http://dx.doi.org/10.1161/01.HYP.22.4.496] [PMID: 8406654]

[27] Dzau VJ, Ellison KE, Brody T, Ingelfinger J, Pratt RE. A comparative study of the distributions of renin and angiotensinogen messenger ribonucleic acids in rat and mouse tissues. Endocrinology 1987; 120(6): 2334-8.
[http://dx.doi.org/10.1210/endo-120-6-2334] [PMID: 3552634]

[28] Sherrod M, Liu X, Zhang X, Sigmund CD. Nuclear localization of angiotensinogen in astrocytes. Am J Physiol Regul Integr Comp Physiol 2005; 288(2): R539-46.
[http://dx.doi.org/10.1152/ajpregu.00594.2004] [PMID: 15388495]

[29] Singh VP, Le B, Bhat VB, Baker KM, Kumar R. High-glucose-induced regulation of intracellular ANG II synthesis and nuclear redistribution in cardiac myocytes. Am J Physiol Heart Circ Physiol 2007; 293(2): H939-48.

[http://dx.doi.org/10.1152/ajpheart.00391.2007] [PMID: 17483239]

[30] Vidotti DB, Casarini DE, Cristovam PC, Leite CA, Schor N, Boim MA. High glucose concentration stimulates intracellular renin activity and angiotensin II generation in rat mesangial cells. Am J Physiol Renal Physiol 2004; 286(6): F1039-45.
[http://dx.doi.org/10.1152/ajprenal.00371.2003] [PMID: 14722017]

[31] Camargo de Andrade MC, Di Marco GS, de Paulo Castro Teixeira V, *et al.* Expression and localization of N-domain ANG I-converting enzymes in mesangial cells in culture from spontaneously hypertensive rats. Am J Physiol Renal Physiol 2006; 290(2): F364-75.
[http://dx.doi.org/10.1152/ajprenal.00110.2005] [PMID: 16106038]

[32] Lucero HA, Kintsurashvili E, Marketou ME, Gavras H. Cell signaling, internalization, and nuclear localization of the angiotensin converting enzyme in smooth muscle and endothelial cells. J Biol Chem 2010; 285(8): 5555-68.
[http://dx.doi.org/10.1074/jbc.M109.074740] [PMID: 20022959]

[33] Shen XZ, Lukacher AE, Billet S, Williams IR, Bernstein KE. Expression of angiotensin-converting enzyme changes major histocompatibility complex class I peptide presentation by modifying C termini of peptide precursors. J Biol Chem 2008; 283(15): 9957-65.
[http://dx.doi.org/10.1074/jbc.M709574200] [PMID: 18252713]

[34] Réaux A, de Mota N, Zini S, *et al.* PC18, a specific aminopeptidase N inhibitor, induces vasopressin release by increasing the half-life of brain angiotensin III. Neuroendocrinology 1999; 69(5): 370-6.
[http://dx.doi.org/10.1159/000054439] [PMID: 10343178]

[35] Reaux A, Iturrioz X, Vazeux G, *et al.* Aminopeptidase A, which generates one of the main effector peptides of the brain renin-angiotensin system, angiotensin III, has a key role in central control of arterial blood pressure. Biochem Soc Trans 2000; 28(4): 435-40.
[PMID: 10961935]

[36] González A, López B, Díez J. Fibrosis in hypertensive heart disease: role of the renin-angiotensi--aldosterone system. Med Clin North Am 2004; 88(1): 83-97.
[http://dx.doi.org/10.1016/S0025-7125(03)00125-1] [PMID: 14871052]

[37] Pérez-Díaz I, Guzmán C, Olivares-Reyes JA, *et al.* Evidence of an intracellular angiotensin-generating system and non-AT1, non-AT2 binding site in a human pancreatic cell line. Pancreas 2011; 40(5): 701-7.
[http://dx.doi.org/10.1097/MPA.0b013e318215a891] [PMID: 21602736]

[38] Cook JL, Zhang Z, Re RN. *In vitro* evidence for an intracellular site of angiotensin action. Circ Res 2001; 89(12): 1138-46.
[http://dx.doi.org/10.1161/hh2401.101270] [PMID: 11739278]

[39] Cook JL, Re RN. Lessons from *in vitro* studies and a related intracellular angiotensin II transgenic mouse model. Am J Physiol Regul Integr Comp Physiol 2012; 302(5): R482-93.
[http://dx.doi.org/10.1152/ajpregu.00493.2011] [PMID: 22170617]

[40] Deliu E, Tica AA, Motoc D, Brailoiu GC, Brailoiu E. Intracellular angiotensin II activates rat myometrium. Am J Physiol Cell Physiol 2011; 301(3): C559-65.
[http://dx.doi.org/10.1152/ajpcell.00123.2011] [PMID: 21613610]

[41] McEuen AR, Sharma B, Walls AF. Regulation of the activity of human chymase during storage and release from mast cells: the contributions of inorganic cations, pH, heparin and histamine. Biochim Biophys Acta 1995; 1267(2-3): 115-21. [http://dx.doi.org/10.1016/0167-4889(95)00066-2] [PMID: 7612663]

[42] Dzau VJ, Re RN. Evidence for the existence of renin in the heart. Circulation 1987; 75(1 Pt 2): I134-6. [PMID: 3539402]

[43] Dostal DE, Baker KM. The cardiac renin-angiotensin system: conceptual, or a regulator of cardiac function? Circ Res 1999; 85(7): 643-50. [http://dx.doi.org/10.1161/01.RES.85.7.643] [PMID: 10506489]

[44] Peters J, Farrenkopf R, Clausmeyer S, *et al.* Functional significance of prorenin internalization in the rat heart. Circ Res 2002; 90(10): 1135-41. [http://dx.doi.org/10.1161/01.RES.0000019242.51541.99] [PMID: 12039805]

[45] Maru I, Ohta Y, Murata K, Tsukada Y. Molecular cloning and identification of N-acyl-D-glucosamine 2-epimerase from porcine kidney as a renin-binding protein. J Biol Chem 1996; 271(27): 16294-9. [http://dx.doi.org/10.1074/jbc.271.27.16294] [PMID: 8663114]

[46] Danser AH, Saris JJ, Schuijt MP, van Kats JP. Is there a local renin-angiotensin system in the heart? Cardiovasc Res 1999; 44(2): 252-65. [http://dx.doi.org/10.1016/S0008-6363(99)00202-3] [PMID: 10690302]

[47] Nguyen G, Delarue F, Burcklé C, Bouzhir L, Giller T, Sraer JD. Pivotal role of the renin/prorenin receptor in angiotensin II production and cellular responses to renin. J Clin Invest 2002; 109(11): 1417-27. [http://dx.doi.org/10.1172/JCI0214276] [PMID: 12045255]

[48] Nguyen G, Burcklé CA, Sraer JD. Renin/prorenin-receptor biochemistry and functional significance. Curr Hypertens Rep 2004; 6(2): 129-32. [http://dx.doi.org/10.1007/s11906-004-0088-3] [PMID: 15010017]

[49] Sawa H, Tokuchi F, Mochizuki N, *et al.* Expression of the angiotensinogen gene and localization of its protein in the human heart. Circulation 1992; 86(1): 138-46. [http://dx.doi.org/10.1161/01.CIR.86.1.138] [PMID: 1377612]

[50] van Kats JP, Danser AH, van Meegen JR, Sassen LM, Verdouw PD, Schalekamp MA. Angiotensin production by the heart: a quantitative study in pigs with the use of radiolabeled angiotensin infusions. Circulation 1998; 98(1): 73-81. [http://dx.doi.org/10.1161/01.CIR.98.1.73] [PMID: 9665063]

[51] Lindpaintner K, Jin MW, Niedermaier N, Wilhelm MJ, Ganten D. Cardiac angiotensinogen and its local activation in the isolated perfused beating heart. Circ Res 1990; 67(3): 564-73. [http://dx.doi.org/10.1161/01.RES.67.3.564] [PMID: 2204498]

[52] Müller DN, Bohlender J, Hilgers KF, *et al.* Vascular angiotensin-converting enzyme expression regulates local angiotensin II. Hypertension 1997; 29(1 Pt 1): 98-104. [http://dx.doi.org/10.1161/01.HYP.29.1.98] [PMID: 9039087]

[53] Uehara Y, Miura SI, Yahiro E, *et al.* Non-ACE pathway-induced angiotensin II production. Curr Pharm Des 2012.

[PMID: 23176219]

[54] Vijan SG. Angiotensin-converting enzyme inhibitors (ACEIs), not angiotensin receptor blockers (ARBs), are preferred and effective mode of therapy in high cardiovascular risk patients. J Indian Med Assoc 2009; 107(3): 178-82.
[PMID: 19810392]

[55] Urata H, Nishimura H, Ganten D. Chymase-dependent angiotensin II forming systems in humans. Am J Hypertens 1996; 9(3): 277-84.
[http://dx.doi.org/10.1016/0895-7061(95)00349-5] [PMID: 8695029]

[56] Hilgers KF, Veelken R, Müller DN, *et al.* Renin uptake by the endothelium mediates vascular angiotensin formation. Hypertension 2001; 38(2): 243-8.
[http://dx.doi.org/10.1161/01.HYP.38.2.243] [PMID: 11509484]

[57] Singh VP, Baker KM, Kumar R. Activation of the intracellular renin-angiotensin system in cardiac fibroblasts by high glucose: role in extracellular matrix production. Am J Physiol Heart Circ Physiol 2008; 294(4): H1675-84.
[http://dx.doi.org/10.1152/ajpheart.91493.2007] [PMID: 18296558]

[58] Tamura J, Konno A, Hashimoto Y, Kon Y. Upregulation of renal renin-angiotensin system in mouse diabetic nephropathy. Jpn J Vet Res 2005; 53(1-2): 13-26.
[PMID: 16190318]

[59] Crabos M, Roth M, Hahn AW, Erne P. Characterization of angiotensin II receptors in cultured adult rat cardiac fibroblasts. Coupling to signaling systems and gene expression. J Clin Invest 1994; 93(6): 2372-8.
[http://dx.doi.org/10.1172/JCI117243] [PMID: 8200970]

[60] Lévy BI. Can angiotensin II type 2 receptors have deleterious effects in cardiovascular disease? Implications for therapeutic blockade of the renin-angiotensin system. Circulation 2004; 109(1): 8-13.
[http://dx.doi.org/10.1161/01.CIR.0000096609.73772.C5] [PMID: 14707017]

[61] Kumar R, Yong QC, Thomas CM, Baker KM. Intracardiac intracellular angiotensin system in diabetes. Am J Physiol Regul Integr Comp Physiol 2012; 302(5): R510-7.
[http://dx.doi.org/10.1152/ajpregu.00512.2011] [PMID: 22170614]

[62] Burns KD, Homma T, Harris RC. The intrarenal renin-angiotensin system. Semin Nephrol 1993; 13(1): 13-30.
[PMID: 8434183]

[63] Wolf G, Ziyadeh FN. The role of angiotensin II in diabetic nephropathy: emphasis on nonhemodynamic mechanisms. Am J Kidney Dis 1997; 29(1): 153-63.
[http://dx.doi.org/10.1016/S0272-6386(97)90023-8] [PMID: 9002545]

[64] Quinto BM, Juliano MA, Hirata I, Carmona AK, Juliano L, Casarini DE. Specificity comparison of a serine endopeptidase (SH1) and a serine thiol endopeptidase (STH2) purified from human urine. Int J Biochem Cell Biol 2004; 36(10): 1933-44.
[http://dx.doi.org/10.1016/j.biocel.2004.02.011] [PMID: 15203108]

[65] Taugner R, Hackenthal E, Rix E, Nobiling R, Poulsen K. Immunocytochemistry of the renin-angiotensin system: renin, angiotensinogen, angiotensin I, angiotensin II, and converting enzyme in

the kidneys of mice, rats, and tree shrews. Kidney Int Suppl 1982; 12: S33-43.
[PMID: 6290746]

[66] Leyssac PP. Changes in single nephron renin release are mediated by tubular fluid flow rate. Kidney Int 1986; 30(3): 332-9.
[http://dx.doi.org/10.1038/ki.1986.189] [PMID: 3537444]

[67] Kobori H, Nangaku M, Navar LG, Nishiyama A. The intrarenal renin-angiotensin system: from physiology to the pathobiology of hypertension and kidney disease. Pharmacol Rev 2007; 59(3): 251-87.
[http://dx.doi.org/10.1124/pr.59.3.3] [PMID: 17878513]

[68] Navar LG, Harrison-Bernard LM, Nishiyama A, Kobori H. Regulation of intrarenal angiotensin II in hypertension. Hypertension 2002; 39(2 Pt 2): 316-22.
[http://dx.doi.org/10.1161/hy0202.103821] [PMID: 11882566]

[69] Burns KD. The emerging role of angiotensin-converting enzyme-2 in the kidney. Curr Opin Nephrol Hypertens 2007; 16(2): 116-21.
[http://dx.doi.org/10.1097/MNH.0b013e3280123c0e] [PMID: 17293686]

[70] Takao T, Horino T, Kagawa T, *et al.* Possible involvement of intracellular angiotensin II receptor in high-glucose-induced damage in renal proximal tubular cells. J Nephrol 2011; 24(2): 218-24.
[http://dx.doi.org/10.5301/JN.2010.5785] [PMID: 20890878]

[71] Pohl M, Kaminski H, Castrop H, *et al.* Intrarenal renin angiotensin system revisited: role of megalin-dependent endocytosis along the proximal nephron. J Biol Chem 2010; 285(53): 41935-46.
[http://dx.doi.org/10.1074/jbc.M110.150284] [PMID: 20966072]

[72] Nguyen Dinh Cat A, Touyz RM. Cell signaling of angiotensin II on vascular tone: novel mechanisms. Curr Hypertens Rep 2011; 13(2): 122-8.
[http://dx.doi.org/10.1007/s11906-011-0187-x] [PMID: 21274755]

[73] Navar LG, Prieto MC, Satou R, Kobori H. Intrarenal angiotensin II and its contribution to the genesis of chronic hypertension. Curr Opin Pharmacol 2011; 11(2): 180-6.
[http://dx.doi.org/10.1016/j.coph.2011.01.009] [PMID: 21339086]

[74] Ma LJ, Fogo AB. Modulation of glomerulosclerosis. Semin Immunopathol 2007; 29(4): 385-95.
[http://dx.doi.org/10.1007/s00281-007-0087-y] [PMID: 17828397]

[75] Wenzel RR. Renal protection in hypertensive patients: selection of antihypertensive therapy. Drugs 2005; 65 (Suppl. 2): 29-39.
[http://dx.doi.org/10.2165/00003495-200565002-00005] [PMID: 16398060]

[76] NIDDK. Glomerular Disease. NIH Publication 2006.

[77] Wolf G. Renal injury due to renin-angiotensin-aldosterone system activation of the transforming growth factor-beta pathway. Kidney Int 2006; 70(11): 1914-9.
[http://dx.doi.org/10.1038/sj.ki.5001846] [PMID: 16985515]

[78] Rüster C, Wolf G. Renin-angiotensin-aldosterone system and progression of renal disease. J Am Soc Nephrol 2006; 17(11): 2985-91.
[http://dx.doi.org/10.1681/ASN.2006040356] [PMID: 17035613]

[79] Kohan DE. Angiotensin II and endothelin in chronic glomerulonephritis. Kidney Int 1998; 54(2): 646-7.
[http://dx.doi.org/10.1046/j.1523-1755.1998.00038.x] [PMID: 9690233]

[80] Urushihara M, Kobori H. Angiotensinogen expression is enhanced in the progression of glomerular disease. Int J Clin Med 2011; 2(1): 378-87.
[http://dx.doi.org/10.4236/ijcm.2011.24064] [PMID: 22247811]

[81] Ahmed A, Rich MW, Zile M, *et al.* Renin-angiotensin inhibition in diastolic heart failure and chronic kidney disease. Am J Med 2013; 126(2): 150-61.
[http://dx.doi.org/10.1016/j.amjmed.2012.06.031] [PMID: 23331442]

[82] Ruggenenti P, Cravedi P, Remuzzi G. Mechanisms and treatment of CKD. J Am Soc Nephrol 2012; 23(12): 1917-28.
[http://dx.doi.org/10.1681/ASN.2012040390] [PMID: 23100218]

[83] Nickenig G, Harrison DG. The AT(1)-type angiotensin receptor in oxidative stress and atherogenesis: part I: oxidative stress and atherogenesis. Circulation 2002; 105(3): 393-6.
[http://dx.doi.org/10.1161/hc0302.102618] [PMID: 11804998]

[84] Hollenberg NK, Fisher ND, Nussberger J, Moukarbel GV, Barkoudah E, Danser AH. Renal responses to three types of renin-angiotensin system blockers in patients with diabetes mellitus on a high-salt diet: a need for higher doses in diabetic patients? J Hypertens 2011; 29(12): 2454-61.
[http://dx.doi.org/10.1097/HJH.0b013e32834c627a] [PMID: 22002336]

[85] Azizi M, Menard J. Renin inhibitors and cardiovascular and renal protection: An endless quest? Cardiovasc Drugs Ther 2011.

[86] Volpe M, Danser AH, Menard J, *et al.* Inhibition of the renin-angiotensin-aldosterone system: is there room for dual blockade in the cardiorenal continuum? J Hypertens 2012; 30(4): 647-54.
[http://dx.doi.org/10.1097/HJH.0b013e32834f6e00] [PMID: 22278139]

[87] Turnbull F. Effects of different blood-pressure-lowering regimens on major cardiovascular events: results of prospectively-designed overviews of randomised trials. Lancet 2003; 362(9395): 1527-35.
[http://dx.doi.org/10.1016/S0140-6736(03)14739-3] [PMID: 14615107]

[88] Azizi M, Ménard J. Combined blockade of the renin-angiotensin system with angiotensin-converting enzyme inhibitors and angiotensin II type 1 receptor antagonists. Circulation 2004; 109(21): 2492-9.
[http://dx.doi.org/10.1161/01.CIR.0000131449.94713.AD] [PMID: 15173039]

[89] Lewis EJ, Hunsicker LG, Clarke WR, *et al.* Renoprotective effect of the angiotensin-receptor antagonist irbesartan in patients with nephropathy due to type 2 diabetes. N Engl J Med 2001; 345(12): 851-60.
[http://dx.doi.org/10.1056/NEJMoa011303] [PMID: 11565517]

[90] Brenner BM, Cooper ME, de Zeeuw D, *et al.* Effects of losartan on renal and cardiovascular outcomes in patients with type 2 diabetes and nephropathy. N Engl J Med 2001; 345(12): 861-9.
[http://dx.doi.org/10.1056/NEJMoa011161] [PMID: 11565518]

[91] Ruggenenti P, Perna A, Gherardi G, *et al.* Renoprotective properties of ACE-inhibition in non-diabetic nephropathies with non-nephrotic proteinuria. Lancet 1999; 354(9176): 359-64.
[http://dx.doi.org/10.1016/S0140-6736(98)10363-X] [PMID: 10437863]

[92] Agodoa LY, Appel L, Bakris GL, *et al.* Effect of ramipril vs amlodipine on renal outcomes in hypertensive nephrosclerosis: a randomized controlled trial. JAMA 2001; 285(21): 2719-8.

[93] Jafar TH, Schmid CH, Landa M, *et al.* Angiotensin-converting enzyme inhibitors and progression of nondiabetic renal disease. A meta-analysis of patient-level data. Ann Intern Med 2001; 135(2): 73-87. [http://dx.doi.org/10.7326/0003-4819-135-2-200107170-00007] [PMID: 11453706]

[94] Pfeffer MA, McMurray JJ, Velazquez EJ, *et al.* Valsartan, captopril, or both in myocardial infarction complicated by heart failure, left ventricular dysfunction, or both. N Engl J Med 2003; 349(20): 1893-906.
[http://dx.doi.org/10.1056/NEJMoa032292] [PMID: 14610160]

[95] Wright JT Jr, Bakris G, Greene T, *et al.* Effect of blood pressure lowering and antihypertensive drug class on progression of hypertensive kidney disease: results from the AASK trial. JAMA 2002; 288(19): 2421-31.
[http://dx.doi.org/10.1001/jama.288.19.2421] [PMID: 12435255]

[96] Dzau VJ, Bernstein K, Celermajer D, *et al.* The relevance of tissue angiotensin-converting enzyme: manifestations in mechanistic and endpoint data. Am J Cardiol 2001; 88(9A): 1L-20L.
[http://dx.doi.org/10.1016/S0002-9149(01)01878-1] [PMID: 11694220]

[97] Remuzzi A, Perico N, Sangalli F, *et al.* ACE inhibition and ANG II receptor blockade improve glomerular size-selectivity in IgA nephropathy. Am J Physiol 1999; 276(3 Pt 2): F457-66.
[PMID: 10070170]

[98] Ruggenenti P, Perna A, Mosconi L, Pisoni R, Remuzzi G. Urinary protein excretion rate is the best independent predictor of ESRF in non-diabetic proteinuric chronic nephropathies. "Gruppo Italiano di Studi Epidemiologici in Nefrologia" (GISEN). Kidney Int 1998; 53(5): 1209-16.
[http://dx.doi.org/10.1046/j.1523-1755.1998.00874.x] [PMID: 9573535]

[99] Nakao N, Yoshimura A, Morita H, Takada M, Kayano T, Ideura T. Combination treatment of angiotensin-II receptor blocker and angiotensin-converting-enzyme inhibitor in non-diabetic renal disease (COOPERATE): a randomised controlled trial. Lancet 2003; 361(9352): 117-24.
[http://dx.doi.org/10.1016/S0140-6736(03)12229-5] [PMID: 12531578]

[100] Remuzzi G, Bertani T. Pathophysiology of progressive nephropathies. N Engl J Med 1998; 339(20): 1448-56.
[http://dx.doi.org/10.1056/NEJM199811123392007] [PMID: 9811921]

[101] Weber MA. The angiotensin II receptor blockers: opportunities across the spectrum of cardiovascular disease. Rev Cardiovasc Med 2002; 3(4): 183-91.
[PMID: 12556752]

[102] Schmieder RE. Mechanisms for the clinical benefits of angiotensin II receptor blockers. Am J Hypertens 2005; 18(5 Pt 1): 720-30.
[http://dx.doi.org/10.1016/j.amjhyper.2004.11.032] [PMID: 15882557]

[103] Linz W, Wiemer G, Gohlke P, Unger T, Schölkens BA. Contribution of kinins to the cardiovascular actions of angiotensin-converting enzyme inhibitors. Pharmacol Rev 1995; 47(1): 25-49.
[PMID: 7784479]

[104] Iyer SN, Ferrario CM, Chappell MC. Angiotensin-(1-7) contributes to the antihypertensive effects of

blockade of the renin-angiotensin system. Hypertension 1998; 31(1 Pt 2): 356-61.
[http://dx.doi.org/10.1161/01.HYP.31.1.356] [PMID: 9453328]

[105] Israili ZH, Hall WD. Cough and angioneurotic edema associated with angiotensin-converting enzyme inhibitor therapy. A review of the literature and pathophysiology. Ann Intern Med 1992; 117(3): 234-42.
[http://dx.doi.org/10.7326/0003-4819-117-3-234] [PMID: 1616218]

[106] Timmermans PB, Wong PC, Chiu AT, *et al.* Angiotensin II receptors and angiotensin II receptor antagonists. Pharmacol Rev 1993; 45(2): 205-51.
[PMID: 8372104]

[107] Carey RM, Wang ZQ, Siragy HM. Role of the angiotensin type 2 receptor in the regulation of blood pressure and renal function. Hypertension 2000; 35(1 Pt 2): 155-63.
[http://dx.doi.org/10.1161/01.HYP.35.1.155] [PMID: 10642292]

[108] Martin J, Krum H. Role of valsartan and other angiotensin receptor blocking agents in the management of cardiovascular disease. Pharmacol Res 2002; 46(3): 203-12.
[http://dx.doi.org/10.1016/S1043-6618(02)00092-0] [PMID: 12220962]

[109] Navar LG, Kobori H, Prieto-Carrasquero M. Intrarenal angiotensin II and hypertension. Curr Hypertens Rep 2003; 5(2): 135-43.
[http://dx.doi.org/10.1007/s11906-003-0070-5] [PMID: 12642013]

[110] Nishiyama A, Yoshizumi M, Rahman M, *et al.* Effects of AT1 receptor blockade on renal injury and mitogen-activated protein activity in Dahl salt-sensitive rats. Kidney Int 2004; 65(3): 972-81.
[http://dx.doi.org/10.1111/j.1523-1755.2004.00476.x] [PMID: 14871417]

[111] Prieto-Carrasquero MC, Kobori H, Ozawa Y, Gutiérrez A, Seth D, Navar LG. AT1 receptor-mediated enhancement of collecting duct renin in angiotensin II-dependent hypertensive rats. Am J Physiol Renal Physiol 2005; 289(3): F632-7.
[http://dx.doi.org/10.1152/ajprenal.00462.2004] [PMID: 15870381]

[112] Zhuo JL, Imig JD, Hammond TG, Orengo S, Benes E, Navar LG. Ang II accumulation in rat renal endosomes during Ang II-induced hypertension: role of AT(1) receptor. Hypertension 2002; 39(1): 116-21.
[http://dx.doi.org/10.1161/hy0102.100780] [PMID: 11799089]

[113] Fisher ND, Hollenberg NK. Renin inhibition: what are the therapeutic opportunities? J Am Soc Nephrol 2005; 16(3): 592-9.
[http://dx.doi.org/10.1681/ASN.2004100874] [PMID: 15703270]

[114] Gradman AH, Schmieder RE, Lins RL, Nussberger J, Chiang Y, Bedigian MP. Aliskiren, a novel orally effective renin inhibitor, provides dose-dependent antihypertensive efficacy and placebo-like tolerability in hypertensive patients. Circulation 2005; 111(8): 1012-8.
[http://dx.doi.org/10.1161/01.CIR.0000156466.02908.ED] [PMID: 15723979]

[115] Nadeem S, Batisky DL. Aliskiren, the first direct renin inhibitor: assessing a role in pediatric hypertension and kidney diseases. Pediatr Nephrol 2013.
[PMID: 24337365]

[116] Pilz B, Shagdarsuren E, Wellner M, *et al.* Aliskiren, a human renin inhibitor, ameliorates cardiac and

renal damage in double-transgenic rats. Hypertension 2005; 46(3): 569-76. [http://dx.doi.org/10.1161/01.HYP.0000179573.91016.3f] [PMID: 16103264]

[117] Sen S, Sabırlı S, Ozyiğit T, Uresin Y. Aliskiren: review of efficacy and safety data with focus on past and recent clinical trials. Ther Adv Chronic Dis 2013; 4(5): 232-41. [http://dx.doi.org/10.1177/2040622313495288] [PMID: 23997927]

[118] Azizi M, Webb R, Nussberger J, Hollenberg NK. Renin inhibition with aliskiren: where are we now, and where are we going? J Hypertens 2006; 24(2): 243-56. [http://dx.doi.org/10.1097/01.hjh.0000202812.72341.99] [PMID: 16508564]

[119] Nussberger J, Wuerzner G, Jensen C, Brunner HR. Angiotensin II suppression in humans by the orally active renin inhibitor Aliskiren (SPP100): comparison with enalapril. Hypertension 2002; 39(1): E1-8. [http://dx.doi.org/10.1161/hy0102.102293] [PMID: 11799102]

[120] Azizi M, Ménard J, Bissery A, *et al.* Pharmacologic demonstration of the synergistic effects of a combination of the renin inhibitor aliskiren and the AT1 receptor antagonist valsartan on the angiotensin II-renin feedback interruption. J Am Soc Nephrol 2004; 15(12): 3126-33. [http://dx.doi.org/10.1097/01.ASN.0000146686.35541.29] [PMID: 15579516]

[121] Alan H. Gradman PaP. Evolving understanding of the renin-angiotensin-aldosterone system: Pathophysiology and targets for therapeutic intervention. Am Heart J 2009; 157(6)

[122] Wolf G, Ritz E. Combination therapy with ACE inhibitors and angiotensin II receptor blockers to halt progression of chronic renal disease: pathophysiology and indications. Kidney Int 2005; 67(3): 799-812. [http://dx.doi.org/10.1111/j.1523-1755.2005.00145.x] [PMID: 15698420]

[123] Christian Werner MB, Koon K. Teo, Roland Schmieder, Johannes Mann, Thomas Unger, Salim Yusuf, Michael Böhm. RAS blockade with ARB and ACE inhibitors: current perspective on rationale and patient selection. Clin Res Cardiol 2008; 97(7)

[124] Unger T, Stoppelhaar M. Rationale for double renin-angiotensin-aldosterone system blockade. Am J Cardiol 2007; 100(3A): 25J-31J. [http://dx.doi.org/10.1016/j.amjcard.2007.05.011] [PMID: 17666194]

[125] Slagman MC, Navis G, Laverman GD. Dual blockade of the renin-angiotensin-aldosterone system in cardiac and renal disease. Curr Opin Nephrol Hypertens 2010; 19(2): 140-52. [http://dx.doi.org/10.1097/MNH.0b013e3283361887] [PMID: 20051849]

[126] Burnier M, Brunner HR. Angiotensin II receptor antagonists. Lancet 2000; 355(9204): 637-45. [http://dx.doi.org/10.1016/S0140-6736(99)10365-9] [PMID: 10696996]

[127] Müller DN, Luft FC. Direct renin inhibition with aliskiren in hypertension and target organ damage. Clin J Am Soc Nephrol 2006; 1(2): 221-8. [http://dx.doi.org/10.2215/CJN.01201005] [PMID: 17699210]

[128] Locatelli F, Del Vecchio L, Cavalli A. Inhibition of the renin-angiotensin system in chronic kidney disease: a critical look to single and dual blockade. Nephron Clin Pract 2009; 113(4): c286-93. [http://dx.doi.org/10.1159/000235946] [PMID: 19729963]

[129] Weber MA. Telmisartan in high-risk cardiovascular patients. Am J Cardiol 2010; 105(1) (Suppl.): 36A-43A.

[http://dx.doi.org/10.1016/j.amjcard.2009.10.008] [PMID: 20102972]

[130] Haynes R, Mason P, Rahimi K, Landray MJ. Dual blockade of the renin-angiotensin system: are two better than one? Nephrol Dial Transplant 2009; 24(12): 3602-7. [http://dx.doi.org/10.1093/ndt/gfp458] [PMID: 19762601]

[131] Arici M, Erdem Y. Dual blockade of the renin-angiotensin system for cardiorenal protection: an update. Am J Kidney Dis 2009; 53(2): 332-45. [http://dx.doi.org/10.1053/j.ajkd.2008.11.021] [PMID: 19166800]

[132] Ferrario CM. Addressing the theoretical and clinical advantages of combination therapy with inhibitors of the renin-angiotensin-aldosterone system: antihypertensive effects and benefits beyond BP control. Life Sci 2010; 86(9-10): 289-99. [http://dx.doi.org/10.1016/j.lfs.2009.11.020] [PMID: 19958778]

[133] Volpe M, Danser AH, Menard J, *et al.* Inhibition of the renin-angiotensin-aldosterone system: is there room for dual blockade in the cardiorenal continuum? J Hypertens 2012; 30(4): 647-54. [http://dx.doi.org/10.1097/HJH.0b013e32834f6e00] [PMID: 22278139]

[134] Toto R, Palmer BF. Rationale for combination angiotensin receptor blocker and angiotensin-converting enzyme inhibitor treatment and end-organ protection in patients with chronic kidney disease. Am J Nephrol 2008; 28(3): 372-80. [http://dx.doi.org/10.1159/000112269] [PMID: 18073461]

[135] MacKinnon M, Shurraw S, Akbari A, Knoll GA, Jaffey J, Clark HD. Combination therapy with an angiotensin receptor blocker and an ACE inhibitor in proteinuric renal disease: a systematic review of the efficacy and safety data. Am J Kidney Dis 2006; 48(1): 8-20. [http://dx.doi.org/10.1053/j.ajkd.2006.04.077] [PMID: 16797382]

[136] Dalla Vestra M, Simioni N, Masiero A. Renal effects of dual renin-angiotensin-aldosterone system blockade in patients with diabetic nephropathy. Int Urol Nephrol 2009; 41(1): 119-26. [http://dx.doi.org/10.1007/s11255-008-9490-0] [PMID: 18958580]

[137] Ripley E. Complementary effects of angiotensin-converting enzyme inhibitors and angiotensin receptor blockers in slowing the progression of chronic kidney disease. Am Heart J 2009; 157(6) (Suppl.): S7-S16. [http://dx.doi.org/10.1016/j.ahj.2009.04.008] [PMID: 19450722]

[138] Parfrey PS. Inhibitors of the renin angiotensin system: proven benefits, unproven safety. Ann Intern Med 2008; 148(1): 76-7. [http://dx.doi.org/10.7326/0003-4819-148-1-200801010-00191] [PMID: 17984483]

[139] Pimenta E, Oparil S. Renin inhibitors: novel agents for renoprotection or a better angiotensin receptor blocker for blood pressure lowering? Cardiol Clin 2008; 26(4): 527-35. [http://dx.doi.org/10.1016/j.ccl.2008.06.003] [PMID: 18929229]

[140] Parving HH, Persson F, Lewis JB, Lewis EJ, Hollenberg NK. Aliskiren combined with losartan in type 2 diabetes and nephropathy. N Engl J Med 2008; 358(23): 2433-46. [http://dx.doi.org/10.1056/NEJMoa0708379] [PMID: 18525041]

[141] Santos PC, Krieger JE, Pereira AC. Renin-angiotensin system, hypertension, and chronic kidney disease: pharmacogenetic implications. J Pharmacol Sci 2012; 120(2): 77-88.

[http://dx.doi.org/10.1254/jphs.12R03CR] [PMID: 23079502]

[142] Gheorghiade M, Böhm M, Greene SJ, *et al.* Effect of aliskiren on postdischarge mortality and heart failure readmissions among patients hospitalized for heart failure: the ASTRONAUT randomized trial. JAMA 2013; 309(11): 1125-35.
[http://dx.doi.org/10.1001/jama.2013.1954] [PMID: 23478743]

[143] Michel Azizi JM. Renin inhibitors and cardiovascular and renal protection: An endless quest? Cardiovasc Drugs Ther 2012.
[PMID: 22392185]

CHAPTER 3

Renin-Angiotensin System and Cardiovascular Physiology

Maria Cláudia Irigoyen[1,*], **Kátia De Angelis**[2], **Ivana Cinthya de Moraes da Silva**[1], **Silvia Lacchini**[3], **Janaina Barcellos Ferreira**[1], **Kátia Bilhar Scapini**[1] and **Fernanda Marciano Consolim-Colombo**[1]

[1] *University of Sao Paulo Medical School, Heart Institute (InCor), Hypertension Unit, Sao Paulo, Brazil*

[2] *Nove de Julho University, Sao Paulo, Brazil*

[3] *University of Sao Paulo, Institute of Biomedical Science, Department of Anatomy, Sao Paulo, Brazil*

Abstract: Since the discovery of renin at the end of 19th century and the identification of angiotensin I (Ang I) and Angiotensin II (Ang II) seven decades ago, renin-angiotensin system (RAS) has been widely studied. The RAS is an important endocrine system that regulates blood pressure and fluid homeostasis. This system is composed of peptides, enzymes and receptors. The RAS plays a key role in the development and progression of cardiovascular diseases. In this sense, Ang II is an important peptide of this system, presenting vasoconstrictor and salt-retaining properties and, at cellular level, promoting proliferation, fibrosis and hypertrophy. This chapter focuses on RAS and cardiovascular physiology addressing to an overview about RAS and cardiovascular disease, RAS and its relation with elevated blood pressure, sympathetic overactivity, cardiac hypertrophy, endothelial and vascular dysfunctions, and immune response activation, as well as the physiological basis of RAS inhibitors and cardiovascular disease treatment.

Keywords: Angiotensin-converting enzyme inhibitors, Angiotensin receptor antagonists, Angiotensin II receptor blockers, Autonomic nervous system,

[*] **Corresponding author Maria Claudia Irigoyen:** Laboratory of Experimental Hypertension, Hypertension Unit, Heart Institute [InCor], University of Sao Paulo. Av. Dr Eneas de Carvalho Aguiar 44, Sao Paulo, SP CEP 05403-000, Brazil; E-mail: maria.irigoyen@incor.usp.br.

Dulce Elena Casarini, Danielle Yuri Arita, Tatiana Sousa Cunha & Juliana Almada Colucci (Eds.)

Baroreflex, Blood pressure, Cardiac hypertrophy, Cardiovascular diseases, Endothelial dysfunction, Hypertension, Inflammation, Sympathetic nervous system, Vascular resistance.

RAS & CARDIOVASCULAR SYSTEM: AN OVERVIEW

The renin–angiotensin system (RAS) plays a key role in regulating the systemic volume and vascular resistance; thus, influencing both the cardiac output and the blood pressure (BP). In this sense, it is well known that renin secretion by the juxtaglomerular cells depends on the increase of sodium concentration in the macula densa, the decrease in the perfusion pressure and the enhancement of the sympathetic activity. In addition, the production of renin by different tissues has been studied [1 - 4]. The cleavage of the angiotensinogen by renin action produces the inactive decapeptide, *i.e.,* Angiotensin I (Ang I). On the other hand, the *angiotensin converting enzyme (ACE)* cleaves Ang I, forming Angiotensin II (Ang II) and can promote the bradykinin degradation (Fig. **1**). Ang II can act directly on the AT1 receptors on the smooth muscle cells of the vessel [5], inducing vasoconstrictor effect as well as increasing the vascular tone by sympathetic nervous system interaction [6, 7]. Moreover, Ang II may induce volume expansion [8] and cellular proliferation and hypertrophy [9, 10].

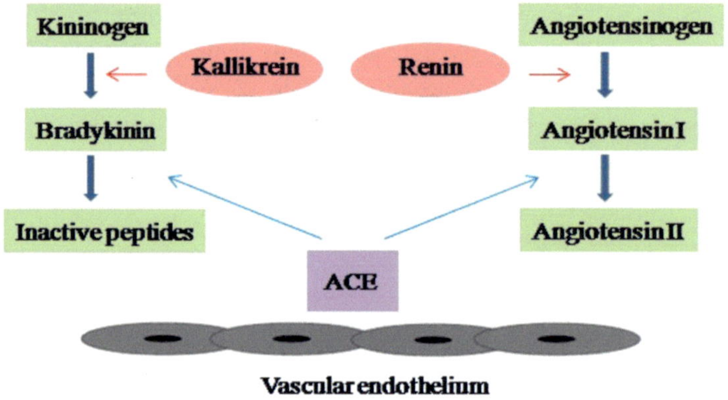

Fig. (1). Schematic of the classical RAS and the kallikrein-kinin system. ACE regulates the balance between Ang II and bradykinin. (*Modified of Brown and Vaughan* [11]).

In brief, the balance between natriuretic and vasodilatory characteristics of bradykinin and the vasoconstrictor and salt-retaining properties of Ang II are regulated by ACE. ACE inhibitors decrease bradykinin degradation and Ang II formation (Fig. **1**).

It is important to emphasize that Ang II is the most studied molecule of the RAS and can act as a systemic hormone (endocrine) or as a locally generated factor (paracrine and autocrine). Ang II is also an omnipresent factor in several cardiovascular disorders, having an absolutely important influence on the pathophysiology and progression of cardiovascular diseases and on several cardiovascular risk factors (Fig. **2**).

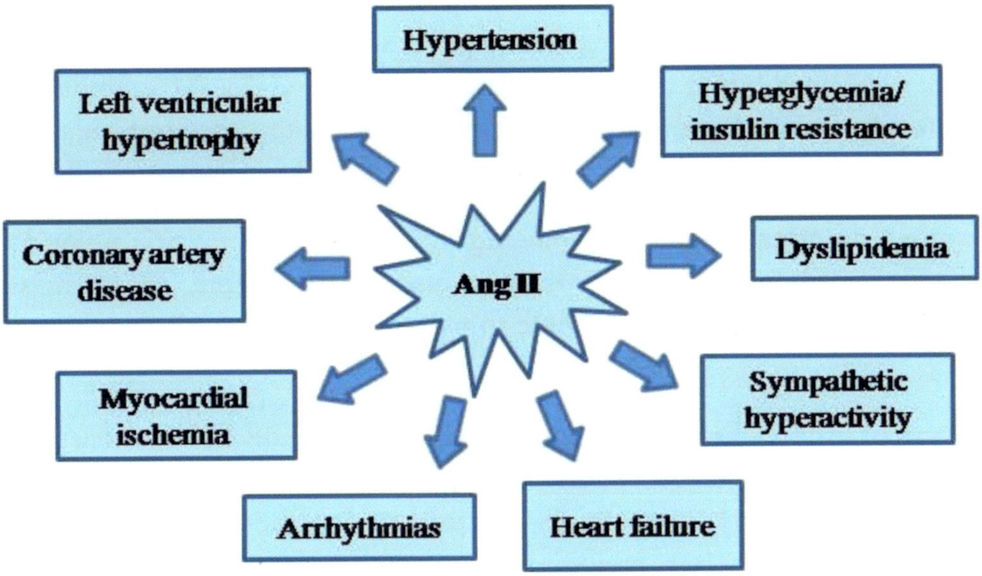

Fig. (2). Angiotensin II and its influences on several cardiometabolic disturbances.

Over the last decades, the view of the RAS has expanded to a more complex concept. The Ang II arm, classically known for its "harmful" responses through the interaction with AT1 receptor, can be counterbalanced by the Ang-(1- 7)-ACE2-Mas receptors axis, which can exert beneficial effects in the cardiovascular homeostasis in physiological and pathological conditions. Furthermore, recently was discovered a new element of RAS, the alamandine, which is derivative of Ang-(1-7), and its receptor, the Mas-related G-coupled receptor type D (MrgD) [12]. Alamandine is a vasoactive peptide that produces similar physiological actions of Ang (1-7), including vasodilation, antifibrosis, antihypertensive, and central effects [12, 13]. However, evidence of the actions and effectiveness of this new arm of the RAS system is still emerging in the literature.

RAS & ELEVATED BLOOD PRESSURE

Recent studies have shown that the RAS is a much more complex hormonal cascade than initially thought. However, the RAS remain an important regulator of the BP and fluid homeostasis. ACE and ACE2 provide a refined control of Ang II levels and its metabolites downstream and Ang II is an important effector molecule of this system. However, other RAS mediators, like the renin and Ang (1-7), have independent functions of Ang II, which may influence on the regulation of BP and target organ damage. Indeed, Ang (1-7), for example, has become the focus of studies because of its effects on the cardiovascular and baroreflex systems, which are counter-regulatory Ang II [14].

ACE can act on other substrates, including the vasodilator bradykinin peptide, which is degraded by ACE in an inactive peptide. Therefore, the increased bradykinin activity appears to contribute to the lowering of the BP by inhibiting ACE [15].

The effects of Ang II in cardiovascular regulation include its vasoconstrictor action, its ability to potentiate the effects of noradrenaline released at the nerve endings. In fact, it may increase the synthesis of noradrenaline release by facilitating the nerve impulses, inhibiting the neuronal reuptake and increasing the concentration of the neurotransmitter in the synaptic cleft. Ang II also enhances the ganglionic transmission, the release of adrenal catecholamines and still stimulates the various regions of the central nervous system that can increase the sympathetic tone. In parallel, it stimulates the release of vasopressin from the neurohypophysis, reduces the sensitivity of the baroreceptor reflex and stimulates the synthesis and the release of aldosterone. All of these Ang II effects stimulate the increase of the BP (increased peripheral resistance and blood volume). In addition, Ang II has actions at multiple levels of cardiac function, including the trophic effect, increased inotropic and pro-arrhythmogenic effects. The effects of Ang II in cardiac hypertrophy and apoptosis of cardiomyocytes appear to involve both AT1 and AT2 [16, 17].

In contrast, it has been observed that the central effects of Ang (1-7) are opposed to those of Ang II. The sensitivity of the baroreflex bradycardia in response to the increased BP is increased under microinjection of Ang (1-7) in the nucleus of the solitary tract (NTS) [18 - 20]. Moreover, approximately 40% of reduction in the bradycardia reflex can be seen after the injection of Mas receptor antagonist, A-779. Further, in rats with renovascular hypertension (2-kidney-1-clip), A-779 inhibits the baroreflex sensitivity improvement produced by the treatment with an ACE inhibitor (orally or intracerebroventricular) [21]. It was recently shown that transgenic mice (with overexpression of ACE2, a promoter derived from neuronal) are protected against the increases in the BP caused by Ang II infusion. overexpression of ACE2 in the ventral medulla of SHR, *via* gene transfer, has also been associated with the lowering of BP. These data suggest a role for endogenous peptides in the modulation of baroreceptor reflex [22]. On the other hand, the Ang (1-7) is anti arrhythmogenic, preserving the cardiac function, coronary perfusion and endothelial function [23].

Besides the classic vasoconstrictor effects, known for over a century, the RAS modulates the vascular function in several ways. Ang II has a vasoconstrictor effect generally identified as an AT1 mediated action [23]. However, both the activation of AT1 receptors and AT2 in the endothelium can produce a vasodilator effect which counteracts the vasoconstrictor effect by a direct action on the smooth muscle cells (*via* AT1 receptor activation) [24]. The same vasodilator effect is produced by Ang (1-7) [23].

Thus, an overactive RAS is markedly associated with high BP. The RAS controls the volume and electrolyte balance in the circulation contributing to hemodynamic function [25].

In this way, RAS is a budget in the treatment of the hypertension and cardiovascular disease and the suppression of this system protects against the target organ damage. Thus, drugs blocking Ang II action (by inhibiting its synthesis or it's receptor ligation dependent action) are effective and widely used as antihypertensive agents [26] that can improve morbidity and mortality in cardiovascular diseases, such as congestive heart failure [27, 28], delaying the progression of a variety of kidney chronic diseases, including diabetic nephropathy [29].

ACE2 has been associated with several disorders, including atherosclerosis, hypertension, heart failure, and diabetic nephropathy [30 - 33]. ACE2 may influence the RAS activity, at least, by two different ways. Firstly, Ang II is a substrate to ACE2 action so ACE2 is a metabolic pathway to extinguish Ang II activity [31]. Secondly, the removal of an aminoacid from the carboxy terminus of Ang II leads to Ang (1- 7) formation, which has a number of biological actions [34] as already described in this text, like vasodilation and, natriuresis, promoting the reduction of the BP [35] by activating the Mas receptor [14].

RAS & SYMPATHETIC OVERACTIVITY

As already written previously in this text, it is well known that Ang II (Ang II) facilitates sympathetic neurotransmission by several mechanisms, most of them associated with Ang II receptors. Ang II can increase sympathetic nerve outflow by directly acting on central nervous system as well as by reducing the reflex inhibition of sympathetic activity that accompanies BP increase. Other influence, like the increase in the ganglionic transmission and in the release of norepinephrine by acting on the presynaptic site are also well documented, especially in animal models. However, in humans these evidence are not so clear, probably associated with the limitations of measurements of autonomic activity [36].

Indeed, the brain RAS seems to be enrolled in the action of the endocrine RAS, probably by a positive biofeedback. Although the brain RAS is separated from the endocrine RAS by the blood brain barrier there are some areas (the circumventricular organs) that lack this barrier, allowing circulating Ang II to act into the brain. Centrally acting Ang II can modulate baroreflex control of heart rate and sympathetic outflow [37, 38].

The contribution of the brain RAS to several pathological states associated with sympathetic overactivity was clarified by experiments using a transgenic rat [TGR (ASr AOGEN)] that presents the production of brain angiotensinogen inhibited

[39] due to an antisense RNA expressed against angiotensinogen. This rat was investigated in experimental conditions of hypertension and other heart pathology conditions and it was demonstrated that brain RAS contributes to hypertensive state [39]. In other words, the permanent inhibition of brain RAS, as observed in this transgenic rat, may induce a decreased basal sympathetic outflow [40] associated with an increased sensitivity to B- receptor agonists [41].

In this sense, it is important to highlight the role of Ang II in arterial baroreflex control. An inhibitory central action of Ang II in baroreflex control of heart rate [42, 43] and renal sympathetic activity [44] are well demonstrated.

The contribution of endogenous brain Ang II in the modulation of arterial baroreflex control of renal sympathetic activity is regulated by changes in dietary sodium that may induce physiological changes in the activity of the RAS. In addition, in other condition as heart failure the increased Ang II activity in specific brain sites may contribute to the tonic increase of basal renal sympathetic activity as well as its impaired arterial baroreflex control [45]. In fact, these and other findings give support to the idea that brain origin angiotensin peptides may have actions (paracrine and autocrine) on sites that control the basal and reflex changes of renal sympathetic activity [46].

The interaction of sympathetic activity and RAS on the kidney production of renin can be understood in experiments that have shown that the effects of sympathetic on renin secretion rate are increased when BP is decreased [47]. However, in experimental high renin hypertension the renal denervation procedure was able to reduce BP and to reduce significantly the plasma renin activity [48].

The RAS-sympathetic connection is important in other pathophysiological conditions, as myocardial infarction [49]. In addition, brain RAS influences the development of cardiac hypertrophy and fibrosis through sympathetic activation [50]. Currently RAS- targeting drugs are mandatory therapy for heart failure patients. By acting in both endocrine and local tissue components, RAS inhibiting drugs are being improved to obtain increased tissue penetrability and volume of distribution.

Regarding, renal denervation it is necessary to remember the procedure as a new treatment tool for resistant hypertension patients. Increased renal sympathetic activity increases renal vasoconstriction, renin secretion rate and renal tubular sodium reabsorption, as well as anti-natriuretic effect. On the other hand, decreased renal sympathetic activity elicits opposite responses. Considering that renal dysfunction can contribute to development of hypertension, impairing pressure diuresis and natriuresis, renal denervation was demonstrated to be efficient in BP controlling in several hypertensive states [51, 52]. According to the evidence obtained by several experimental studies, a growing interest in the minimally invasive devices-based approaches to renal nerves ablation in hypertensive humans has been observed in the last years [53, 54]. However, it seems that current evidence is consistent to justify the use of this therapy only to patients with pharmacotherapy resistant hypertension which cannot be extrapolated to other conditions or hypertensive states.

RAS & ENDOTHELIAL AND VASCULAR DYSFUNCTIONS

In the last two decades, many studies have shown the involvement of the RAS in the regulation of vascular function and structure. In this sense is important to remind that the arteries are complex structures made up of a number of integrated active and endothelial cells, smooth muscle cells and fibroblasts, and a complex extracellular matrix. All these components are connected to each other by a network of autocrine and paracrine interactions, being able to adapt actively to hemodynamic and mechanical variations [55]. The vascular wall is characterized by the presence of three tunicas, with their own characteristics, and these are called the tunica intima, tunica media and tunica adventitia, and the general configuration of these is different from the arterial and venous network [56]. The endothelium lies in a strategic position, internally lining the entire cardiovascular system, detecting hemodynamic and humoral signals, and it also works as an effector of biological responses that may possibly affect the vessel structure [56 - 58]. The endothelial cell is exposed to the blood components and constituents, such as leukocytes, platelets, cytokines, hormones, lipids, signaling molecules, oxygen tension, concentration of protein, as well as the hemodynamic factors, such as shear stress, blood flow and wall tension [59]. Thus, the endothelium is able to detect and respond appropriately to any mechanical, physical or chemical stimulus processing information and releasing factors that modify the vascular tone, as well as coagulation, thrombolysis, vascular remodeling and inflammatory and immune response.

In this context, a series of studies has shown that the endothelial cells regulate the proliferation of monocytes [60], vascular tone [61], inflammation and lipid metabolism [55], cell growth, cell migration, and integration with extracellular matrix [62] through receptor-mediated mechanisms. Changes in the endothelial function may be considered an indication of a process that modifies the vascular function, which may be momentary or triggering a vascular pathology. An important consequence of this process leads to the migration of the smooth muscle cells into the intima and the deposition of extracellular matrix, which becomes thicker and so-called neointima [63]. When the arterial endothelium is in contact with certain risk factors, it modifies its operation, turning molecules into adhesion, promoting leukocyte migration into the arterial wall [63]. Among these factors, it might be highlighted the following: dyslipidemia, vasoconstrictor hormones, products of glycoxidation associated with hyperglycemia [64], reactive oxygen species [65] and pro-inflammatory cytokines derived from adipose tissue. The transmigration of leukocytes into the subendothelial space depends mainly on the expression of chemotherapy attractive cytokines (such as MCP-1).

In 1993, an experimental study, evaluating arteries undergoing vascular injury by balloon, described the increased expression of angiotensinogen in the tunica media and neointima [66]. Shortly after, it was observed an increased expression of ACE I in atherosclerotic lesions [67], which should directly participate in the local production of Ang II during the atherosclerotic process [68]. ACE is important not only in the vascular smooth muscle contractility, but also in the growth of muscles, contributing to the development of intimal hyperplasia and medial hypertrophy [69]. More recently, the importance of ACE was shown in genetically modified mice undergoing vascular injury and containing an increasing number of copies of the ACE gene, which can be regarded as a susceptibility factor for vascular injury. It was observed that both the degree of injury and ACE activity in the exact location of the injury increased simultaneously with the largest number of copies of the gene [70].

Ang II is produced in the vascular wall [69] and is capable of generating intimal hyperplasia independently of hemodynamic or neurohumoral effects [71]. In addition to the functions characterized above, the Ang II has been considered a multifunctional cytokine with non-hemodynamic properties, including the growth factor, pro- inflammatory and pro-fibrogenic cytokines [72] and an immune response modulator, leading to the chemotaxis, proliferation and differentiation of monocytes into macrophages [73]. Moreover, it stimulates the activation of transcription programs for several genes that lead to changes in the vascular function, such as matrix metalloproteinases (MMPs), monocyte chemoattractant protein-1 (MCP-1), vascular cell adhesion molecule (VCAM), vascular endothelial growth factor (VEGF), plasminogen activator inhibitor (PAI-1), among others [74]. Another factor that reinforces this idea of Ang II participation in the vascular injury is the fact that it has been observed that the production of Ang II is increased in atheroma, aortic atherosclerosis and restenosis after angioplasty or stenting.

Further, it has also been shown that the AT1 receptor antagonism reduces the endothelial dysfunction and intimal thickening in atherosclerotic vessels [67, 75]. The mechanisms involved in the formation of atherosclerotic plaque include the release of proinflammatory cytokines, lipoprotein oxidation and the activation of metalloproteinases of extracellular matrix [76]. In this context, Ang II is known to induce the production of vascular pro-inflammatory cytokines such as IL-6 and TNF-α [77]. In this case, Ang II leads to an increased production of reactive oxygen species, which in turn leads to an increased production of IL-6 [78], creating a vicious cycle in response to Ang II, promoting an increase in IL-6, oxidative stress and vascular injury. Thus, it can be stated that IL-6 synthesized and stored in the cell can be quickly released if the AT1 receptor activation may lead to a rapid increase in the intracellular calcium. In this sense, the phospholipase C (PLC) pathway to inositol triphosphate (IP3) leads ultimately to the release of intracellular calcium, functioning as *via* of action of a series of membrane receptors, including the AT1 [79]. This route is considered important in cell survival, metabolism, and cytoskeletal reorganization, having also an important role in promoting growth and anti-apoptosis [80], and it may be related not only to the process of intimal hyperplasia, but also to the neointimal formation during the atherosclerotic process. The TGFβ is another important inflammatory cytokine observed in the acute response to Ang II. It is known that the TGFβ is a protein with multifunctional actions, participating in the regulation of cell division, differentiation, migration, cell adhesion, extracellular matrix production, among other things, involved in several diseases, including the cardiovascular diseases [81]. Importantly, the TGFβ is synthesized as an inactive protein, having the latency-associated peptide (LAP) in its structure, which interacts with the latent TGFβ binding protein (LTBP), anchoring it to the extracellular matrix. This latent TGFβ is activated by proteolytic cleavage by plasmin, microenvironment acid and matrix metalloproteinases (MMP-2 and 9), among others [82 - 84]. The final production of plasmin occurs through the conversion of plasminogen by the enzymes called serine proteases tissue type plasminogen activator (t-PA) and urokinase type plasminogen activator (u-PA) (plasminogen activator system or fibrinolytic system) and is regulated by plasminogen activator inhibitor (PAI-1) [85].

Considering that Ang II acts on the vascular fibrinolytic balance, it can be postulated that the manner in which Ang II, by acting on its AT1 receptor, is capable of increasing the u-PA [86, 87], leading to the rapid release of TGFβ. In addition, another protein involved in the anchoring of TGFβ, the LTBP (Latent TGFβ Binding Protein) plays a fundamental role in the secretion of TGFβ [84]. Recently, Huby and colleagues [88] have shown indirect evidence of the action of Ang II on a variant of the LTBP, LTBP-4, where the blockade of AT1 receptor leads to the reduction in both LTBP-4 and in active TGFβ. These studies demonstrate a critical role of Ang II not only in preserving the vascular structural integrity, but also in the initiation and progression of degenerative processes, such as aortic aneurysms.

RAS & CARDIAC HYPERTROPHY

The heart is able to respond to hemodynamic stimuli, for instance, the alterations in workload, pressure and volume. These hemodynamic alterations are imposed by certain pathophysiological determinants, such as arterial hypertension and myocardial infarction, and also by physiological conditions, such as exercise training. When chronically exposed to these hemodynamic regimens, the heart adapts its structure, through a complex cellular and molecular process, by increasing the myocardial mass; thus, characterizing cardiac hypertrophy (CH).

Hypertension is one of the main contributing factors to pathological CH. The increased afterload imposed upon the left ventricle due to the chronic increase of the BP levels leads to the process of hypertrophy, characterized by an augment above 2.5 to 5% in the left ventricle mass [89]. Although it is a compensatory adaptation of the heart in an attempt to reduce the stress in the left ventricle wall imposed by the increased BP levels, hypertension-induced cardiac hypertrophy brings important consequences to the cardiovascular health, being considered an independent risk factor for cardiovascular events [89, 90].

Nevertheless, the determinant mechanisms leading to CH go beyond the hemodynamic alterations. Several factors, such as the sympathetic hyperactivity [91, 92], insulin [93], growth [94] and sexual hormones [95, 96], are examples of non-hemodynamic stimuli that may influence the increase of the cardiac mass. One of the first triggers of the hypertrophic process is the mechanical stretch in the ventricle wall, which stimulates the cardiac angiotensinogen expression, the precursor of the RAS cascade [97]. Therefore, it increases the local production of Ang II from cardiac myocytes, an initial mediator of the hypertrophic process [98].

During the complex process of CH, the re-expression of fetal genes is characteristic of the cardiomyocytes [99]. The release of Ang II can optimize this process by inducing the rapid activation of immediate-early genes in the cardiac cells, such as the skeletal α- actin in the ventricle, β-myosin heavy chain and atrial natriuretic factor [100].

At vascular and cardiac levels, Ang II can exert a direct effect on the smooth muscle and cardiac cells [100, 101]. Also, it induces fibroblasts proliferation in the heart, thus contributing to the increased interstitial fibrosis [102, 103].

Other important direct effects of Ang II contributing to CH are related to the responses induced by the interactions of this peptide in the heart. For instance, Ang II interaction with cardiac nerves modulates the catecholamine release, which is a potent hypertrophy inducer. Ang II can also influence on the cardiac cell metabolism by its interaction with intracellular receptors, and it can also influence on the endothelial factors release by interacting with the vascular endothelial cells [104].

It is noticeable that RAS local activation contributing to CH is independent of the BP levels, as demonstrated by Mazzolai *et al.* [105]. The authors used transgenic mice with cardiac angiotensinogen overexpression, which, in turn, presented an increased cardiac Ang II production. When comparing the transgenic *versus* control mice, all within normotensive level of BP, the transgenic ones presented an increase in the left ventricular mass.

Other RAS components also participate in the CH pathological process. Plasmatic renin activity, the precursor of the RAS, is also related to the degree of CH [105]. Although the study of Solomon *et al.* [106] showed that renin inhibition can be as effective as the AT1 blocker losartan in reducing the left ventricle mass in hypertensive patients, investigations on the renin inhibitors effectiveness or superiority are still on the way to become evidence. Additionally, aldosterone has been reported to be involved in the myocardial fibroblasts metabolic regulation and growth [107].

RAS & IMMUNE RESPONSE ACTIVATION

It is well known that AT_1 receptors found in different tissues may regulate regulate water and sodium homeostasis but other actions of Ang II influencing immune responses can also participate in BP regulation and target organ damage in hypertension. Indeed, AT1 receptors and other RAS peptides were described in mononuclear cell populations by gene expression and ligand-binding studies [108, 109]. In this way RAS immune system and cardiovascular disease pathophysiology link was highlighted only recently.

Thus, it has been observed in Rag1-deficient mice that chronic infusion of Ang II did not increase BP in these animals. This finding is probably due to the absence of functional lymphocytes in these animals, since the administration of T cells, but not B cells, could recover the BP elevation response to Ang II [110]. It is not well understood why T cells can influence Ang II-induced hypertension, but changes in the water and sodium control mechanisms and in vasculature may be considered [110, 111].

It is not clear what kind of antigens could activate the adaptive immune response in hypertension, but it is possible that T cell stimulation by antigen-specific mechanism may be involved [112]. The role of AT1 receptors in this response is controversial as suggested by AT1 receptor-deficienct mice experiments [111], as well as by the possibility to activate indirectly T cells by Ang II actions in the central nervous system [113]. Indeed, the induction of immunosuppression can reduce albuminuria, and the renal damage during Ang II induced hypertension independently of changes in BP [114]. It seems that Ang II dependent kidney lesions may be associated with increased expression of pro-inflammatory cytokines in the kidney as for example tumor necrosis factor-α (TNF-α) [115], since the blockade of TNF-α is able to abolish Ang II-induced renal injury [114]. Although Ang II is linked to tissue damage in hypertension it is now some evidence that, Ang II can also induce some cardioprotection by inducing immunosuppressive T regulatory cells [116, 117].

Thus, the functions of the immune system and RAS in cardiovascular and renal disease are complex, including other elements of the system and will require further elucidation.

RAS INHIBITORS & CARDIOVASCULAR DISEASE TREATMENT: PHYSIOLOGICAL BASIS

The most widely prescribed class of medications for the control of BP in hypertensive subjects are RAS inhibitors. ACE inhibitors and the Ang II type 1 (AT1) receptor blockers (ARBs) are the most clinically important drugs that block the RAS. Recently, a new compound has been introduced in the market, aliskiren, a direct renin inhibitor.

ACE inhibitors are considered a breakthrough in the management of hypertension and cardiovascular diseases. They are among the most effective antihypertensive drugs with the combination of efficacy, low incidence of adverse events and maintenance of quality of life, by protecting the target organs such as the heart, kidneys and blood vessels [118].

When ACE inhibitors are taken in the short term, there is a decrease in the endogenous levels of Ang II and aldosterone, whereas there is an increase in the plasma renin activity and in Ang I levels [118 - 120]. With the chronic ACE inhibition, Ang II and aldosterone levels may return to the pre-treatment levels while the hemodynamic effect is maintained [121, 122]. The role of bradykinin in the hemodynamic effects of ACE inhibitors in humans remains uncertain [122, 123]. In fact, ACE inhibitors reduce the systemic vascular resistance without causing a compensatory increase in the heart rate [124] and have little effect on cardiac output and pulmonary capillary wedge pressure in individuals with a normal left ventricular function [125] and may reduce the after- load, pre-load and systolic wall stress, increasing the cardiac output in patients with systolic dysfunction [126 - 128]. In addition, ACE Inhibitors can cause salt excretion by increasing the renal blood flow and by decreasing the production of aldosterone and antidiuretic hormone, can reduce the glomerular capillary pressure by selectively dilating the efferent arterioles [129, 130]; and can decrease the sympathetic nervous activity improving the autonomic reflex control of the circulation [131, 132]. It has been proposed that ACE inhibitors have beneficial effects on different tissues, independently of hemodynamic alterations. In animal models, ACE inhibitors act on ventricular remodeling by blocking the effects of Ang II on cardiac myocytes [124, 133]; and may have beneficial effects on vascular structure and function [134, 135]. Furthermore, in models of renal injury, ACE inhibitors reduce the mesangial cell growth and the production of extracellular matrix [136].

ACE inhibitors can cause hypotension, especially under low sodium intake and during the use of diuretics [137]; in patients with impaired renal function or taking potassium supplements (including salt substitutes), or potassium-sparing diuretics hyperkalemia, may occur [138]. In bilateral renal artery stenosis [139], with decreased renal perfusion or in severe congestive heart failure, or depletion in volume, ACE inhibitors may cause a reversible decrease in the renal function [140 - 142]. Cough is a frequent side effect of ACE inhibitors. The rate reaches 10% in white populations, but in Asian populations it can be as high as 44% [143 - 145]. The mechanism may involve an increase in the levels of bradykinin or substance P and a stimulation of vagal pulmonary C-fibers [143]. Angioedema is a rare, but potentially fatal side effect of ACE inhibitors, especially in Afro – descendants [146]. ACE inhibitors can cause a number of fetal abnormalities, including oligohydramnios, pulmonary hypoplasia, growth retardation, fetal death, neonatal anuria and stillbirth if administered in the second or third trimester of pregnancy [147, 148]. Consequently, these drugs must be used carefully in childbearing-aged women, and should immediately be discontinued in any woman whose pregnancy has been diagnosed. Rare adverse effects potentially related to the presence of a sulfhydryl group are: neutropenic syndrome, nephritic syndrome, and skin rash [149].

However, it is important to highlight that is well established in the literature that ACE inhibitors decrease cardiovascular events, such as myocardial infarction, stroke, heart failure, and cardiovascular death as shown in several clinical trials [150 - 153]. Furthermore, ACE inhibitors reduce surrogate end points, including the left ventricular hypertrophy [154]. Diabetic hypertensive patients have a preferential indication for the use of ACE inhibitors, since these drugs have at least a neutral effect in the carbohydrate metabolism and a positive impact on the renal function. Also, it is stated that ACE inhibitors may have additional benefits beyond the reduction in the BP levels, especially, in diabetic patients [155]. In the congestive heart failure, the combination of ACE inhibitors and diuretics is the first line of treatment. ACE inhibitors improve exercise tolerance, reducing the risk of death and recurrence of hospitalization due to heart failure [27, 156].

Ang II receptor blockers (ARBs) represent a class of effective and well tolerated orally active antihypertensive agents. The ARBs reduce BP by blocking of AT1 receptor, inducing smooth cell relaxation, increasing water and salt excretion and reducing plasma volume and cellular hypertrophy. These effects are most due to the decrease in peripheral vascular resistance than in changes in heart rate. In the recommended doses, all current available ARBs have comparable antihypertensive efficacy, and most of the drugs have a good maintenance of action through 24-hour Ambulatory BP Monitoring [157]. More recently, these drugs have been presented in combination with diuretics or calcium channel blockers, and have shown an additive effect in dropping the high levels of BP.

The AT1 receptor blockers are different in their pharmacological properties and clinical efficacy. Losartan shifts the dose-response curve for Ang II to the right but did not change the maximal response, acting as a surmountable antagonist. In contrast, other agents suppress the maximal response to Ang II which cannot be overcome by increasing the Ang II concentrations and, hence, these agents are insurmountable antagonists [158]. The antihypertensive potency of the ARBs on the basis of the daily mg dose, follows the sequence: candesartan cilexetil > telmisartan approximately = losartan > irbesartan approximately = valsartan > eprosartan. As a consequence of the displacement of Ang II from AT1 receptor, all of its known effects are antagonized, resulting in the fall of the peripheral resistance and little change in the heart rate and cardiac output [159]. It has been suggested that the stimulation of AT2 receptors may have a beneficial effect on neuroprotection, however, this issue needs further attention [160].

Other potential effects are improvement in the endothelial function, anti-inflammatory effects, suppression of reactive oxygen species and a variety of cytokines [161]. Among the well-known ancillary properties of ARBs are their peculiar effectiveness in reducing proteinuria in renal diseases and improving outcomes in chronic heart failure.

Recently, focus has been placed on another mechanism of ARBs: the increase in angiotensin I and II that may promote an increase in Ang (1-7). This peptide stimulates Mas receptors with functional effects similar to those observed with AT2 stimulation [35].

A potentially salient and serious adverse event, angioedema, was reported in very few studies with ARBs, with a lesser incidence compared to ACEi [162]. Furthermore, the ARB telmisartan was well tolerated in patients who have been intolerant to an ACEi [163]. Among the other side effects of ARBs, a report from a recent meta-analysis has demonstrated a mean occurrence of: 3% cough; 6,3 % headache; 4,3% dizziness. Regarding a hypothesis of an association of ARBs and cancer onset, [164] a larger meta-analysis, of randomized trials demonstrated any evidence of increased cancer incidence [165]. Less frequently adverse effects, like fatigue, upper respiratory infection, back pain and muscle clamps are less incidents with ARBs, even in elderly population [166]. Compelling and possible contra-indications of ARBs are similar to the ones of ACEIs: pregnancy and women with child bearing potential, hypercalcemia and bilateral renal artery stenosis [167].

It is important to highlight that ARBs and ACEIs are among those widely used in hypertensive therapy as a single agent or in combination with diuretics and calcium antagonists [167]. Direct comparison of ACEIs and ARBs reviewed in a recent meta-analysis, had shown little difference in antihypertensive efficacy and other outcomes, including death, cardiovascular events, quality of life, lipid and glucose levels, left ventricular mass and kidney disease [168]. However, other meta-analysis, including the ONTARGET study, suggested that ARB telmisartan may be inferior to ACEI ramipril in preventing myocardial infarction [169]. The only combination that cannot be recommended on the basis of the trials results is that between the two different blockers of RAS (ARBs and ACEIs) [170, 171].

More recently, a direct renin inhibitors (DRI), aliskiren, has been approved for the treatment of hypertension, both as monotherapy and combined with other antihypertensive agents [172, 173]. Prolonged administration in combined treatment can have a favorable effect on urinary protein excretion [174] and biomarkers of heart failure [175]. No trial has been available on the effect of aliskiren on cardiovascular or renal morbid and fatal events in hypertension.

Aliskiren binds to intracellular stored renin, inhibiting renin´s catalytic site. Therefore, aliskiren inhibits rennin activity before its secretion. Despite aliskiren has a low absorption and bioavailability (3%), it has a high specificity for the enzymatically active site of human renin, a long half-life (40h) and it is minimally metabolized [176]. This drug reduces the formation of Ang I formation and its generation of Ang II, resulting in a fall of BP. As a consequence of the removal of the normal inhibition of pro rennin secretion from the juxtaglomerular apparatus, the level of prorenin and renin are markedly increased. Whether or not there are hazards from prorenin action on its own receptor, deserves to be fully understood in further studies.

A meta-analysis comparing the efficacy between DRI and ARBs has shown similar antihypertensive effects. Also, regarding the adverse effects, Aliskiren has been reported to be similar to ARBs except for rises in serum potassium, and diarrhea [177]. Moreover, Aliskiren is contraindicated in pregnancy.

In diabetic patients, Aliskiren administered on top of an RAS blocker increased the risk of cardiovascular and renal events [178]. Consequently, this treatment strategy (combination of the two RAS blockers), is therefore contra-indicated in such conditions. Furthermore, no beneficial effect on mortality and hospitalization has been shown by adding Aliskiren to standard treatment in heart failure [179].

CONFLICT OF INTEREST

The authors certify that they have NO affiliations with or involvement in any organization or entity with any financial interest or non-financial interest in the subject matter or materials discussed in this chapter.

ACKNOWLEDGEMENTS

The authors would like to thank Isabel Cristina Lameirinhas for technical support.

REFERENCES

[1] Danser AH, van Kats JP, Admiraal PJ, *et al.* Cardiac renin and angiotensins. Uptake from plasma *versus in situ* synthesis. Hypertension 1994; 24(1): 37-48. [http://dx.doi.org/10.1161/01.HYP.24.1.37] [PMID: 8021006]

[2] Dzau VJ. Vascular renin-angiotensin system and vascular protection. J Cardiovasc Pharmacol 1993; 22 (Suppl. 5): S1-9. [http://dx.doi.org/10.1097/00005344-199322005-00002] [PMID: 7508045]

[3] Krop M, Danser AH. Circulating *versus* tissue renin-angiotensin system: on the origin of (pro)renin. Curr Hypertens Rep 2008; 10(2): 112-8. [http://dx.doi.org/10.1007/s11906-008-0022-1] [PMID: 18474177]

[4] Cassis LA, Police SB, Yiannikouris F, Thatcher SE. Local adipose tissue renin-angiotensin system. Curr Hypertens Rep 2008; 10(2): 93-8. [http://dx.doi.org/10.1007/s11906-008-0019-9] [PMID: 18474174]

[5] Folkow B, Johansson B, Mellander S. The comparative effects of angiotensin and noradrenaline on consecutive vascular sections. Acta Physiol Scand 1961; 53: 99-104. [http://dx.doi.org/10.1111/j.1748-1716.1961.tb02267.x] [PMID: 13893844]

[6] Zimmerman BG, Sybertz EJ, Wong PC. Interaction between sympathetic and renin-angiotensin system. J Hypertens 1984; 2(6): 581-7. [http://dx.doi.org/10.1097/00004872-198412000-00002] [PMID: 6098607]

[7] Reid IA. Interactions between ANG II, sympathetic nervous system, and baroreceptor reflexes in regulation of blood pressure. Am J Physiol 1992; 262(6 Pt 1): E763-78. [PMID: 1616014]

[8] Padfield PL, Morton JJ. Effects of angiotensin II on arginine-vasopressin in physiological and pathological situations in man. J Endocrinol 1977; 74(2): 251-9.

[http://dx.doi.org/10.1677/joe.0.0740251] [PMID: 302301]

[9] Daemen MJ, Lombardi DM, Bosman FT, Schwartz SM. Angiotensin II induces smooth muscle cell proliferation in the normal and injured rat arterial wall. Circ Res 1991; 68(2): 450-6. [http://dx.doi.org/10.1161/01.RES.68.2.450] [PMID: 1991349]

[10] Yaghini FA, Song CY, Lavrentyev EN, *et al.* Angiotensin II-induced vascular smooth muscle cell migration and growth are mediated by cytochrome P450 1B1-dependent superoxide generation. Hypertension 2010; 55(6): 1461-7. [http://dx.doi.org/10.1161/HYPERTENSIONAHA.110.150029] [PMID: 20439821]

[11] Brown NJ, Vaughan DE. Angiotensin-converting enzyme inhibitors. Circulation 1998; 97(14): 1411-20. [http://dx.doi.org/10.1161/01.CIR.97.14.1411] [PMID: 9577953]

[12] Lautner RQ, Villela DC, Fraga-Silva RA, *et al.* Discovery and characterization of alamandine: a novel component of the renin-angiotensin system. Circ Res 2013; 112(8): 1104-11. [http://dx.doi.org/10.1161/CIRCRESAHA.113.301077] [PMID: 23446738]

[13] Villela DC, Passos-Silva DG, Santos RA. Alamandine: a new member of the angiotensin family. Curr Opin Nephrol Hypertens 2014; 23(2): 130-4. [http://dx.doi.org/10.1097/01.mnh.0000441052.44406.92] [PMID: 24389733]

[14] Santos RA, Simoes e Silva AC, Maric C, *et al.* Angiotensin-(1-7) is an endogenous ligand for the G protein-coupled receptor Mas. Proc Natl Acad Sci USA 2003; 100(14): 8258-63. [http://dx.doi.org/10.1073/pnas.1432869100] [PMID: 12829792]

[15] Gainer JV, Morrow JD, Loveland A, King DJ, Brown NJ. Effect of bradykinin-receptor blockade on the response to angiotensin-converting-enzyme inhibitor in normotensive and hypertensive subjects. N Engl J Med 1998; 339(18): 1285-92. [http://dx.doi.org/10.1056/NEJM199810293391804] [PMID: 9791144]

[16] De Mello WC, Frohlich ED. On the local cardiac renin angiotensin system. Basic and clinical implications. Peptides 2011; 32(8): 1774-9. [http://dx.doi.org/10.1016/j.peptides.2011.06.018] [PMID: 21729730]

[17] Sun Y. Intracardiac renin-angiotensin system and myocardial repair/remodeling following infarction. J Mol Cell Cardiol 2010; 48(3): 483-9. [http://dx.doi.org/10.1016/j.yjmcc.2009.08.002] [PMID: 19682461]

[18] Britto RR, Santos RA, Fagundes-Moura CR, Khosla MC, Campagnole-Santos MJ. Role of angiotensin-(1-7) in the modulation of the baroreflex in renovascular hypertensive rats. Hypertension 1997; 30(3 Pt 2): 549-56. [http://dx.doi.org/10.1161/01.HYP.30.3.549] [PMID: 9322980]

[19] Silva LC, Fontes MA, Campagnole-Santos MJ, *et al.* Cardiovascular effects produced by micro-injection of angiotensin-(1-7) on vasopressor and vasodepressor sites of the ventrolateral medulla. Brain Res 1993; 613(2): 321-5. [http://dx.doi.org/10.1016/0006-8993(93)90920-I] [PMID: 8186985]

[20] Gironacci MM, Cerniello FM, Longo Carbajosa NA, Goldstein J, Cerrato BD. Protective axis of the renin-angiotensin system in the brain. Clin Sci 2014; 127(5): 295-306.

[http://dx.doi.org/10.1042/CS20130450] [PMID: 24827941]

[21] Cangussu LM, de Castro UG, do Pilar Machado R, *et al.* Angiotensin-(1-7) antagonist, A-779, microinjection into the caudal ventrolateral medulla of renovascular hypertensive rats restores baroreflex bradycardia. Peptides 2009; 30(10): 1921-7. [http://dx.doi.org/10.1016/j.peptides.2009.06.028] [PMID: 19577603]

[22] Sriramula S, Cardinale JP, Lazartigues E, Francis J. ACE2 overexpression in the paraventricular nucleus attenuates angiotensin II-induced hypertension. Cardiovasc Res 2011; 92(3): 401-8. [http://dx.doi.org/10.1093/cvr/cvr242] [PMID: 21952934]

[23] Santos RA, Ferreira AJ, Simões E Silva AC. Recent advances in the angiotensin-converting enzyme 2-angiotensin(1-7)-Mas axis. Exp Physiol 2008; 93(5): 519-27. [http://dx.doi.org/10.1113/expphysiol.2008.042002] [PMID: 18310257]

[24] de Gasparo M, Catt KJ, Inagami T, Wright JW, Unger T. International union of pharmacology. XXIII. The angiotensin II receptors. Pharmacol Rev 2000; 52(3): 415-72. [PMID: 10977869]

[25] Skeggs LT, Dorer FE, Kahn JR, Lentz KE, Levine M. The biochemistry of the renin-angiotensin system and its role in hypertension. Am J Med 1976; 60(6): 737-48. [http://dx.doi.org/10.1016/0002-9343(76)90888-3] [PMID: 190880]

[26] Hussain A, Graham R. Drugs, Enzymes and Receptors of the Renin-Angiotensin System: Celebrating a Century of Discovery Amsterdam. Harwood Academic Publishers 2000.

[27] The SOLVD Investigators. Effect of enalapril on survival in patients with reduced left ventricular ejection fractions and congestive heart failure. N Engl J Med 1991; 325(5): 293-302. [http://dx.doi.org/10.1056/NEJM199108013250501] [PMID: 2057034]

[28] Effect of enalapril on mortality and the development of heart failure in asymptomatic patients with reduced left ventricular ejection fractions. The SOLVD Investigattors. N Engl J Med 1992; 327(10): 685-91. [http://dx.doi.org/10.1056/NEJM199209033271003] [PMID: 1463530]

[29] Lewis EJ, Hunsicker LG, Bain RP, Rohde RD. The Collaborative Study Group. The effect of angiotensin-converting-enzyme inhibition on diabetic nephropathy. N Engl J Med 1993; 329(20): 1456-62. [http://dx.doi.org/10.1056/NEJM199311113292004] [PMID: 8413456]

[30] Crackower MA, Sarao R, Oudit GY, *et al.* Angiotensin-converting enzyme 2 is an essential regulator of heart function. Nature 2002; 417(6891): 822-8. [http://dx.doi.org/10.1038/nature00786] [PMID: 12075344]

[31] Gurley SB, Allred A, Le TH, *et al.* Altered blood pressure responses and normal cardiac phenotype in ACE2-null mice. J Clin Invest 2006; 116(8): 2218-25. [http://dx.doi.org/10.1172/JCI16980] [PMID: 16878172]

[32] Thomas MC, Pickering RJ, Tsorotes D, *et al.* Genetic Ace2 deficiency accentuates vascular inflammation and atherosclerosis in the ApoE knockout mouse. Circ Res 2010; 107(7): 888-97. [http://dx.doi.org/10.1161/CIRCRESAHA.110.219279] [PMID: 20671240]

[33] Wong DW, Oudit GY, Reich H, *et al.* Loss of angiotensin-converting enzyme-2 (Ace2) accelerates

diabetic kidney injury. Am J Pathol 2007; 171(2): 438-51.
[http://dx.doi.org/10.2353/ajpath.2007.060977] [PMID: 17600118]

[34] Vickers C, Hales P, Kaushik V, *et al.* Hydrolysis of biological peptides by human angiotensin-converting enzyme-related carboxypeptidase. J Biol Chem 2002; 277(17): 14838-43.
[http://dx.doi.org/10.1074/jbc.M200581200] [PMID: 11815627]

[35] Ferrario CM, Brosnihan KB, Diz DI, *et al.* Angiotensin-(1-7): a new hormone of the angiotensin system. Hypertension 1991; 18(5) (Suppl.): III126-33.
[PMID: 1937675]

[36] Saxena PR. Interaction between the renin-angiotensin-aldosterone and sympathetic nervous systems. J Cardiovasc Pharmacol 1992; 19 (Suppl. 6): S80-8.
[http://dx.doi.org/10.1097/00005344-199219006-00013] [PMID: 1382170]

[37] Dampney RA, Tan PS, Sheriff MJ, Fontes MA, Horiuchi J. Cardiovascular effects of angiotensin II in the rostral ventrolateral medulla: the push-pull hypothesis. Curr Hypertens Rep 2007; 9(3): 222-7.
[http://dx.doi.org/10.1007/s11906-007-0040-4] [PMID: 17519129]

[38] Carlson SH, Wyss JM. Neurohormonal regulation of the sympathetic nervous system: new insights into central mechanisms of action. Curr Hypertens Rep 2008; 10(3): 233-40.
[http://dx.doi.org/10.1007/s11906-008-0044-8] [PMID: 18765096]

[39] Schinke M, Baltatu O, Böhm M, *et al.* Blood pressure reduction and diabetes insipidus in transgenic rats deficient in brain angiotensinogen. Proc Natl Acad Sci USA 1999; 96(7): 3975-80.
[http://dx.doi.org/10.1073/pnas.96.7.3975] [PMID: 10097148]

[40] Campos LA, Iliescu R, Fontes MA, Schlegel WP, Bader M, Baltatu OC. Enhanced isoproterenol-induced cardiac hypertrophy in transgenic rats with low brain angiotensinogen. Am J Physiol Heart Circ Physiol 2006; 291(5): H2371-6.
[http://dx.doi.org/10.1152/ajpheart.01145.2005] [PMID: 16731636]

[41] Parrish DC, Gritman K, Van Winkle DM, Woodward WR, Bader M, Habecker BA. Postinfarct sympathetic hyperactivity differentially stimulates expression of tyrosine hydroxylase and norepinephrine transporter. Am J Physiol Heart Circ Physiol 2008; 294(1): H99-H106.
[http://dx.doi.org/10.1152/ajpheart.00533.2007] [PMID: 17951370]

[42] Guo GB, Abboud FM. Angiotensin II attenuates baroreflex control of heart rate and sympathetic activity. Am J Physiol 1984; 246(1 Pt 2): H80-9.
[PMID: 6696093]

[43] Wong LF, Polson JW, Murphy D, Paton JF, Kasparov S. Genetic and pharmacological dissection of pathways involved in the angiotensin II-mediated depression of baroreflex function. FASEB journal : official publication of the Federation of American Societies for Experimental Biology 2002; 16(12): 1595-601.

[44] Irigoyen MC, Moreira ED, Cestari IA, Krieger EM. The relationship between renal sympathetic nerve activity and arterial pressure after selective denervation of baroreceptors and chemoreceptors. Brazilian journal of medical and biological research = Revista brasileira de pesquisas medicas e biologicas / Sociedade Brasileira de Biofisica (et al) 1991; 24(2): 219-2.

[45] DiBona GF. Central angiotensin modulation of baroreflex control of renal sympathetic nerve activity

in the rat: influence of dietary sodium. Acta Physiol Scand 2003; 177(3): 285-9.
[http://dx.doi.org/10.1046/j.1365-201X.2003.01074.x] [PMID: 12608998]

[46] DiBona GF. Nervous kidney. Interaction between renal sympathetic nerves and the renin-angiotensin system in the control of renal function. Hypertension 2000; 36(6): 1083-8.
[http://dx.doi.org/10.1161/01.HYP.36.6.1083] [PMID: 11116129]

[47] DiBona GF, Kopp UC. Neural control of renal function. Physiol Rev 1997; 77(1): 75-197.
[PMID: 9016301]

[48] Oliveira VL, Irigoyen MC, Moreira ED, Strunz C, Krieger EM. Renal denervation normalizes pressure and baroreceptor reflex in high renin hypertension in conscious rats. Hypertension 1992; 19(2) (Suppl.): II17-21.
[PMID: 1735574]

[49] Huang BS, Leenen FH. The brain renin-angiotensin-aldosterone system: a major mechanism for sympathetic hyperactivity and left ventricular remodeling and dysfunction after myocardial infarction. Curr Heart Fail Rep 2009; 6(2): 81-8.
[http://dx.doi.org/10.1007/s11897-009-0013-9] [PMID: 19486591]

[50] Campos LA, Bader M, Baltatu OC. Brain Renin-Angiotensin system in hypertension, cardiac hypertrophy, and heart failure. Front Physiol 2011; 2: 115.
[PMID: 22291657]

[51] DiBona GF, Esler M. Translational medicine: the antihypertensive effect of renal denervation. Am J Physiol Regul Integr Comp Physiol 2010; 298(2): R245-53.
[http://dx.doi.org/10.1152/ajpregu.00647.2009] [PMID: 19955493]

[52] Ram CV, Kumar AS. Renal denervation therapy for resistant hypertension: a clinical update. J Hum Hypertens 2014; 28(12): 699-704.
[http://dx.doi.org/10.1038/jhh.2014.6] [PMID: 24599151]

[53] Schlaich MP, Hering D, Sobotka PA, Krum H, Esler MD. Renal denervation in human hypertension: mechanisms, current findings, and future prospects. Curr Hypertens Rep 2012; 14(3): 247-53.
[http://dx.doi.org/10.1007/s11906-012-0264-9] [PMID: 22457244]

[54] Esler MD, Krum H, Sobotka PA, Schlaich MP, Schmieder RE, Böhm M. Symplicity HTN-2 Investigators. Renal sympathetic denervation in patients with treatment-resistant hypertension (The Symplicity HTN-2 Trial): a randomised controlled trial. Lancet 2010; 376(9756): 1903-9.
[http://dx.doi.org/10.1016/S0140-6736(10)62039-9] [PMID: 21093036]

[55] Gimbrone MA Jr. Vascular endothelium, hemodynamic forces, and atherogenesis. Am J Pathol 1999; 155(1): 1-5.
[http://dx.doi.org/10.1016/S0002-9440(10)65090-0] [PMID: 10393828]

[56] Wilting J. Integrated Vascular Anatomy. In: Lanzer P, Topol E, Eds. Pan Vascular Medicine: Springer Berlin Heidelberg. 2002; pp. 50-75.
[http://dx.doi.org/10.1007/978-3-642-56225-9_4]

[57] Gimbrone MA. Vascular endothelium in health and disease. In: Haber E, Ed. Molecular Cardiovascular Medicine. New York: Scientific American Inc. 1995; pp. 49-62.

[58] Lüscher TF, Noll G. The Endothelium as a Regulator of Vascular Tone and Growth. In: Lüscher T,

Ed. The Endothelium in Cardiovascular Disease: Springer Berlin Heidelberg. 1995; pp. 1-24. [http://dx.doi.org/10.1007/978-3-642-79803-0_1]

[59] Viegas KA, Lacchini S. Injúria vascular e reestenose. In: Krieger JE, Ed. Bases Moleculares das Doenças Cardiovasculares: a integração entre a pesquisa e a prática clínica. São Paulo: Atheneu 2008; pp. 415-32.

[60] Pakala R, Benedict CR. Endothelial cells regulate the proliferation of monocytes *in vitro*. Atherosclerosis 1999; 147(1): 25-32. [http://dx.doi.org/10.1016/S0021-9150(99)00144-6] [PMID: 10525121]

[61] Moncada S, Palmer RM, Higgs EA. Nitric oxide: physiology, pathophysiology, and pharmacology. Pharmacol Rev 1991; 43(2): 109-42. [PMID: 1852778]

[62] Weissberg P. Mechanisms modifying atherosclerotic disease - from lipids to vascular biology. Atherosclerosis 1999; 147 (Suppl. 1): S3-S10. [http://dx.doi.org/10.1016/S0021-9150(99)00249-X] [PMID: 10575056]

[63] Libby P, Theroux P. Pathophysiology of coronary artery disease. Circulation 2005; 111(25): 3481-8. [http://dx.doi.org/10.1161/CIRCULATIONAHA.105.537878] [PMID: 15983262]

[64] Goldin A, Beckman JA, Schmidt AM, Creager MA. Advanced glycation end products: sparking the development of diabetic vascular injury. Circulation 2006; 114(6): 597-605. [http://dx.doi.org/10.1161/CIRCULATIONAHA.106.621854] [PMID: 16894049]

[65] Ellis A, Triggle CR. Endothelium-derived reactive oxygen species: their relationship to endothelium-dependent hyperpolarization and vascular tone. Can J Physiol Pharmacol 2003; 81(11): 1013-28. [http://dx.doi.org/10.1139/y03-106] [PMID: 14719036]

[66] Rakugi H, Jacob HJ, Krieger JE, Ingelfinger JR, Pratt RE. Vascular injury induces angiotensinogen gene expression in the media and neointima. Circulation 1993; 87(1): 283-90. [http://dx.doi.org/10.1161/01.CIR.87.1.283] [PMID: 8419017]

[67] Ohishi M, Ueda M, Rakugi H, *et al.* Enhanced expression of angiotensin-converting enzyme is associated with progression of coronary atherosclerosis in humans. J Hypertens 1997; 15(11): 1295-302. [http://dx.doi.org/10.1097/00004872-199715110-00014] [PMID: 9383179]

[68] Ohishi M, Ueda M, Rakugi H, *et al.* Relative localization of angiotensin-converting enzyme, chymase and angiotensin II in human coronary atherosclerotic lesions. J Hypertens 1999; 17(4): 547-53. [http://dx.doi.org/10.1097/00004872-199917040-00013] [PMID: 10404957]

[69] Dzau VJ, Krieger JE, Hutchinson HG. Molecular mechanisms of hypertension. In: Haber E, Ed. Molecular cardiovascular medicine. New York: Scientific American Inc 1995; pp. 225-442.

[70] Lacchini S, Heimann AS, Evangelista FS, Cardoso L, Silva GJ, Krieger JE. Cuff-induced vascular intima thickening is influenced by titration of the Ace gene in mice. Physiol Genomics 2009; 37(3): 225-30. [http://dx.doi.org/10.1152/physiolgenomics.90288.2008] [PMID: 19258495]

[71] Ross R. Atherosclerosis--an inflammatory disease. N Engl J Med 1999; 340(2): 115-26. [http://dx.doi.org/10.1056/NEJM199901143400207] [PMID: 9887164]

[72] Wolf G, Butzmann U, Wenzel UO. The renin-angiotensin system and progression of renal disease: from hemodynamics to cell biology. Nephron, Physiol 2003; 93(1): 3-13. [http://dx.doi.org/10.1159/000066656] [PMID: 12411725]

[73] Ruiz-Ortega M, Lorenzo O, Rupérez M, *et al.* Role of the renin-angiotensin system in vascular diseases: expanding the field. Hypertension 2001; 38(6): 1382-7. [http://dx.doi.org/10.1161/hy1201.100589] [PMID: 11751722]

[74] Dzau VJ, Lopez-Ilasaca M. Searching for transcriptional regulators of Ang II-induced vascular pathology. J Clin Invest 2005; 115(9): 2319-22. [http://dx.doi.org/10.1172/JCI26384] [PMID: 16138186]

[75] Ribichini F, Pugno F, Ferrero V, *et al.* Angiotensin-converting enzyme tissue activity in the diffuse in-stent restenotic plaque. Circulation 2000; 101(2): E33-5. [http://dx.doi.org/10.1161/01.CIR.101.2.e33] [PMID: 10637219]

[76] Schuett H, Luchtefeld M, Grothusen C, Grote K, Schieffer B. How much is too much? Interleukin-6 and its signalling in atherosclerosis. Thromb Haemost 2009; 102(2): 215-22. [PMID: 19652871]

[77] Schieffer B, Luchtefeld M, Braun S, Hilfiker A, Hilfiker-Kleiner D, Drexler H. Role of NAD(P)H oxidase in angiotensin II-induced JAK/STAT signaling and cytokine induction. Circ Res 2000; 87(12): 1195-201. [http://dx.doi.org/10.1161/01.RES.87.12.1195] [PMID: 11110778]

[78] Wassmann S, Stumpf M, Strehlow K, *et al.* Interleukin-6 induces oxidative stress and endothelial dysfunction by overexpression of the angiotensin II type 1 receptor. Circ Res 2004; 94(4): 534-41. [http://dx.doi.org/10.1161/01.RES.0000115557.25127.8D] [PMID: 14699015]

[79] Touyz RM. Reactive oxygen species as mediators of calcium signaling by angiotensin II: implications in vascular physiology and pathophysiology. Antioxidants & redox signaling 2005; 7(9-10): 1302-4. [http://dx.doi.org/10.1089/ars.2005.7.1302]

[80] Touyz RM, Berry C. Recent advances in angiotensin II signaling. Brazilian journal of medical and biological research = Revista brasileira de pesquisas medicas e biologicas / Sociedade Brasileira de Biofisica (et al) 2002; 35(9): 1001-5. [http://dx.doi.org/10.1590/S0100-879X2002000900001]

[81] Ruiz-Ortega M, Rodríguez-Vita J, Sanchez-Lopez E, Carvajal G, Egido J. TGF-beta signaling in vascular fibrosis. Cardiovasc Res 2007; 74(2): 196-206. [http://dx.doi.org/10.1016/j.cardiores.2007.02.008] [PMID: 17376414]

[82] Gibbons GH, Pratt RE, Dzau VJ. Vascular smooth muscle cell hypertrophy *vs.* hyperplasia. Autocrine transforming growth factor-beta 1 expression determines growth response to angiotensin II. J Clin Invest 1992; 90(2): 456-61. [http://dx.doi.org/10.1172/JCI115881] [PMID: 1644917]

[83] Khalil N, Corne S, Whitman C, Yacyshyn H. Plasmin regulates the activation of cell-associated latent TGF-beta 1 secreted by rat alveolar macrophages after *in vivo* bleomycin injury. Am J Respir Cell Mol Biol 1996; 15(2): 252-9. [http://dx.doi.org/10.1165/ajrcmb.15.2.8703482] [PMID: 8703482]

[84] Annes JP, Munger JS, Rifkin DB. Making sense of latent TGFbeta activation. J Cell Sci 2003; 116(Pt 2): 217-24.
[http://dx.doi.org/10.1242/jcs.00229] [PMID: 12482908]

[85] Vaughan DE. Angiotensin and vascular fibrinolytic balance. Am J Hypertens 2002; 15(1 Pt 2): 3S-8S.
[http://dx.doi.org/10.1016/S0895-7061(01)02273-7] [PMID: 11824873]

[86] Wang YX, Martin-McNulty B, Freay AD, *et al.* Angiotensin II increases urokinase-type plasminogen activator expression and induces aneurysm in the abdominal aorta of apolipoprotein E-deficient mice. Am J Pathol 2001; 159(4): 1455-64.
[http://dx.doi.org/10.1016/S0002-9440(10)62532-1] [PMID: 11583973]

[87] Daugherty A, Manning MW, Cassis LA. Antagonism of AT2 receptors augments angiotensin II-induced abdominal aortic aneurysms and atherosclerosis. Br J Pharmacol 2001; 134(4): 865-70.
[http://dx.doi.org/10.1038/sj.bjp.0704331] [PMID: 11606327]

[88] Huby AC, Rastaldi MP, Caron K, Smithies O, Dussaule JC, Chatziantoniou C. Restoration of podocyte structure and improvement of chronic renal disease in transgenic mice overexpressing renin. PLoS One 2009; 4(8): e6721.
[http://dx.doi.org/10.1371/journal.pone.0006721] [PMID: 19696925]

[89] Levy D, Anderson KM, Savage DD, Kannel WB, Christiansen JC, Castelli WP. Echocardiographically detected left ventricular hypertrophy: prevalence and risk factors. The Framingham Heart Study. Ann Intern Med 1988; 108(1): 7-13.
[http://dx.doi.org/10.7326/0003-4819-108-1-7] [PMID: 2962527]

[90] Devereux RB, Wachtell K, Gerdts E, *et al.* Prognostic significance of left ventricular mass change during treatment of hypertension. JAMA 2004; 292(19): 2350-6.
[http://dx.doi.org/10.1001/jama.292.19.2350] [PMID: 15547162]

[91] Grassi G. Sympathetic overdrive as an independent predictor of left ventricular hypertrophy: prospective evidence. J Hypertens 2006; 24(5): 815-7.
[http://dx.doi.org/10.1097/01.hjh.0000222748.37078.2d] [PMID: 16612240]

[92] Moraes-Silva IC, De La Fuente RN, Mostarda C, *et al.* Baroreflex deficit blunts exercise training-induced cardiovascular and autonomic adaptations in hypertensive rats. Clin Exp Pharmacol Physiol 2010; 37(3): e114-20.
[http://dx.doi.org/10.1111/j.1440-1681.2009.05333.x] [PMID: 19930428]

[93] Phillips RA, Krakoff LR, Dunaif A, Finegood DT, Gorlin R, Shimabukuro S. Relation among left ventricular mass, insulin resistance, and blood pressure in nonobese subjects. J Clin Endocrinol Metab 1998; 83(12): 4284-8.
[PMID: 9851765]

[94] Lim MJ, Barkan AL, Buda AJ. Rapid reduction of left ventricular hypertrophy in acromegaly after suppression of growth hormone hypersecretion. Ann Intern Med 1992; 117(9): 719-26.
[http://dx.doi.org/10.7326/0003-4819-117-9-719] [PMID: 1416573]

[95] Marcus R, Krause L, Weder AB, Dominguez-Meja A, Schork NJ, Julius S. Sex-specific determinants of increased left ventricular mass in the Tecumseh Blood Pressure Study. Circulation 1994; 90(2): 928-36.

[http://dx.doi.org/10.1161/01.CIR.90.2.928] [PMID: 8044964]

[96] de Simone G, Devereux RB, Daniels SR, Meyer RA. Gender differences in left ventricular growth. Hypertension 1995; 26(6 Pt 1): 979-83. [http://dx.doi.org/10.1161/01.HYP.26.6.979] [PMID: 7490158]

[97] Lindpaintner K, Jin MW, Niedermaier N, Wilhelm MJ, Ganten D. Cardiac angiotensinogen and its local activation in the isolated perfused beating heart. Circ Res 1990; 67(3): 564-73. [http://dx.doi.org/10.1161/01.RES.67.3.564] [PMID: 2204498]

[98] Sadoshima J, Xu Y, Slayter HS, Izumo S. Autocrine release of angiotensin II mediates stretch-induced hypertrophy of cardiac myocytes *in vitro*. Cell 1993; 75(5): 977-84. [http://dx.doi.org/10.1016/0092-8674(93)90541-W] [PMID: 8252633]

[99] Ames EG, Lawson MJ, Mackey AJ, Holmes JW. Sequencing of mRNA identifies re-expression of fetal splice variants in cardiac hypertrophy. J Mol Cell Cardiol 2013; 62: 99-107. [http://dx.doi.org/10.1016/j.yjmcc.2013.05.004] [PMID: 23688780]

[100] Sadoshima J, Izumo S. Molecular characterization of angiotensin II--induced hypertrophy of cardiac myocytes and hyperplasia of cardiac fibroblasts. Critical role of the AT1 receptor subtype. Circ Res 1993; 73(3): 413-23. [http://dx.doi.org/10.1161/01.RES.73.3.413] [PMID: 8348686]

[101] Baker KM, Chernin MI, Wixson SK, Aceto JF. Renin-angiotensin system involvement in pressure-overload cardiac hypertrophy in rats. Am J Physiol 1990; 259(2 Pt 2): H324-32. [PMID: 2143633]

[102] Weber KT, Sun Y, Tyagi SC, Cleutjens JP. Collagen network of the myocardium: function, structural remodeling and regulatory mechanisms. J Mol Cell Cardiol 1994; 26(3): 279-92. [http://dx.doi.org/10.1006/jmcc.1994.1036] [PMID: 8028011]

[103] Bouzegrhane F, Thibault G. Is angiotensin II a proliferative factor of cardiac fibroblasts? Cardiovasc Res 2002; 53(2): 304-12. [http://dx.doi.org/10.1016/S0008-6363(01)00448-5] [PMID: 11827680]

[104] Re RN. Cellular mechanisms of growth in cardiovascular tissue. Am J Cardiol 1987; 60(17): 104I-9I. [http://dx.doi.org/10.1016/0002-9149(87)90469-3] [PMID: 2961244]

[105] Mazzolai L, Nussberger J, Aubert JF, *et al.* Blood pressure-independent cardiac hypertrophy induced by locally activated renin-angiotensin system. Hypertension 1998; 31(6): 1324-30. [http://dx.doi.org/10.1161/01.HYP.31.6.1324] [PMID: 9622149]

[106] Solomon SD, Appelbaum E, Manning WJ, *et al.* Aliskiren in Left Ventricular Hypertrophy (ALLAY) Trial Investigators. Effect of the direct Renin inhibitor aliskiren, the Angiotensin receptor blocker losartan, or both on left ventricular mass in patients with hypertension and left ventricular hypertrophy. Circulation 2009; 119(4): 530-7. [http://dx.doi.org/10.1161/CIRCULATIONAHA.108.826214] [PMID: 19153265]

[107] Weber KT, Brilla CG. Pathological hypertrophy and cardiac interstitium. Fibrosis and renin-angiotensin-aldosterone system. Circulation 1991; 83(6): 1849-65. [http://dx.doi.org/10.1161/01.CIR.83.6.1849] [PMID: 1828192]

[108] Jurewicz M, McDermott DH, Sechler JM, *et al.* Human T and natural killer cells possess a functional

renin-angiotensin system: further mechanisms of angiotensin II-induced inflammation. J Am Soc Nephrol 2007; 18(4): 1093-102.
[http://dx.doi.org/10.1681/ASN.2006070707] [PMID: 17329576]

[109] Nataraj C, Oliverio MI, Mannon RB, *et al.* Angiotensin II regulates cellular immune responses through a calcineurin-dependent pathway. J Clin Invest 1999; 104(12): 1693-701.
[http://dx.doi.org/10.1172/JCI7451] [PMID: 10606623]

[110] Guzik TJ, Hoch NE, Brown KA, *et al.* Role of the T cell in the genesis of angiotensin II induced hypertension and vascular dysfunction. J Exp Med 2007; 204(10): 2449-60.
[http://dx.doi.org/10.1084/jem.20070657] [PMID: 17875676]

[111] Crowley SD, Song YS, Lin EE, Griffiths R, Kim HS, Ruiz P. Lymphocyte responses exacerbate angiotensin II-dependent hypertension. Am J Physiol Regul Integr Comp Physiol 2010; 298(4): R1089-97.
[http://dx.doi.org/10.1152/ajpregu.00373.2009] [PMID: 20147609]

[112] Vinh A, Chen W, Blinder Y, *et al.* Inhibition and genetic ablation of the B7/CD28 T-cell costimulation axis prevents experimental hypertension. Circulation 2010; 122(24): 2529-37.
[http://dx.doi.org/10.1161/CIRCULATIONAHA.109.930446] [PMID: 21126972]

[113] Marvar PJ, Thabet SR, Guzik TJ, *et al.* Central and peripheral mechanisms of T-lymphocyte activation and vascular inflammation produced by angiotensin II-induced hypertension. Circ Res 2010; 107(2): 263-70.
[http://dx.doi.org/10.1161/CIRCRESAHA.110.217299] [PMID: 20558826]

[114] Muller DN, Shagdarsuren E, Park JK, *et al.* Immunosuppressive treatment protects against angiotensin II-induced renal damage. Am J Pathol 2002; 161(5): 1679-93.
[http://dx.doi.org/10.1016/S0002-9440(10)64445-8] [PMID: 12414515]

[115] Crowley SD, Frey CW, Gould SK, *et al.* Stimulation of lymphocyte responses by angiotensin II promotes kidney injury in hypertension. Am J Physiol Renal Physiol 2008; 295(2): F515-24.
[http://dx.doi.org/10.1152/ajprenal.00527.2007] [PMID: 18495795]

[116] Barhoumi T, Kasal DA, Li MW, *et al.* T regulatory lymphocytes prevent angiotensin II-induced hypertension and vascular injury. Hypertension 2011; 57(3): 469-76.
[http://dx.doi.org/10.1161/HYPERTENSIONAHA.110.162941] [PMID: 21263125]

[117] Kvakan H, Kleinewietfeld M, Qadri F, *et al.* Regulatory T cells ameliorate angiotensin II-induced cardiac damage. Circulation 2009; 119(22): 2904-12.
[http://dx.doi.org/10.1161/CIRCULATIONAHA.108.832782] [PMID: 19470887]

[118] van Vark LC, Bertrand M, Akkerhuis KM, *et al.* Angiotensin-converting enzyme inhibitors reduce mortality in hypertension: a meta-analysis of randomized clinical trials of renin-angiotensi--aldosterone system inhibitors involving 158,998 patients. Eur Heart J 2012; 33(16): 2088-97.
[http://dx.doi.org/10.1093/eurheartj/ehs075] [PMID: 22511654]

[119] Vander AJ, Geelhoed GW. Inhibition of renin secretion by angiotensin. II. Proc Soc Exp Biol Med 1965; 120(2): 399-403.
[http://dx.doi.org/10.3181/00379727-120-30547] [PMID: 4285454]

[120] Brunner HR, Gavras H, Waeber B, *et al.* Oral angiotensin-converting enzyme inhibitor in long-term

treatment of hypertensive patients. Ann Intern Med 1979; 90(1): 19-23.
[http://dx.doi.org/10.7326/0003-4819-90-1-19] [PMID: 217289]

[121] MacFadyen RJ, Lee AF, Morton JJ, Pringle SD, Struthers AD. How often are angiotensin II and aldosterone concentrations raised during chronic ACE inhibitor treatment in cardiac failure? Heart 1999; 82(1): 57-61.
[http://dx.doi.org/10.1136/hrt.82.1.57] [PMID: 10377310]

[122] Cruden NL, Witherow FN, Webb DJ, Fox KA, Newby DE. Bradykinin contributes to the systemic hemodynamic effects of chronic angiotensin-converting enzyme inhibition in patients with heart failure. Arterioscler Thromb Vasc Biol 2004; 24(6): 1043-8.
[http://dx.doi.org/10.1161/01.ATV.0000129331.21092.1d] [PMID: 15105283]

[123] Hornig B, Kohler C, Drexler H. Role of bradykinin in mediating vascular effects of angiotensin-converting enzyme inhibitors in humans. Circulation 1997; 95(5): 1115-8.
[http://dx.doi.org/10.1161/01.CIR.95.5.1115] [PMID: 9054837]

[124] Dunn FG, Oigman W, Ventura HO, Messerli FH, Kobrin I, Frohlich ED. Enalapril improves systemic and renal hemodynamics and allows regression of left ventricular mass in essential hypertension. Am J Cardiol 1984; 53(1): 105-8.
[http://dx.doi.org/10.1016/0002-9149(84)90692-1] [PMID: 6318542]

[125] Fagard R, Amery A, Reybrouck T, Lijnen P, Billiet L. Acute and chronic systemic and pulmonary hemodynamic effects of angiotensin converting enzyme inhibition with captopril in hypertensive patients. Am J Cardiol 1980; 46(2): 295-300.
[http://dx.doi.org/10.1016/0002-9149(80)90074-0] [PMID: 6250392]

[126] Davis R, Ribner HS, Keung E, Sonnenblick EH, LeJemtel TH. Treatment of chronic congestive heart failure with captopril, an oral inhibitor of angiotensin-converting enzyme. N Engl J Med 1979; 301(3): 117-21.
[http://dx.doi.org/10.1056/NEJM197907193010301] [PMID: 221810]

[127] Dzau VJ, Colucci WS, Williams GH, Curfman G, Meggs L, Hollenberg NK. Sustained effectiveness of converting-enzyme inhibition in patients with severe congestive heart failure. N Engl J Med 1980; 302(25): 1373-9.
[http://dx.doi.org/10.1056/NEJM198006193022501] [PMID: 6246425]

[128] Sharpe DN, Douglas JE, Coxon RJ, Long B. Low-dose captopril in chronic heart failure: acute haemodynamic effects and long-term treatment. Lancet 1980; 2(8205): 1154-7.
[http://dx.doi.org/10.1016/S0140-6736(80)92593-3] [PMID: 6107767]

[129] Ichikawa I, Brenner BM. Glomerular actions of angiotensin II. Am J Med 1984; 76(5B): 43-9.
[http://dx.doi.org/10.1016/0002-9343(84)90882-9] [PMID: 6203406]

[130] Anderson S, Rennke HG, Brenner BM. Therapeutic advantage of converting enzyme inhibitors in arresting progressive renal disease associated with systemic hypertension in the rat. J Clin Invest 1986; 77(6): 1993-2000.
[http://dx.doi.org/10.1172/JCI112528] [PMID: 3011863]

[131] Giannattasio C, Grassi G, Seravalle G, Morganti A, Zanchetti A, Mancia G. Investigation of reflexes from volume and baroreceptors during converting-enzyme inhibition in humans. Am Heart J 1989; 117(3): 740-5.

[http://dx.doi.org/10.1016/0002-8703(89)90764-3] [PMID: 2645757]

[132] Grassi G, Cattaneo BM, Seravalle G, *et al.* Effects of chronic ACE inhibition on sympathetic nerve traffic and baroreflex control of circulation in heart failure. Circulation 1997; 96(4): 1173-9. [http://dx.doi.org/10.1161/01.CIR.96.4.1173] [PMID: 9286946]

[133] Nakashima Y, Fouad FM, Tarazi RC. Regression of left ventricular hypertrophy from systemic hypertension by enalapril. Am J Cardiol 1984; 53(8): 1044-9. [http://dx.doi.org/10.1016/0002-9149(84)90634-9] [PMID: 6322566]

[134] Hayek T, Attias J, Coleman R, *et al.* The angiotensin-converting enzyme inhibitor, fosinopril, and the angiotensin II receptor antagonist, losartan, inhibit LDL oxidation and attenuate atherosclerosis independent of lowering blood pressure in apolipoprotein E deficient mice. Cardiovasc Res 1999; 44(3): 579-87. [http://dx.doi.org/10.1016/S0008-6363(99)00239-4] [PMID: 10690290]

[135] Ridker PM, Gaboury CL, Conlin PR, Seely EW, Williams GH, Vaughan DE. Stimulation of plasminogen activator inhibitor *in vivo* by infusion of angiotensin II. Evidence of a potential interaction between the renin-angiotensin system and fibrinolytic function. Circulation 1993; 87(6): 1969-73. [http://dx.doi.org/10.1161/01.CIR.87.6.1969] [PMID: 8504511]

[136] Ruiz-Ortega M, Gomez-Garre D, Alcazar R, Palacios I, Bustos C, Gonzalez S, *et al.* Involvement of angiotensin II and endothelin in matrix protein production and renal sclerosis. Journal of hypertension Supplement : official journal of the International Society of Hypertension 1994; 12(4): S51-8.

[137] Hodsman GP, Isles CG, Murray GD, Usherwood TP, Webb DJ, Robertson JI. Factors related to first dose hypotensive effect of captopril: prediction and treatment. Br Med J (Clin Res Ed) 1983; 286(6368): 832-4. [http://dx.doi.org/10.1136/bmj.286.6368.832] [PMID: 6403103]

[138] Warren SE, O'Connor DT. Hyperkalemia resulting from captopril administration. JAMA 1980; 244(22): 2551-2. [http://dx.doi.org/10.1001/jama.1980.03310220049028] [PMID: 7001073]

[139] Hricik DE, Browning PJ, Kopelman R, Goorno WE, Madias NE, Dzau VJ. Captopril-induced functional renal insufficiency in patients with bilateral renal-artery stenoses or renal-artery stenosis in a solitary kidney. N Engl J Med 1983; 308(7): 373-6. [http://dx.doi.org/10.1056/NEJM198302173080706] [PMID: 6337327]

[140] Textor SC, Bravo EL, Fouad FM, Tarazi RC. Hyperkalemia in azotemic patients during angiotensin-converting enzyme inhibition and aldosterone reduction with captopril. Am J Med 1982; 73(5): 719-25. [http://dx.doi.org/10.1016/0002-9343(82)90415-6] [PMID: 6291388]

[141] Murphy BF, Whitworth JA, Kincaid-Smith P. Renal insufficiency with combinations of angiotensin converting enzyme inhibitors and diuretics. Br Med J (Clin Res Ed) 1984; 288(6420): 844-5. [Clin Res Ed]. [http://dx.doi.org/10.1136/bmj.288.6420.844] [PMID: 6322905]

[142] Kastner PR, Hall JE, Guyton AC. Control of glomerular filtration rate: role of intrarenally formed angiotensin II. Am J Physiol 1984; 246(6 Pt 2): F897-906.

[PMID: 6377913]

[143] Israili ZH, Hall WD. Cough and angioneurotic edema associated with angiotensin-converting enzyme inhibitor therapy. A review of the literature and pathophysiology. Ann Intern Med 1992; 117(3): 234-42.
[http://dx.doi.org/10.7326/0003-4819-117-3-234] [PMID: 1616218]

[144] Woo KS, Nicholls MG. High prevalence of persistent cough with angiotensin converting enzyme inhibitors in Chinese. Br J Clin Pharmacol 1995; 40(2): 141-4.
[PMID: 8562296]

[145] Visser LE, Stricker BH, van der Velden J, Paes AH, Bakker A. Angiotensin converting enzyme inhibitor associated cough: a population-based case-control study. J Clin Epidemiol 1995; 48(6): 851-7.
[http://dx.doi.org/10.1016/0895-4356(94)00231-E] [PMID: 7769416]

[146] Slater EE, Merrill DD, Guess HA, *et al.* Clinical profile of angioedema associated with angiotensin converting-enzyme inhibition. JAMA 1988; 260(7): 967-70.
[http://dx.doi.org/10.1001/jama.1988.03410070095035] [PMID: 2840522]

[147] Pryde PG, Sedman AB, Nugent CE, Barr M Jr. Angiotensin-converting enzyme inhibitor fetopathy. J Am Soc Nephrol 1993; 3(9): 1575-82.
[PMID: 8507813]

[148] Sedman AB, Kershaw DB, Bunchman TE. Recognition and management of angiotensin converting enzyme inhibitor fetopathy. Pediatr Nephrol 1995; 9(3): 382-5.
[http://dx.doi.org/10.1007/BF02254221] [PMID: 7632538]

[149] DiBianco R. Adverse reactions with angiotensin converting enzyme (ACE) inhibitors. Med Toxicol 1986; 1(2): 122-41.
[http://dx.doi.org/10.1007/BF03259832] [PMID: 3023783]

[150] Maldonado J. Recommended article of the month: Effects of intensive blood-pressure lowering and low-dose aspirin in patients with hypertension: principal results of the hypertension optimal treatment (HOT randomised trial).. Revista portuguesa de cardiologia : orgao oficial da Sociedade Portuguesa de Cardiologia = Portuguese journal of cardiology : an official journal of the Portuguese Society of Cardiology 1998; 17(10): 843-4.

[151] Hansson L, Zanchetti A, Carruthers SG, *et al.* HOT Study Group. Effects of intensive blood-pressure lowering and low-dose aspirin in patients with hypertension: principal results of the Hypertension Optimal Treatment (HOT) randomised trial. Lancet 1998; 351(9118): 1755-62.
[http://dx.doi.org/10.1016/S0140-6736(98)04311-6] [PMID: 9635947]

[152] Hansson L, Lindholm LH, Niskanen L, *et al.* Effect of angiotensin-converting-enzyme inhibition compared with conventional therapy on cardiovascular morbidity and mortality in hypertension: the Captopril Prevention Project (CAPPP) randomised trial. Lancet 1999; 353(9153): 611-6.
[http://dx.doi.org/10.1016/S0140-6736(98)05012-0] [PMID: 10030325]

[153] ALLHAT Officers and Coordinators for the ALLHAT Collaborative Research Group. The Antihypertensive and Lipid-Lowering Treatment to Prevent Heart Attack Trial. Major outcomes in high-risk hypertensive patients randomized to angiotensin-converting enzyme inhibitor or calcium channel blocker vs diuretic: The Antihypertensive and Lipid-Lowering Treatment to Prevent Heart

Attack Trial (ALLHAT). JAMA 2002; 288(23): 2981-97. [ALLHAT]. [http://dx.doi.org/10.1001/jama.288.23.2981] [PMID: 12479763]

[154] Schmieder RE, Martus P, Klingbeil A. Reversal of left ventricular hypertrophy in essential hypertension. A meta-analysis of randomized double-blind studies. JAMA 1996; 275(19): 1507-13. [http://dx.doi.org/10.1001/jama.1996.03530430051039] [PMID: 8622227]

[155] Tight blood pressure control and risk of macrovascular and microvascular complications in type 2 diabetes: UKPDS 381998. 1998; 703-13.

[156] The Acute Infarction Ramipril Efficacy (AIRE) Study Investigators. Effect of ramipril on mortality and morbidity of survivors of acute myocardial infarction with clinical evidence of heart failure. Lancet 1993; 342(8875): 821-8. [AIRE]. [PMID: 8104270]

[157] Fabia MJ, Abdilla N, Oltra R, Fernandez C, Redon J. Antihypertensive activity of angiotensin II AT1 receptor antagonists: a systematic review of studies with 24 h ambulatory blood pressure monitoring. J Hypertens 2007; 25(7): 1327-36. [http://dx.doi.org/10.1097/HJH.0b013e3280825625] [PMID: 17563549]

[158] Gradman AH. AT(1)-receptor blockers: differences that matter. J Hum Hypertens 2002; 16 (Suppl. 3): S9-S16. [http://dx.doi.org/10.1038/sj.jhh.1001434] [PMID: 12140723]

[159] Burnier M. Angiotensin II type 1 receptor blockers. Circulation 2001; 103(6): 904-12. [http://dx.doi.org/10.1161/01.CIR.103.6.904] [PMID: 11171802]

[160] Thöne-Reineke C, Zimmermann M, Neumann C, *et al.* Are angiotensin receptor blockers neuroprotective? Curr Hypertens Rep 2004; 6(4): 257-66. [http://dx.doi.org/10.1007/s11906-004-0019-3] [PMID: 15257859]

[161] Kaplan NM, Victor RG. Treatment of hypertension: drug therapy. 2014.

[162] Sica DA, Black HR. Current concepts of pharmacotherapy in hypertension: ACE inhibitor-related angioedema: can angiotensin-receptor blockers be safely used? J Clin Hypertens (Greenwich) 2002; 4(5): 375-80. [http://dx.doi.org/10.1111/j.1524-6175.2002.01509.x] [PMID: 12368584]

[163] Yusuf S, Teo K, Anderson C, *et al.* Telmisartan Randomised AssessmeNt Study in ACE iNtolerant subjects with cardiovascular Disease (TRANSCEND) Investigators. Effects of the angiotensin-receptor blocker telmisartan on cardiovascular events in high-risk patients intolerant to angiotensin-converting enzyme inhibitors: a randomised controlled trial. Lancet 2008; 372(9644): 1174-83. [http://dx.doi.org/10.1016/S0140-6736(08)61242-8] [PMID: 18757085]

[164] Sipahi I, Debanne SM, Rowland DY, Simon DI, Fang JC. Angiotensin-receptor blockade and risk of cancer: meta-analysis of randomised controlled trials. Lancet Oncol 2010; 11(7): 627-36. [http://dx.doi.org/10.1016/S1470-2045(10)70106-6] [PMID: 20542468]

[165] ARB Trialists Collaboration. Effects of telmisartan, irbesartan, valsartan, candesartan, and losartan on cancers in 15 trials enrolling 138,769 individuals. J Hypertens 2011; 29(4): 623-35. [PMID: 21358417]

[166] Israili ZH. Clinical pharmacokinetics of angiotensin II (AT1) receptor blockers in hypertension. J Hum

Hypertens 2000; 14 (Suppl. 1): S73-86.
[http://dx.doi.org/10.1038/sj.jhh.1000991] [PMID: 10854085]

[167] Taylor J. 2013 ESH/ESC guidelines for the management of arterial hypertension. Eur Heart J 2013; 34(28): 2108-9.
[PMID: 24040671]

[168] Matchar DB, McCrory DC, Orlando LA, *et al.* Systematic review: comparative effectiveness of angiotensin-converting enzyme inhibitors and angiotensin II receptor blockers for treating essential hypertension. Ann Intern Med 2008; 148(1): 16-29.
[http://dx.doi.org/10.7326/0003-4819-148-1-200801010-00189] [PMID: 17984484]

[169] Strauss MH, Hall AS. Angiotensin receptor blockers may increase risk of myocardial infarction: unraveling the ARB-MI paradox. Circulation 2006; 114(8): 838-54.
[http://dx.doi.org/10.1161/CIRCULATIONAHA.105.594986] [PMID: 16923768]

[170] Mann JF, Schmieder RE, McQueen M, *et al.* ONTARGET investigators. Renal outcomes with telmisartan, ramipril, or both, in people at high vascular risk (the ONTARGET study): a multicentre, randomised, double-blind, controlled trial. Lancet 2008; 372(9638): 547-53.
[http://dx.doi.org/10.1016/S0140-6736(08)61236-2] [PMID: 18707986]

[171] Yusuf S, Teo KK, Pogue J, *et al.* ONTARGET Investigators. Telmisartan, ramipril, or both in patients at high risk for vascular events. N Engl J Med 2008; 358(15): 1547-59.
[http://dx.doi.org/10.1056/NEJMoa0801317] [PMID: 18378520]

[172] Gradman AH, Schmieder RE, Lins RL, Nussberger J, Chiang Y, Bedigian MP. Aliskiren, a novel orally effective renin inhibitor, provides dose-dependent antihypertensive efficacy and placebo-like tolerability in hypertensive patients. Circulation 2005; 111(8): 1012-8.
[http://dx.doi.org/10.1161/01.CIR.0000156466.02908.ED] [PMID: 15723979]

[173] Musini VM, Fortin PM, Bassett K, Wright JM. Blood pressure lowering efficacy of renin inhibitors for primary hypertension: a Cochrane systematic review. J Hum Hypertens 2009; 23(8): 495-502.
[http://dx.doi.org/10.1038/jhh.2008.162] [PMID: 19158826]

[174] Parving HH, Persson F, Lewis JB, Lewis EJ, Hollenberg NK. AVOID Study Investigators. Aliskiren combined with losartan in type 2 diabetes and nephropathy. N Engl J Med 2008; 358(23): 2433-46.
[http://dx.doi.org/10.1056/NEJMoa0708379] [PMID: 18525041]

[175] McMurray JJ, Pitt B, Latini R, *et al.* Aliskiren Observation of Heart Failure Treatment (ALOFT) Investigators. Effects of the oral direct renin inhibitor aliskiren in patients with symptomatic heart failure. Circ Heart Fail 2008; 1(1): 17-24.
[http://dx.doi.org/10.1161/CIRCHEARTFAILURE.107.740704] [PMID: 19808266]

[176] Krop M, Garrelds IM, de Bruin RJ, *et al.* Aliskiren accumulates in Renin secretory granules and binds plasma prorenin. Hypertension 2008; 52(6): 1076-83.
[http://dx.doi.org/10.1161/HYPERTENSIONAHA.108.123042] [PMID: 18981317]

[177] Zheng Z, Lin S, Shi H. A systematic review and meta-analysis of telmisartan *versus* valsartan in the management of essential hypertension. J Clin Hypertens (Greenwich) 2010; 12(6): 414-21.
[http://dx.doi.org/10.1111/j.1751-7176.2010.00287.x] [PMID: 20591086]

[178] McMurray JJ, Abraham WT, Dickstein K, Køber L, Massie BM, Krum H. Aliskiren, ALTITUDE, and

the implications for ATMOSPHERE. Eur J Heart Fail 2012; 14(4): 341-3. [http://dx.doi.org/10.1093/eurjhf/hfs033] [PMID: 22431404]

[179] Gheorghiade M, Böhm M, Greene SJ, *et al.* ASTRONAUT Investigators and Coordinators. Effect of aliskiren on postdischarge mortality and heart failure readmissions among patients hospitalized for heart failure: the ASTRONAUT randomized trial. JAMA 2013; 309(11): 1125-35. [http://dx.doi.org/10.1001/jama.2013.1954] [PMID: 23478743]

CHAPTER 4

Cardiac Intracellular Renin-Angiotensin System

Rajesh Kumar*, Kenneth M. Baker, Wen Chen, Larissa Miranda Pereira, Candice M. Thomas and **Qian Chen Yong**

Division of Molecular Cardiology, Department of Medicine, Texas A&M Health Science Center, College of Medicine; Scott & White; Central Texas Veterans Health Care System, Temple, Texas, USA

Abstract: As a hormonal system, the renin-angiotensin system (RAS) is known for endocrine and autocrine/paracrine physiological functions. An intracrine role of the RAS has been proposed long ago; however, evidence for this function has started accumulating only recently. Angiotensin (Ang) II is the major hormone of the RAS and is the focus of research for the intracrine nature of this system. The intracrine functionality is characterized by intracellular actions of the hormone within the cell of synthesis or following internalization. Intracellular synthesis and actions of Ang II have been demonstrated in several cell types and tissues, with a significant amount of work in the heart. This review focuses on the cardiac intracellular RAS, delineating differences from the extracellular RAS that further consists of the circulatory and local RASs. The pathophysiological significance of the intracellular cardiac RAS has been discussed.

Keywords: Angiotensin converting enzyme, Angiotensin II, Angiotensinogen, Autocrine, Chymase, Diabetes, Diabetic cardiomyopathy, Heart, Hormone, Intracrine, Nucleus, Paracrine, Renin, Renin-angiotensin system.

INTRODUCTION

Hormones

Hormones, by definition, are factors released by cells in one part of the body that

* **Corresponding author Rajesh Kumar:** 1901 South First Street, Building 205 Temple, Texas 76504; Phone: 254-743-1203; Fax: 254-743-0165; E-mail: kumar@medicine.tamhsc.edu.

Dulce Elena Casarini, Danielle Yuri Arita, Tatiana Sousa Cunha & Juliana Almada Colucci (Eds.)

modulate the function of cells in other parts of the organism. Thus, hormones represent long distance control mechanisms to maintain proper coordination between different organs of an organism. Generally, hormones are carried from one part of the body to the other through the bloodstream. Sometimes, hormones affect the function of cells in close proximity to their cell of synthesis immediately after release. Depending on whether the hormone travels through the bloodstream to target distant organs or acts on neighboring cells through simple diffusion, their functions are categorized as endocrine and autocrine/paracrine functions, respectively (Fig. **1**). A single hormone may have one or both types of functionality. In either case, hormones act by interaction with specific receptors located generally on the plasma membrane of the target cells, for peptide hormones, or inside the cell, for steroid hormones.

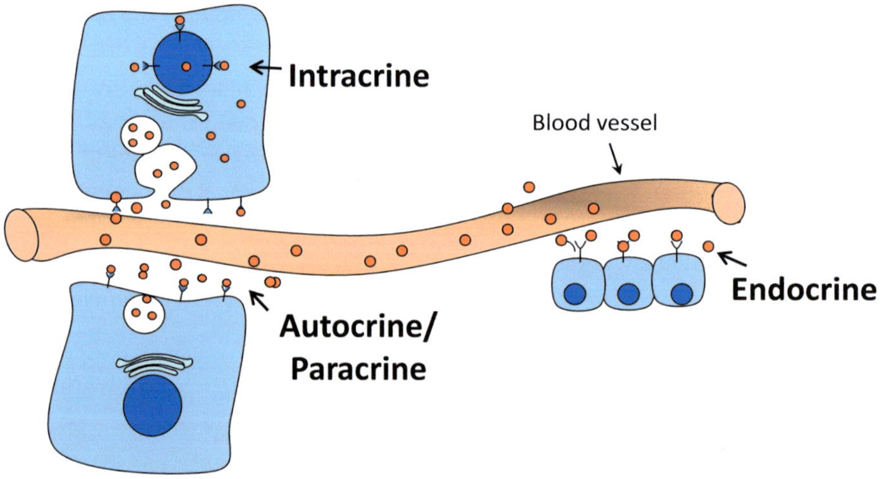

Fig. (1). Modes of peptide hormone action: Peptide hormones mainly act in two modes. One is endocrine mode, where the hormone released into circulation by endocrine glands targets distant organs. Another is autocrine/paracrine mode where the target site is on the same or adjacent cells. In both modes, the hormone binds to specific receptors on the cell surface, triggering intracellular signaling events. The third, mainly known for steroid hormones, is intracrine mode where the hormone acts intracellularly by binding to same receptors as on plasma membrane or other binding sites.

Another term, intracrine, has been used to describe certain hormone functions. According to a recent proposal, intracrine refers to intracellular actions of peptide hormones after internalization or within cells of their synthesis [1]. The latter part of the definition fits better with the definition of endocrine and autocrine/paracrine functionality that is based on the relationship between the site of synthesis and that of action of the hormone. Thus, a peptide hormone that also acts from an intracellular location is called an intracrine hormone; however, this term is used more commonly in relation to steroid hormones, as these generally act through intracellular receptors.

The significance of categorizing hormone functions, as described above, is not limited to the convenience of organization or the variety of physiological effects due to differences in the type of target cells at different locations. Recent evidence has shown that intracrine effects of peptide hormones can be similar or different than endocrine or autocrine/paracrine effects, in the same tissue or type of cells, due to differences in the intracellular and cell membrane receptors or in the signaling pathways activated by these receptors. Therefore, it is important to study all aspects of the hormone action to fully understand their physiological functions.

The Renin-Angiotensin System

The renin-angiotensin system (RAS) comprises of several peptide hormones generated as a result of cleavage of angiotensinogen (AGT) by renin, followed by actions of various other enzymes. AGT and renin are secretory proteins produced in the liver and kidneys, respectively. Therefore, the peptide hormones of the RAS are believed not to be synthesized in a particular cell type of the body, rather in the bloodstream or interstitial space within tissues where AGT and renin encounter each other. Angiotensin (Ang) peptide hormones include Ang II, Ang III, Ang IV, and Ang (1-7). Although structurally similar, differing from Ang II by lack of only one or two N- or C- terminal amino acids, these peptides have distinct receptor affinities and biological functions. Given the multicomponent nature and different tissue origin of the circulating components, resulting in Ang peptide production in the blood, the RAS is primarily known as an endocrine system. Ang peptides are also generated at tissue sites, thereby affecting neighboring cells and acting as autocrine/paracrine hormones. Based on the above described site of synthesis of Ang II, the major peptide of the system, the RAS has been characterized as the circulating or the tissue/local RAS.

THE INTRACRINE RAS

Early Studies with Isolated Nuclei

Recently, evidence has been presented for intracrine actions of Ang II in several types of cells and tissues [2 - 4]. The initial evidence came from studies in which radiolabeled Ang II injected into the myocardium of rats was localized in the nuclei and mitochondria of cardiac muscle cells, suggesting specific intracellular function [5]. Later, Re *et al.* demonstrated high affinity Ang II receptors in association with chromatin, which upregulated transcription in isolated hepatic nuclei following exposure to Ang II [6, 7]. Further studies on Ang II binding in hepatocyte nuclei revealed AT_1-like sites, using specific AT_1 antagonists and other Ang peptides [8, 9]. AT_1 is one of the two specific receptors of Ang II known as type 1 (AT_1) and type 2 (AT_2). These AT_1-like nuclear receptors caused increased RNA transcription in general and a several fold increase in the expression of AGT and renin, when isolated nuclei were exposed to Ang II [10]. Together, these studies presented the proof of concept for intracrine actions of Ang II.

Studies with Intact Isolated Cells

Later studies, by several investigators, demonstrated direct functional effects of intracellular Ang II in isolated cells (reviewed in [11]). They observed that intracellular Ang II increased cytosolic and nuclear calcium levels, had an effect on cardiac myocyte conductance, induced rat aorta contraction and cell proliferation in vascular smooth muscle cells and hepatocytes. We also demonstrated that intracellular Ang II increases protein synthesis and cell growth in neonatal rat ventricular myocytes. In these studies, Ang II was either introduced by microinjection or liposome-mediated internalization into cells or was produced intracellularly using recombinant DNA approaches.

Whereas the above studies in intact cells unequivocally demonstrated intracellular actions of Ang II, these differed in their conclusion regarding the nature of intracellular Ang II receptors. Both AT_1-like and AT_1-independent binding sites were shown to be responsible for intracellular Ang II actions, depending on the cell types used in these experiments, which included vascular smooth muscle cells, Chinese hamster ovary K1 cell line, hepatocytes, and cardiac myocytes.

Studies with Animals

We produced Ang II intracellularly in mouse hearts by injecting them with a plasmid that expressed the mature Ang II peptide sequence under the control of α-myosin heavy chain promoter [12]. Animals expressing intracellular Ang II in the heart developed significant cardiac hypertrophy compared to control animals. In another study, transgenic mice, which expressed intracellular Ang II in fusion with a fluorescent protein in multiple tissues under the control of metallothionein promoter, were generated. These mice developed hypertension and thrombotic microangiopathy [13]. When the same Ang II fusion construct was expressed specifically in the proximal tubule of the kidney under the sodium and glucose co-transporter promoter using intrarenal adenovirus infection, an increase in blood pressure and decrease in fractional sodium expression was observed [14]. These effects were ameliorated by AT_1 antagonist and were not observed in AT_1 knockout animals.

Thus, comprehensive studies using isolated nuclei, isolated cells of different types, and animal models have clearly demonstrated that Ang II can produce cellular and physiological effects from an intracellular location.

THE INTRACELLULAR RAS IN THE HEART

Intracrine functionality requires that the hormone be internalized or synthesized in the cell of action. In the studies described above, Ang II was introduced intracellularly by various artificial means. Though Ang II is internalized following binding to AT_1 receptor, microinjection or liposome-mediated delivery techniques were used to separate Ang II effects from extracellular and intracellular locations. Effectiveness of receptor internalized Ang II in producing intracrine effects was doubted due to possible compartmentalization in lysosomes for degradation in physiological settings. Thus, demonstration of intracellular synthesis of Ang II would provide a more convincing argument in favor of the intracrine nature of the RAS.

Intracellular RAS

The intracellular RAS is defined as I) existence of a complete machinery required to produce Ang II, II) synthesis of Ang II and, III) presence of Ang II receptors or other binding partners inside the cell. The classical RAS consists of the following components: the precursor AGT, enzymes renin and ACE, and receptors AT_1 and AT_2. In certain circumstances, functions of renin and ACE may be performed by other enzymes, such as cathepsin D and chymase. In the following paragraphs, we will review the evidence of intracellular presence of these components in the two major types of heart cells, cardiac myocytes and fibroblasts.

AGT: Both cardiac myocytes and fibroblasts express AGT. However, AGT is a secretory protein owing to the presence of the signal peptide sequence in the mRNA that causes co-translational insertion of the protein into the endoplasmic reticulum. AGT is glycosylated at four potential sites and the level of glycosylation at these sites affects efficiency of AGT secretion. Brain astrocytes produce a non-glycosylated form of AGT, which is not secreted and is targeted to the nucleus [15]. Several natural variants of AGT that are abnormally glycosylated lead to reduced plasma levels of AGT [16]. The presence of multiple glycosylation sites likely provides flexibility in the targeting of proteins, as has been observed with other members of the Serpin family to which AGT belongs [17]. Different cell types and environmental conditions can also have an impact on protein targeting. We have reported that neonatal rat ventricular myocytes, that constitutively secret AGT, retain it intracellularly when exposed to high ambient glucose conditions, whereas fibroblasts continue to secret it [18, 19].

Renin: Prorenin, the inactive precursor of renin, contains a secretory signal and occurs in both glycosylated and non-glycosylated forms. Glycosylation of prorenin determines whether it is constitutively secreted or targeted to secretory granules for conversion into active renin and subsequent regulated secretion. In the heart, uptake of circulatory glycosylated prorenin through the mannose-6-phosphate receptor or that of non-glycosylated prorenin *via* an unidentified mechanism is considered a major source of cardiac renin. Internalization of prorenin by cardiac myocytes has been shown to increase intracellular levels of Ang I and Ang II [20]. Additionally, a truncated isoform of prorenin, that lacks a secretory signal and is thus retained intracellularly, has been shown to be expressed in rat hearts [21]. The truncated prorenin is catalytically active. Significantly, high glucose levels in the culture medium have been shown to significantly enhance intracellular levels of renin in rat mesangial cells and neonatal ventricular myocytes, which are also associated with increased intracellular Ang II levels [18, 22].

ACE: ACE is a membrane bound protein with catalytic sites outside of the cell. Though cytoplasmic ACE staining has been observed in cardiac myocytes and fibroblasts, this is likely depictive of its presence in secretory vesicles. The latter assumption is based on our observations of ACE-inhibitable intracellular Ang II synthesis, which co-localized with actin filaments in cardiac myocytes following stimulation with isoproterenol [18]. Thus, even secretory precursor proteins and enzymes, when co-sorted in secretory vesicles, will produce Ang II intracellularly that may escape from the vesicles owing to its chemical properties.

Chymase: Chymase, an intracellular enzyme, has been demonstrated in mast cells, endothelial cells, and mesenchymal interstitial cells of the heart. Several isoforms of chymase with different substrate specificity occur, which may result in either Ang II formation or degradation. In a transgenic mouse, expression of an Ang II forming human chymase isoform specifically in the heart resulted in a 3-fold increase in cardiac Ang II levels [23]. These observations suggested that chymase had access to its substrate Ang I in the intracellular milieu to generate Ang II. A role of chymase has been suggested in Ang II generation from a novel Ang peptide, Ang-(1-12), following its internalization by rat neonatal cardiac myocytes [24]. We reported that intracellular Ang II formation in response to high glucose levels in rat cardiac myocytes is prevented by inhibiting chymase activity by chymostatin [18]. We also observed increased chymase expression by Western analysis, suggesting that high glucose upregulates the Ang II generating isoform of chymase in rodent cardiac myocytes.

Ang II receptors: Ang II binds to two types of specific G-protein coupled transmembrane receptors, AT_1 and AT_2. With regard to intracellular presence, AT_1 receptor was the first of the two receptors to be identified on the nuclear membrane of hepatocytes. Recent studies have identified both AT_1 and AT_2 receptors on nuclei of renal and cardiac cells [3, 25]. Stimulation of the nuclear Ang receptors increased RNA synthesis in isolated cardiac myocyte nuclei. Further, Ang II activated NF-κB mRNA expression in these nuclei. AT_1 activation also increased [Ca^{2+}] in isolated nuclei [25]. These studies demonstrated that both Ang II receptors are present on the nuclear membrane and couple to cellular effects upon stimulation.

Intracellular Synthesis of Ang II in the Heart

The site of Ang II synthesis, intracellular or extracellular, has been debated for long time. The secretory nature of AGT and renin, and expression of renin in limited tissues, favor the concept of extracellular synthesis of Ang II. However, co-localization of AGT and renin in the same cell and even in the same secretory granule in some tissues suggests that intracellular Ang II synthesis might occur [26, 27].

In the heart, the source of renin could be uptake from the circulation or endogenous synthesis in pathological states. In addition, the truncated non-secretory isoform of prorenin expressed in the heart could lead to intracellular Ang II generation. Both internalized prorenin- and endogenous renin-mediated Ang II synthesis has been demonstrated in isolated cardiac myocytes, isolated perfused hearts, and in adult animal hearts [17]. In adult rat cardiac myocytes, incubation of the cells with non-glycosylated mouse ren-2d prorenin resulted in the generation of intracellular Ang II [20].

Detailed studies on intracellular Ang II formation in neonatal cardiac myocytes and fibroblasts were reported by us recently [18, 19]. We observed that both types of cardiac cells synthesize Ang II intracellularly as well extracellularly in normal physiological conditions (Fig. **2**). The intracellular synthesis likely occurred in secretory granules, as Ang II staining was observed largely along the actin filaments in cardiac myocytes. Synthesis in secretory vesicles was likely the result of co-sorting of RAS components. An increase in intracellular Ang II levels, following RAS stimulation with isoproterenol or high glucose, was also observed in the presence of an AT_1 blocker that prevented internalization of Ang II. The latter observation confirmed that the increase in Ang II was due to intracellular synthesis. However, high glucose caused retention of AGT and renin inside cardiac myocytes resulting in all of the Ang II synthesis intracellularly, part of which trafficked to the nucleus [18]. Exposure of adult mouse cardiac myocytes to high glucose in culture also led to increased intracellular Ang II synthesis [28]. The mechanism of intracellular retention of AGT and renin is not known. Significantly, intracellular Ang II synthesis by cardiac myocytes in high glucose conditions was catalyzed by chymase, which is in contrast to ACE-mediated Ang I cleavage in response to isoproterenol or in cardiac fibroblasts [19]. Similar observations of chymase-mediated intracellular Ang II synthesis in response to high glucose levels have been reported in vascular smooth muscle and mesangial cells [22, 29].

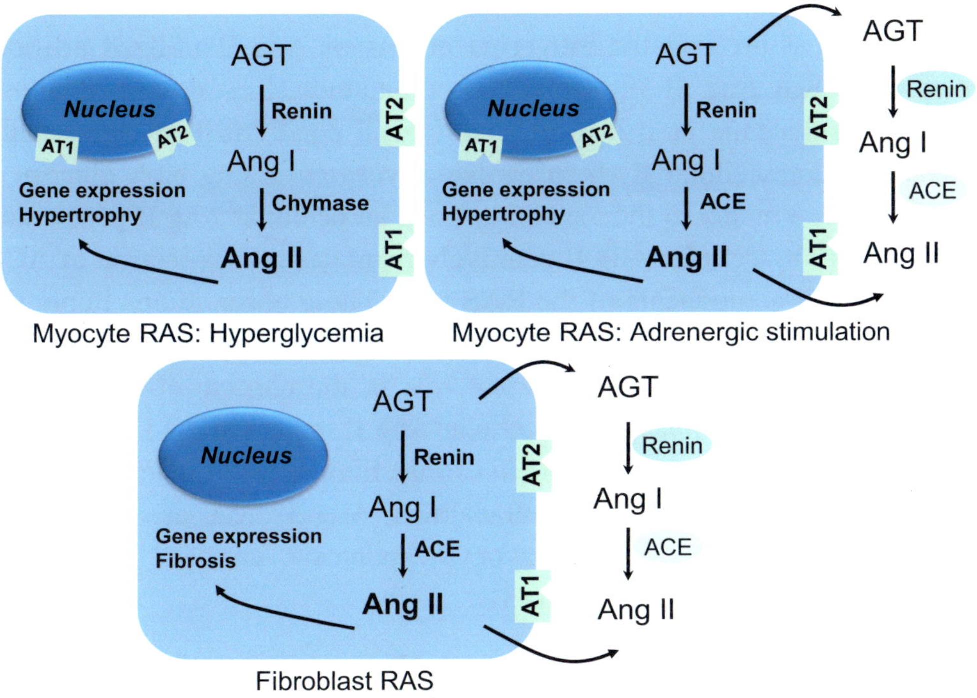

Fig. (2). The intracellular renin-angiotensin system in cardiac myocytes and fibroblasts. Activation of the intracellular cardiac RAS has been observed in response to hyperglycemia or beta-adrenergic stimulation. The two stimuli have significant effect on the RAS in cardiac myocytes with regard to the enzymes involved in Ang I to Ang II conversion and the site of Ang II synthesis. The RAS in fibroblasts is not affected by the nature of stimulus. Presence of functional AT1 and AT2 receptors have been demonstrated on cardiac myocytes, where cardiac fibroblasts have not been studied. Intracellular Ang II produces cellular effects, such as gene expression, in both cardiac myocytes and fibroblasts.

The above *in vitro* findings of high glucose-induced and chymase-mediated intracellular Ang II synthesis by cardiac myocytes were also confirmed in diabetic rat and mouse models. One week of diabetes, induced by destruction of pancreatic β-cells by streptozotocin, significantly upregulated cardiac Ang II levels [30, 31]. That the Ang II was synthesized intracellularly was confirmed by measuring Ang II in animals treated with an AT_1 receptor blocker in isolated cardiac myocytes and using confocal microscopy. Further, an ACE inhibitor only partially prevented the diabetes-induced increase in cardiac Ang II levels, suggesting the involvement of chymase in this process.

Role of the Endogenous Intracellular RAS In Cardiac Function

Earlier studies that investigated intracrine effects of Ang II utilized artificial means to introduce Ang II intracellularly. Our studies, as described above, identified hyperglycemia as a natural pathological condition that significantly upregulated the intracellular RAS in cardiac myocytes. Using high glucose or hyperglycemia as a model to induce endogenous intracellular Ang II production, we reported that intracellular Ang II positively regulates the expression of AGT, renin, and AT_1, all components of the RAS [18]. These observations imply that intracellular Ang II generates a positive feedback loop to upregulate RAS expression, which may have an important role in the chronic effects of RAS activation. In cardiac fibroblasts, intracellular Ang II increased the expression of TGF-β and collagen I, suggesting a role in cardiac fibrosis [19]. In animal studies, we reported that diabetes-induced intracellular Ang II was associated with increased oxidative stress, cardiac myocyte apoptosis, cardiac fibrosis, and diastolic and systolic dysfunction [30, 31].

SIGNIFICANCE OF THE INTRACELLULAR RAS IN THE HEART

The importance of the intracrine function of peptide hormones is that it may constitute a significant part of the overall mechanism of hormone action. In the case of the cardiac intracellular RAS, it is associated with positive feedback regulation and cardiac dysfunction in diabetes, as described above. More significantly, the intracellular Ang II generation mechanism in diabetes, that utilizes chymase, differs from the classical pathway. Additionally, intracellular Ang II does not require AT_1 receptor for its actions. Thus, the above aspect, specific to the cardiac intracellular RAS, needs to be considered when targeting the RAS for therapeutic purpose in diabetes.

CONFLICT OF INTEREST

The authors confirm that they have no conflict of interest to declare for this publication.

ACKNOWLEDGMENTS

This material is the result of work supported with resources and the use of facilities at the Central Texas Veterans Health Care System, Temple, Texas. This work was supported by funding from NIH grant 5R01HL090817.

REFERENCES

[1] Re RN, Cook JL. The intracrine hypothesis: an update. Regul Pept 2006; 133(1-3): 1-9. [http://dx.doi.org/10.1016/j.regpep.2005.09.012] [PMID: 16226324]

[2] Kumar R, Thomas CM, Yong QC, Chen W, Baker KM. The intracrine renin-angiotensin system. Clin Sci 2012; 123(5): 273-84. [http://dx.doi.org/10.1042/CS20120089] [PMID: 22590974]

[3] Gwathmey TM, Alzayadneh EM, Pendergrass KD, Chappell MC. Novel roles of nuclear angiotensin receptors and signaling mechanisms. Am J Physiol Regul Integr Comp Physiol 2012; 302(5): R518-30. [http://dx.doi.org/10.1152/ajpregu.00525.2011] [PMID: 22170620]

[4] Cook JL, Re RN. Lessons from *in vitro* studies and a related intracellular angiotensin II transgenic mouse model. Am J Physiol Regul Integr Comp Physiol 2012; 302(5): R482-93. [http://dx.doi.org/10.1152/ajpregu.00493.2011] [PMID: 22170617]

[5] Robertson AL Jr, Khairallah PA. Angiotensin II: rapid localization in nuclei of smooth and cardiac muscle. Science 1971; 172(3988): 1138-9. [http://dx.doi.org/10.1126/science.172.3988.1138] [PMID: 4324923]

[6] Re R, Parab M. Effect of angiotensin II on RNA synthesis by isolated nuclei. Life Sci 1984; 34(7): 647-51. [http://dx.doi.org/10.1016/0024-3205(84)90228-5] [PMID: 6199638]

[7] Re RN, Vizard DL, Brown J, Bryan SE. Angiotensin II receptors in chromatin fragments generated by micrococcal nuclease. Biochem Biophys Res Commun 1984; 119(1): 220-7. [http://dx.doi.org/10.1016/0006-291X(84)91641-3] [PMID: 6322777]

[8] Booz GW, Conrad KM, Hess AL, Singer HA, Baker KM. Angiotensin-II-binding sites on hepatocyte nuclei. Endocrinology 1992; 130(6): 3641-9. [PMID: 1597161]

[9] Tang SS, Rogg H, Schumacher R, Dzau VJ. Characterization of nuclear angiotensin-II-binding sites in rat liver and comparison with plasma membrane receptors. Endocrinology 1992; 131(1): 374-80. [PMID: 1612017]

[10] Eggena P, Zhu JH, Clegg K, Barrett JD. Nuclear angiotensin receptors induce transcription of renin and angiotensinogen mRNA. Hypertension 1993; 22(4): 496-501. [http://dx.doi.org/10.1161/01.HYP.22.4.496] [PMID: 8406654]

[11] Kumar R, Singh VP, Baker KM. The intracellular renin-angiotensin system in the heart. Curr Hypertens Rep 2009; 11(2): 104-10. [http://dx.doi.org/10.1007/s11906-009-0020-y] [PMID: 19278599]

[12] Baker KM, Chernin MI, Schreiber T, *et al.* Evidence of a novel intracrine mechanism in angiotensin II-induced cardiac hypertrophy. Regul Pept 2004; 120(1-3): 5-13. [http://dx.doi.org/10.1016/j.regpep.2004.04.004] [PMID: 15177915]

[13] Redding KM, Chen BL, Singh A, *et al.* Transgenic mice expressing an intracellular fluorescent fusion of angiotensin II demonstrate renal thrombotic microangiopathy and elevated blood pressure. Am J Physiol Heart Circ Physiol 2010; 298(6): H1807-18. [http://dx.doi.org/10.1152/ajpheart.00027.2010] [PMID: 20363893]

[14] Li XC, Cook JL, Rubera I, Tauc M, Zhang F, Zhuo JL. Intrarenal transfer of an intracellular fluorescent fusion of angiotensin II selectively in proximal tubules increases blood pressure in rats and mice. Am J Physiol Renal Physiol 2011; 300(5): F1076-88. [http://dx.doi.org/10.1152/ajprenal.00329.2010] [PMID: 21307128]

[15] Sherrod M, Liu X, Zhang X, Sigmund CD. Nuclear localization of angiotensinogen in astrocytes. Am J Physiol Regul Integr Comp Physiol 2005; 288(2): R539-46. [http://dx.doi.org/10.1152/ajpregu.00594.2004] [PMID: 15388495]

[16] Nakajima T, Cheng T, Rohrwasser A, *et al.* Functional analysis of a mutation occurring between the two in-frame AUG codons of human angiotensinogen. J Biol Chem 1999; 274(50): 35749-55. [http://dx.doi.org/10.1074/jbc.274.50.35749] [PMID: 10585456]

[17] Kumar R, Singh VP, Baker KM. The intracellular renin-angiotensin system: a new paradigm. Trends Endocrinol Metab 2007; 18(5): 208-14. [http://dx.doi.org/10.1016/j.tem.2007.05.001] [PMID: 17509892]

[18] Singh VP, Le B, Bhat VB, Baker KM, Kumar R. High-glucose-induced regulation of intracellular ANG II synthesis and nuclear redistribution in cardiac myocytes. Am J Physiol Heart Circ Physiol 2007; 293(2): H939-48. [http://dx.doi.org/10.1152/ajpheart.00391.2007] [PMID: 17483239]

[19] Singh VP, Baker KM, Kumar R. Activation of the intracellular renin-angiotensin system in cardiac fibroblasts by high glucose: role in extracellular matrix production. Am J Physiol Heart Circ Physiol 2008; 294(4): H1675-84. [http://dx.doi.org/10.1152/ajpheart.91493.2007] [PMID: 18296558]

[20] Peters J, Farrenkopf R, Clausmeyer S, *et al.* Functional significance of prorenin internalization in the rat heart. Circ Res 2002; 90(10): 1135-41. [http://dx.doi.org/10.1161/01.RES.0000019242.51541.99] [PMID: 12039805]

[21] Clausmeyer S, Reinecke A, Farrenkopf R, Unger T, Peters J. Tissue-specific expression of a rat renin transcript lacking the coding sequence for the prefragment and its stimulation by myocardial infarction. Endocrinology 2000; 141(8): 2963-70.

[PMID: 10919285]

[22] Vidotti DB, Casarini DE, Cristovam PC, Leite CA, Schor N, Boim MA. High glucose concentration stimulates intracellular renin activity and angiotensin II generation in rat mesangial cells. Am J Physiol Renal Physiol 2004; 286(6): F1039-45. [http://dx.doi.org/10.1152/ajprenal.00371.2003] [PMID: 14722017]

[23] Chen LY, Li P, He Q, *et al.* Transgenic study of the function of chymase in heart remodeling. J Hypertens 2002; 20(10): 2047-55. [http://dx.doi.org/10.1097/00004872-200210000-00025] [PMID: 12359984]

[24] Ahmad S, Varagic J, Westwood BM, Chappell MC, Ferrario CM. Uptake and metabolism of the novel peptide angiotensin-(1-12) by neonatal cardiac myocytes. PLoS One 2011; 6(1): e15759. [http://dx.doi.org/10.1371/journal.pone.0015759] [PMID: 21249217]

[25] Tadevosyan A, Maguy A, Villeneuve LR, *et al.* Nuclear-delimited angiotensin receptor-mediated signaling regulates cardiomyocyte gene expression. J Biol Chem 2010; 285(29): 22338-49. [http://dx.doi.org/10.1074/jbc.M110.121749] [PMID: 20463030]

[26] Wang JM, Slembrouck D, Tan J, *et al.* Presence of cellular renin-angiotensin system in chromaffin cells of bovine adrenal medulla. Am J Physiol Heart Circ Physiol 2002; 283(5): H1811-8. [http://dx.doi.org/10.1152/ajpheart.01092.2001] [PMID: 12384458]

[27] Mercure C, Ramla D, Garcia R, Thibault G, Deschepper CF, Reudelhuber TL. Evidence for intracellular generation of angiotensin II in rat juxtaglomerular cells. FEBS Lett 1998; 422(3): 395-9. [http://dx.doi.org/10.1016/S0014-5793(98)00052-0] [PMID: 9498824]

[28] Kumar R, Yong QC, Thomas CM, Baker KM. Intracardiac intracellular angiotensin system in diabetes. Am J Physiol Regul Integr Comp Physiol 2012; 302(5): R510-7. [http://dx.doi.org/10.1152/ajpregu.00512.2011] [PMID: 22170614]

[29] Lavrentyev EN, Estes AM, Malik KU. Mechanism of high glucose induced angiotensin II production in rat vascular smooth muscle cells. Circ Res 2007; 101(5): 455-64. [http://dx.doi.org/10.1161/CIRCRESAHA.107.151852] [PMID: 17626897]

[30] Thomas CM, Yong QC, Seqqat R, *et al.* Direct renin inhibition prevents cardiac dysfunction in a diabetic mouse model: comparison with an angiotensin receptor antagonist and angiotensin-converting enzyme inhibitor. Clin Sci 2013; 124(8): 529-41. [http://dx.doi.org/10.1042/CS20120448] [PMID: 23116220]

[31] Singh VP, Le B, Khode R, Baker KM, Kumar R. Intracellular angiotensin II production in diabetic rats is correlated with cardiomyocyte apoptosis, oxidative stress, and cardiac fibrosis. Diabetes 2008; 57(12): 3297-306. [http://dx.doi.org/10.2337/db08-0805] [PMID: 18829990]

CHAPTER 5

Angiotensin-(1-7) in the Heart

Rodrigo Araújo Fraga-Silva[1], **Anderson José Ferreira**[2] and **Robson Augusto Souza dos Santos**[3,*]

[1] *Institute of Bioengineering, Ecole Polytechnique Fédérale de Lausanne, Lausanne, Switzerland*

[2] *Federal University of Minas Gerais, Departments of Morphology, Brazil*

[3] *Physiology and Biophysics, Biological Sciences Institute, Federal University of Minas Gerais, Belo Horizonte, MG, Brazil*

Abstract: The renin-angiotensin system (RAS) is recognized as one of the most important modulators of the heart function, working intensely on maintaining cardiac homeostasis. Recent advances pointed out that this system is divided into two distinct counter-regulatory axes. The classical axis is well characterized and involves the formation and actions of the octapeptide Angiotensin (Ang) II, while the second axis has emerged in the last decades and has the heptapeptide Ang-(1-7) as the main effector. Ang-(1-7) modulates several aspects of the heart hemostasis, such as cardiac rhythm, contractility, hypertrophy, fibrosis and coronary flow. In this chapter, we will summarize the current literature addressing the role of Ang-(1-7) and its receptor Mas in the heart function and structure, highlighting its beneficial activities under pathological conditions.

Keywords: Angiotensin-converting enzyme, Angiotensin-converting enzyme 2, Angiotensin-(1-7), Angiotensin II, Cardiac homeostasis, Cardiac remodeling, Cardiac rhythm, Heart, Receptor Mas, Renin-angiotensin system.

INTRODUCTION

For many years the renin-angiotensin system (RAS) has been recognized as one of the most important modulator of the cardiovascular system [1, 2]. In fact, great

* **Corresponding author Robson Augusto Souza dos Santos:** Departamento de Fisiologia e Biofísica, Universidade Federal de Minas Gerais, Av. Antonio Carlos, 6627 – UFMG, 31270-901 – Belo Horizonte, MG, Brasil; Tel: +55 31 3409-2956; E-mail: robsonsant@gmail.com.

Dulce Elena Casarini, Danielle Yuri Arita, Tatiana Sousa Cunha & Juliana Almada Colucci (Eds.)

clinical achievements reached by angiotensin converting enzyme (ACE) inhibitors and AT1 blockers underscore the relevance of this system [3, 4]. Moreover, recent advances expanded the understanding of the pathophysiological role of RAS. The discovery of novel components of this system and their function are associated with new pathways which opposes angiotensin (Ang) II effects, thereby opening new avenues to target the RAS in the treatment of cardiovascular diseases [5 - 8].

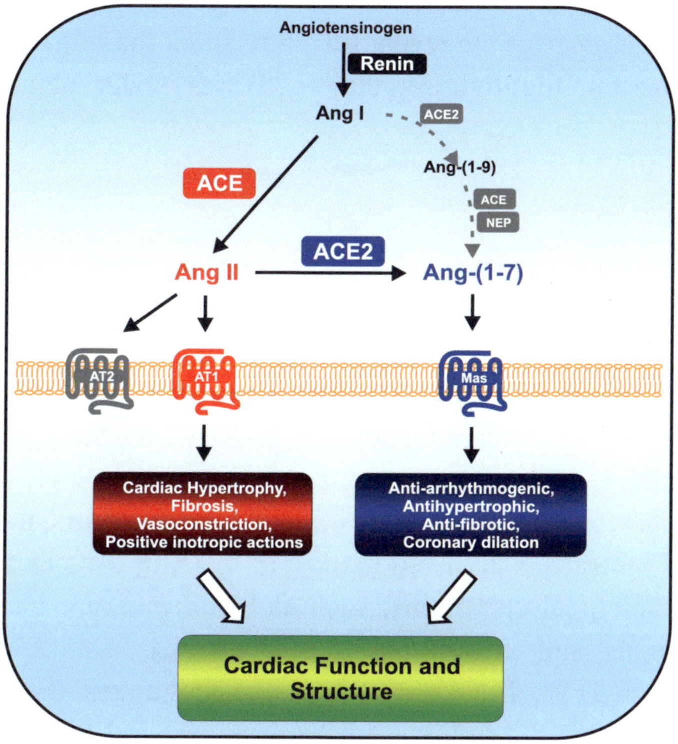

Fig. (1). Schematic representation of the simplified view of the renin-angiotensin system (RAS) cascade. The counterregulatory axes of the RAS are composed by ACE/Ang II/ AT1 and ACE2/Ang-(1–7)/Mas. ACE: angiotensin-converting enzyme; Ang: angiotensin; AT1: Ang II type 1 receptor; AT2: Ang II type 2 receptor; Mas: Ang- (1-7) receptor; NEP: neutral-endopeptidase 24.1.

One of the most important targets of RAS is the heart. This system modulates many features of the cardiac function and structure, such as cardiac rhythm, contractility, coronary perfusion, hypertrophy and fibrosis [9, 10]. Nowadays, the RAS concept consists of two opposite axes (Fig. **1**). One axis composed by ACE forming Ang II, which activates AT1 receptor, and another composed by ACE2 forming Ang-(1-7), which activates Mas receptor [5, 8, 9]. In general terms, ACE/Ang II/AT1 axis evokes deleterious effects under pathological conditions. For instance, Ang II stimulation induces positive inotropic actions, cardiac hypertrophy and fibrosis [8, 11]. Contrarily, ACE2/Ang-(1-7)/Mas axis induces beneficial actions [5, 7]. In the heart, Ang-(1-7) produces antiarrhythmogenic, antihypertrophic and antifibrotic actions [10, 12 - 17].

In this chapter, we summarize the recent literature about the role of Ang-(1-7) and Mas in heart function, highlighting their activities under pathophysiological conditions.

Renin Angiotensin-System Cascade

The RAS is a hormonal system which acts not only in an endocrine manner, but also as a paracrine and autocrine system [8]. Thus, in many organs, this system can be locally modulated and/or disturbed, influencing specific organ functions independent of the circulating system [8, 18]. The system cascade starts with the conversion of the precursor angiotensinogen to Ang I by the enzyme renin [8] (Fig. **1**) Sequentially, ACE cleaves Ang I and forms Ang II [1, 8, 19]. Ang II produces its effects *via* two distinct G-protein coupled receptors, named AT1 and AT2 [1, 20]. AT1 receptor is involved in most of the Ang II-mediated deleterious effects under pathological conditions, such as blood pressure increase, cardiac hypertrophy, fibrosis and arrhythmia [3, 7]. On its turn, AT2 appears to antagonize AT1 actions [4, 21]. Consistent evidences suggest that an augmented AT2 activation is one of the indirect mechanisms implied in the AT1 blockers actions [22, 23]. Moreover, it has been suggested that selective AT2 agonists may represent a potential therapeutic tool against cardiovascular diseases [23, 24]. However, the relevance of AT2 receptor in human pathophysiology still needs to be demonstrated [24].

In the last decades, the classical RAS, described as a linear cascade forming Ang II and promoting deleterious effects, has been expanded and became more complex [5, 7, 8]. A counter-regulatory arm of the RAS mediated by Ang-(1-7) has been established [5, 10]. Ang-(1-7) is a heptapeptide that acts mainly opposing Ang II effects [7, 25, 26]. This peptide acts *via* its own receptor, Mas [27], producing vasodilation, blood pressure decrease, attenuation of cardiac arrhythmia, fibrosis and hypertrophy [12 - 14, 17, 28 - 30]. Ang-(1-7) is predominantly formed *via* Ang II cleavage by ACE2, which acts on the C-terminal phenylalanine of Ang II, promoting Ang-(1-7) formation [31 - 33]. Additionally, this peptide may also be formed by neutral endopeptidase (NEP), such as prolylcarboxypeptidase (PCP) and prolylendopeptidase (PEP) [34 - 36]. Currently, the new concept of two counter-regulatory branches, the deleterious ACE/Ang II/AT1 receptor axis and the protective ACE2/Ang-(1- 7)/Mas receptor axis, is well accepted [5, 7]. In the heart, both branches play fundamental role in the cardiac homeostasis. Importantly, evidences indicate that a imbalance between these two branches is associated with cardiac pathologies [7].

Angiotensin-(1-7) Formation in the Heart

The heart is one of the most important targets for Ang-(1-7). All the major components of RAS (ACE2/Ang-(1- 7)/Mas and ACE/Ang II/AT1 receptor) are locally expressed in the heart [8, 10, 37]. Therefore, this system can influence the cardiac function through circulating peptides carried by the plasma and/or by an intrinsic paracrine system. The local formation of Ang-(1-7) in the myocardium was first reported by Santos *et al.* in right atrium, coronary sinus, and aortic root of canine hearts [38]. In the same study, the treatment with ACE inhibitor CGS-14,831 blocked the Ang-(1-7) production [38]. Interestingly, in a myocardial infarction model induced by left coronary artery occlusion, Ang-(1-7) immunoreactivity was significantly increased in the peri-infarcted area [39], suggesting that Ang-(1-7) is upregulated in a beneficial response against myocardial infarction. Indeed, later on it was shown that a synthetic Mas agonist and an oral formulation of Ang-(1-7) reduced the infarcted area and improved cardiac function after myocardial ischemia induced by left coronary artery occlusion in rats [40 - 42].

Importantly, the expression of Ang-(1-7) in cardiac tissue was also reported in human. Zisman *et al.* reported that Ang-(1-7) is formed in the intact human myocardial circulation [32]. Interestingly, when Ang II formation was suppressed Ang-(1-7) level was also decreased, suggesting that in the intact human heart

Ang-(1-7) generation is dependent on Ang II availability as substrate [32]. The same research group found that Ang-(1-7)-forming activity was increased in failing human heart ventricles [33], which is in accordance with previous animal studies showing an Ang- (1-7) upregulation in myocardial infarction [39]. In a preparation of human cardiac membrane extracts, ACE2 specific inhibitor C16 blocked Ang-(1-7) formation, while inhibitors of ACE, NEP, endothelin-converting enzyme, PEP, carboxypeptidase A, and angiotensinase C had no effect on the hydrolysis of Ang II to Ang-(1-7) [33]. Despite these evidences suggesting ACE2 as the major pathway for Ang-(1-7) formation in the human heart, Campbell *et al.* [36] suggested that Ang-(1-7) is mainly formed by endopeptidase-mediated metabolism of Ang I in human coronary vessels, since ACE inhibition diminished Ang II formation while Ang I and Ang-(1-7) levels were augmented [36]. This finding is in accordance with an earlier study showing that Ang-(1-7) formation derived from Ang I infusion in the coronary bed was not altered by ACE inhibition [43]. Taking these data together and considering the preparations used, it appears that Ang-(1-7) is preferentially formed by endopeptidases in the coronary bed, while ACE2 appears to be the major source in the myocardium. These dissimilarities may have important implications for the actions of emerging compounds such as ACE2 activators [44 - 47]. However, further studies are needed to clarify this issue.

Cardiac Rhythma

Several studies have shown that Ang-(1-7) modulates many aspects of the heart function. This peptide influences the heart rhythm, contractility and coronary flow, usually producing beneficial effects to the cardiac hemostasis [10]. The role of Ang- (1-7) in cardiac rhythm is not completely understood. It may activate both tachycardia and bradycardia responses, which depend on the experimental preparation and influence of others factors, such as autonomic nervous system, ventricular mass and circulating hormonal substances [10]. Mas deficient mice present a significant reduction in heart rate [28, 48], suggesting that the basal interaction between Ang-(1- 7) and Mas is essential to the regulation of the cardiac rhythm. Moreover, a transgenic rat model which presents an increase in the plasma Ang-(1-7) levels has a slight increase in heart rate [49]. On the other hand, cardiomyocytes incubated with Ang-(1- 7) presented a marked reduction in the spontaneously beating rate [50]. Likewise, Ang-(1-7) infusion for 7 days produced a slight bradycardia in Wistar rats [51]. Others studies failed to demonstrate any significant effect of Ang-(1-7) on cardiac rhythm [13]. Despite of these conflicting data regarding the role of Ang-(1-7) in the cardiac rhythm, under pathological conditions Ang-(1-7) appears to produce a positive balance in the heart rate. Indeed, Ang-(1-7) perfusion protected isolated rat hearts against arrhythmia provoked by ischemia/reperfusion [12, 13]. This effect was further confirmed in transgenic rats overexpressing circulating Ang-(1-7), which showed a diminished duration of reperfusion arrhythmias and an improved post-ischemic function in isolated heart preparations [49]. Moreover, local overexpression of Ang-(1-7) in rat hearts caused a slight improvement in the resting cardiac function [17]. Interestingly, Lima *et al.* demonstrated that intravenous injection of Ang-(1-7) attenuated tachycardia induced by stress and isoproterenol, a β-adrenergic agonist [50]. In a canine model of atrial tachycardia induced by paced, Ang-(1-7) prevented atrial tachycardia and fibrillation [52]. In accordance with that, it was shown reduction in the duration and incidence of tachyarrhythmias induced by electrical stimulation in isolated right atria perfused with Ang-(1-7) [37]. In this later study, it was demonstrated that the components of the ACE2/Ang-(1-7)/Mas axis are expressed in the sinoatrial node, suggesting the possibility of local actions of this axis in modulating the cardiac rhythm [37].

The mechanisms involved in the actions of Ang-(1-7) on cardiac rhythm are not fully established. The participation of Mas appears to be essential. For instance, both anti-arrhythmic and anti-tachycardic actions of Ang-(1-7) are antagonized by the selective Mas antagonist, A-779 [37, 50]. It has been suggested that Ang-(1-7) acting through Mas may modulate β-adrenergic responses in cardiomyocytes. In fact, Ang-(1-7) incubation markedly attenuated the increase in cardiomyocytes beating rate induced by isoproterenol [50], which is in accordance with the anti-tachycardic responses caused by intravenous injection of Ang-(1-7) under stress condition and isoproterenol infusion [50].

Evidences also indicate that Ang-(1-7) may modulate cardiomyocytes ionic currents. Ang-(1-7) incubation diminished isolated cardiomyocytes spontaneous beating in absence of chronotropic stimulus [50], indicating an interaction between Mas and ionic channels leading to changes in ionic currents. In fact, it was shown that Ang-(1- 7) prevents alterations in the voltage-dependent L-type calcium current, transient outward current, and expression of Kv4.3 potassium channel induced by atrial fibrillation [52]. Additionally, Ferreira *et al.* have demonstrated that overexpression of Ang-(1-7) in the heart produced an improved calcium handling in cardiomyocytes and increased the expression of SERCA2a [17]. In accordance with these findings, cardiomyocytes from Mas-knockout mice present slower [Ca2 +]i transients accompanied by a lower calcium ATPase expression in the sarcoplasmic reticulum [53, 54].

Also, Ang-(1-7) may modulate the sympathetic neurotransmission in the heart. Gironacci and colleagues reported that Ang-(1-7) enhanced the evoked release of noradrenaline from rat atrial preparations [55]. Moreover, others studies demonstrated that Ang-(1-7) reduces the sympathetic activity in others organs [56]. In addition to the local effects of Ang-(1-7) in the heart, this peptide may modify cardiac rhythm by actions in the central nervous system. Oliveira *et al.* reported a tonic modulatory effect of Ang-(1-7)/Mas axis by intracerebroventricular infusion of A-779, a selective Mas antagonist, that decreases the baroreflex sensitivity in Wistar rats [57, 58]. Furthermore, central administration of Ang-(1-7) in rabbits with chronic heart failure inhibited the sympathetic outflow, increasing vagal outflow [59]. In this line, intracerebroventricular injections of Ang-(1-7) markedly attenuated the tachycardia response induced by acute stress [50], thereby suggesting that Ang-(1-7) reduces the sympathetic load to the heart during situations of emotional stress.

Altogether these findings indicate that Ang-(1-7) holds a significant role in modulating cardiac rhythm. this peptide appears to produce a positive balance in the heart rate under pathological conditions by modulating adrenergic responses and ionic currents in cardiomyocytes.

Coronary Flow

have been reported in many studies using different species, preparations and vascular beds, including coronary arteries [9]. Brosnihan *et al.* showed that Ang-(1-7) produces dose-dependent vasorelaxation in U46619-pre-constricted canine coronary artery rings [60]. In keeping with that, Loot *et al.* demonstrated that chronic infusion of Ang-(1-7) improves coronary perfusion and preserves cardiac function in an experimental rat model of heart failure [15]. Moreover, Ang-(1-7) enhanced coronary perfusion after ischemia/reperfusion injury in isolated rat hearts [13]. Contrarily to these findings, Neves *et al.* reported that Ang-(1-7) perfusion decreases coronary flow in isolated rat hearts, which was not accompanied by consistent alterations of inotropism or cardiac rhythm [61]. Similar results were observed in isolated hamster hearts [62]. Of note, the high concentration of Ang-(1-7) used in those studies may explain these contradictory findings. In fact, different studies report that Ang-(1-7) has a biphasic effect and in higher concentrations it may produce opposite actions [63 - 65].

Similarly to others vascular beds, the vasodilatory effect of Ang-(1-7) in coronary vessels is endothelial–dependent and involves production of NO and/or prostacyclin [10, 60, 66, 67]. Ang-(1-7) binds to Mas and triggers the PI3K/Akt pathway with consequent activation of endothelial NO synthase in endothelial cells [68]. This response culminates in NO release, causing subsequent endothelial-mediated vasorelaxation [27, 68]. Another possible pathway that might be involved in the actions of Ang-(1-7) in the coronary bed is attributed to the potentiation of bradykinin vasodilation [60, 67]. Ang-(1-7) amplifies the vasodilatory effect evoked by bradykinin in isolated perfused rat hearts and isolated canine coronary arteries [60, 67]. Similar results were found in others vascular beds [69, 70]. Although several mechanisms have been proposed to clarify the bradykinin-potentiating activity of Ang-(1-7), it appears that it dependents on Mas activation and intracellular cross-talking [71].

Anti-Hypertrophic and Anti-Fibrotic Actions

It is well reported that Ang II hyperactivity is closely associated with cardiac hypertrophy and extracellular matrix synthesis and deposition, which are key factors in cardiovascular diseases [72, 73]. Oppositely, several studies point out the beneficial effects of Ang-(1-7) in the cardiac structure [8 - 10]. Consistent findings suggest that Mas activation by Ang-(1-7) reduces cardiac hypertrophy and collagen deposition induced by different pathological stimuli [9, 14, 15, 40, 41, 74]. For instance, transgenic rats with augmented plasma Ang-(1-7) levels have a significant attenuation of cardiac fibrosis and hypertrophy induced by isoproterenol [49, 75]. Santiago *et al.* observed that overexpression of Ang-(1-7) protects against cardiac fibrosis and left ventricular hypertrophy induced by blood pressure increase (deoxycorticosterone acetate salt-hypertensive model) [74]. Likewise, local overexpression of Ang-(1-7) in the heart prevented the cardiac remodeling induced by isoproterenol or hypertension [17, 29]. In this line, treatment with an oral formulation based on Ang-(1-7) inclusion in cyclodextrin produced marked reduction in the infarct area induced by coronary occlusion and attenuated cardiac fibrosis and hypertrophy caused by isoproterenol [42]. This data is in accordance with previous reports showing that oral administration of the Mas agonist AVE 0991 significantly decreases the area of infarct induced by coronary ligation [40] and cardiac fibrosis and hypertrophy induced by isoproterenol [41].

The protective effect of Ang-(1-7) on cardiac structure was also confirmed by studies addressing the role of ACE2, the major Ang-(1-7)-forming enzyme. It was shown that pharmacological inhibition of ACE2 exacerbates cardiac hypertrophy and fibrosis in (mRen2)27 transgenic hypertensive rats [76]. Besides, activation of endogenous ACE2 significantly decreased cardiac collagen content in spontaneously hypertensive rats, which was associated with an increase of Ang-(1-7) levels in the heart [46, 77]. These reports are in accordance with early data demonstrating that ACE2 overexpression in the heart prevents hypertension-induced cardiac fibrosis and hypertrophy in spontaneously hypertensive rats and Ang II-infused rats [78, 79]. Similarly, transfection leading to overexpression of ACE2 into the peri-infarcted myocardium was protective against heart failure in a rat model of myocardial infarction [80, 81]. This effect was associated with decreased expression of ACE and Ang II and increased expression of Ang-(1-7) [81]. Evidently, these protective actions of ACE2 are not strictly mediated by an augmented Ang-(1-7) formation and activity, as this enzyme also decreases Ang II levels and activity. However, evidences show that selective Mas blockage significantly attenuates the protective effect of ACE2 activation on cardiac remodeling [82], thereby highlighting the role of Ang-(1-7) on the ACE2 actions.

Different pathways are involved in the modulation of cardiac structure by Ang-(1-7). Grobe *et al.* reported reduction of collagen deposition without any effect on blood pressure after Ang-(1-7) infusion, indicating that this effect is independent of hemodynamic alterations [83]. Indeed, Marques *et al.* observed that the anti-fibrotic and anti- hypertrophic effects of Ang-(1-7) in rat hearts are independent of blood pressure changes [42]. It has been suggested that the anti-fibrotic and anti-trophic effects of Ang-(1-7) in hearts involve attenuation of cytokine signaling cascades [84]. Working with primary cultures of human cardiocytes, Pan *et al.* reported opposite and antagonistic effects of Ang II and Ang-(1-7) on regulation of transcription of MMPs and TIMPs. Ang II stimulation leads to increased ratios of MMPs/TIMPs while Ang-(1-7) stimulation decreased it [85]. These data suggest that Ang-(1-7) has an important regulatory effect on MMP and TIMP expression and activity in cardiac cells [85]. Similar findings were observed *in vivo*, where chronic infusion of Ang-(1-7) attenuated the left ventricular hypertrophy and myocardial fibrosis in spontaneously hypertensive rats, which was associated with associated with an increased MMP and decreased TIMP expression and activity [16].

Similarly to several biological effects produced by Ang-(1-7), the anti-fibrotic role of this peptide in the heart is critically dependent on Mas. Several studies report that the beneficial actions of Ang-(1-7) in cardiac structure are abrogated by the selective Mas antagonist, A-779 [14, 16]. Interestingly, evidences suggest that Mas is crucial for the homeostasis of the cardiac structure, since Mas deficient mice present an increased extracellular matrix deposition in the heart, which is linked to cardiac function impairment [30, 54].

The intracellular pathways involved in the Ang-(1-7) effects on cardiac remodeling are not fully understood. However, consistent evidences indicate that Ang-(1-7) inhibits pro-hypertrophic signaling pathways stimulated by Ang II. In cardiomyocytes, Mas activation by Ang-(1-7) inhibits the ERK1/2 phosphorylation induced by Ang II and Rho kinase activation [86]. Moreover, cardiac overexpression of Ang-(1-7) decreases the Ang II-induced phosphorylation of c-Src and p38 kinase, without effect on ERK1/2 phosphorylation [29]. Moreover, Ang II-induced hypertrophy was prevented by Ang-(1-7) through calcineurin/NFAT signaling cascade. Furthermore, these effects seem to be mediated by NO since they were abolished by NO synthase inhibition and by guanylyl cyclase inhibitors [87]. Together, these finding suggest that Ang-(1-7) plays a protective role in the cardiac structure and function.

Moreover, these actions involve activation of intracellular signaling pathways, which lead to negative crosstalk with Ang II- stimulating cardiac remodeling pathways.

CONCLUSION

Growing evidence indicates that Ang-(1-7) plays a key role in the pathophysiology of cardiac function and structure. Moreover, these findings suggest that Ang-(1-7) or Mas agonists might be an important strategy for new generation of cardiovascular therapeutic agents against cardiac dysfunction and pathological heart remodeling.

CONFLICT OF INTEREST

The authors confirm that they have no conflict of interest to declare for this publication.

ACKNOWLEDGEMENTS

The authors thank CAPES Coordenação de Aperfeiçoamento de Pessoal de nível Superior, CNPq Conselho Nacional de Desenvolvimento Científico e Tecnológico and FAPEMIG Fundação de Amparo a Pesquisa do Estado de Minas Gerais for research grants.

REFERENCES

[1] Unger T. The role of the renin-angiotensin system in the development of cardiovascular disease. Am J Cardiol 2002; 89(2A): 3A-9A. discussion 10A [http://dx.doi.org/10.1016/S0002-9149(01)02321-9]

[2] Nicholls MG, Richards AM, Agarwal M. The importance of the renin-angiotensin system in cardiovascular disease. J Hum Hypertens 1998; 12(5): 295-9. [http://dx.doi.org/10.1038/sj.jhh.1000638] [PMID: 9655650]

[3] Schiffrin EL. Vascular and cardiac benefits of angiotensin receptor blockers. Am J Med 2002; 113(5): 409-18. [http://dx.doi.org/10.1016/S0002-9343(02)01241-X] [PMID: 12401536]

[4] Ma TK, Kam KK, Yan BP, Lam YY. Renin-angiotensin-aldosterone system blockade for cardiovascular diseases: current status. Br J Pharmacol 2010; 160(6): 1273-92. [http://dx.doi.org/10.1111/j.1476-5381.2010.00750.x] [PMID: 20590619]

[5] Fraga-Silva RA, Ferreira AJ, Dos Santos RA. Opportunities for targeting the angiotensin-converting enzyme 2/angiotensin-(1-7)/mas receptor pathway in hypertension. Curr Hypertens Rep 2013; 15(1):

31-8.
[http://dx.doi.org/10.1007/s11906-012-0324-1] [PMID: 23212695]

[6] Santos RA, Ferreira AJ, Simões E Silva AC. Recent advances in the angiotensin-converting enzyme 2-angiotensin(1-7)-Mas axis. Exp Physiol 2008; 93(5): 519-27.
[http://dx.doi.org/10.1113/expphysiol.2008.042002] [PMID: 18310257]

[7] Ferreira AJ, Santos RA, Bradford CN, *et al.* Therapeutic implications of the vasoprotective axis of the renin-angiotensin system in cardiovascular diseases. Hypertension 2010; 55(2): 207-13.
[http://dx.doi.org/10.1161/HYPERTENSIONAHA.109.140145] [PMID: 20038757]

[8] Bader M. Tissue renin-angiotensin-aldosterone systems: Targets for pharmacological therapy. Annu Rev Pharmacol Toxicol 2010; 50: 439-65.
[http://dx.doi.org/10.1146/annurev.pharmtox.010909.105610] [PMID: 20055710]

[9] Ferreira AJ, Murca TM, Fraga-Silva RA, *et al.* New cardiovascular and pulmonary therapeutic strategies based on the Angiotensin-converting enzyme 2/angiotensin-(1-7)/mas receptor axis International journal of hypertension 2012; 2012: 147825.

[10] Ferreira AJ, Santos RA. Cardiovascular actions of angiotensin-(1-7). Braz J Med Biol Res 2005; 38(4): 499-507.
[http://dx.doi.org/10.1590/S0100-879X2005000400003] [PMID: 15962175]

[11] Koch-Weser J. Myocardial Actions of Angiotensin. Circ Res 1964; 14: 337-44.
[http://dx.doi.org/10.1161/01.RES.14.4.337] [PMID: 14135255]

[12] Ferreira AJ, Santos RA, Almeida AP. Angiotensin-(1-7): cardioprotective effect in myocardial ischemia/reperfusion. Hypertension 2001; 38(3 Pt 2): 665-8.
[http://dx.doi.org/10.1161/01.HYP.38.3.665] [PMID: 11566952]

[13] Ferreira AJ, Santos RA, Almeida AP. Angiotensin-(1-7) improves the post-ischemic function in isolated perfused rat hearts. Brazilian journal of medical and biological research = Revista brasileira de pesquisas medicas e biologicas / Sociedade Brasileira de Biofisica [et al] 2002; 35(9): 1083-90.

[14] Grobe JL, Mecca AP, Lingis M, *et al.* Prevention of angiotensin II-induced cardiac remodeling by angiotensin-(1-7). Am J Physiol Heart Circ Physiol 2007; 292(2): H736-42.
[http://dx.doi.org/10.1152/ajpheart.00937.2006] [PMID: 17098828]

[15] Loot AE, Roks AJ, Henning RH, *et al.* Angiotensin-(1-7) attenuates the development of heart failure after myocardial infarction in rats. Circulation 2002; 105(13): 1548-50.
[http://dx.doi.org/10.1161/01.CIR.0000013847.07035.B9] [PMID: 11927520]

[16] Pei Z, Meng R, Li G, *et al.* Angiotensin-(1-7) ameliorates myocardial remodeling and interstitial fibrosis in spontaneous hypertension: role of MMPs/TIMPs. Toxicol Lett 2010; 199(2): 173-81.
[http://dx.doi.org/10.1016/j.toxlet.2010.08.021] [PMID: 20837116]

[17] Ferreira AJ, Castro CH, Guatimosim S, *et al.* Attenuation of isoproterenol-induced cardiac fibrosis in transgenic rats harboring an angiotensin-(1-7)-producing fusion protein in the heart. Ther Adv Cardiovasc Dis 2010; 4(2): 83-96.
[http://dx.doi.org/10.1177/1753944709353426] [PMID: 20051448]

[18] Fraga-Silva RA, Montecucco F, Mach F, Santos RA, Stergiopulos N. Pathophysiological role of the renin-angiotensin system on erectile dysfunction. Eur J Clin Invest 2013; 43(9): 978-85.

[http://dx.doi.org/10.1111/eci.12117] [PMID: 23909886]

[19] Kokubu T, Ueda E, Joh T, Nishimura K. Purification and properties of angiotensin I-converting enzyme in human lung and its role on the metabolism of vasoactive peptides in pulmonary circulation. Adv Exp Med Biol 1979; 120B: 467-75.
[PMID: 229710]

[20] Touyz RM, Berry C. Recent advances in angiotensin II signaling. Brazilian journal of medical and biological research = Revista brasileira de pesquisas medicas e biologicas / Sociedade Brasileira de Biofisica (et al) 2002; 35(15): 1001-5.
[http://dx.doi.org/10.1590/S0100-879X2002000900001]

[21] Matsusaka T, Ichikawa I. Biological functions of angiotensin and its receptors. Annu Rev Physiol 1997; 59: 395-412.
[http://dx.doi.org/10.1146/annurev.physiol.59.1.395] [PMID: 9074770]

[22] Steckelings UM, Unger T. Angiotensin II type 2 receptor agonists--where should they be applied? Expert Opin Investig Drugs 2012; 21(6): 763-6.
[http://dx.doi.org/10.1517/13543784.2012.681046] [PMID: 22519550]

[23] Widdop RE, Matrougui K, Levy BI, Henrion D. AT2 receptor-mediated relaxation is preserved after long-term AT1 receptor blockade. Hypertension 2002; 40(4): 516-20.
[http://dx.doi.org/10.1161/01.HYP.0000033224.99806.8A] [PMID: 12364356]

[24] Savoia C, D'Agostino M, Lauri F, Volpe M. Angiotensin type 2 receptor in hypertensive cardiovascular disease. Curr Opin Nephrol Hypertens 2011; 20(2): 125-32.
[http://dx.doi.org/10.1097/MNH.0b013e3283437fcd] [PMID: 21245762]

[25] Ferrario CM, Chappell MC, Tallant EA, Brosnihan KB, Diz DI. Counterregulatory actions of angiotensin-(1-7). Hypertension 1997; 30(3 Pt 2): 535-41. [1-7].
[http://dx.doi.org/10.1161/01.HYP.30.3.535] [PMID: 9322978]

[26] Santos RA, Campagnole-Santos MJ, Andrade SP. Angiotensin-(1-7): an update. Regul Pept 2000; 91(1-3): 45-62.
[http://dx.doi.org/10.1016/S0167-0115(00)00138-5] [PMID: 10967201]

[27] Di Marco GS, Naffah-Mazzacoratti Md MdaG, Vio CP, Dos Santos OF, Schor N, Casarini DE. Mesangial cells are able to produce catecholamines *in vitro.* J Cell Biochem 2003; 89(1): 144-51.
[http://dx.doi.org/10.1002/jcb.10485] [PMID: 12682915]

[28] Xu P, Costa-Goncalves AC, Todiras M, *et al.* Endothelial dysfunction and elevated blood pressure in MAS gene-deleted mice. Hypertension 2008; 51(2): 574-80.
[http://dx.doi.org/10.1161/HYPERTENSIONAHA.107.102764] [PMID: 18180400]

[29] Mercure C, Yogi A, Callera GE, *et al.* Angiotensin(1-7) blunts hypertensive cardiac remodeling by a direct effect on the heart. Circ Res 2008; 103(11): 1319-26.
[http://dx.doi.org/10.1161/CIRCRESAHA.108.184911] [PMID: 18845809]

[30] Castro CH, Santos RA, Ferreira AJ, Bader M, Alenina N, Almeida AP. Effects of genetic deletion of angiotensin-(1-7) receptor Mas on cardiac function during ischemia/reperfusion in the isolated perfused mouse heart. Life Sci 2006; 80(3): 264-8.
[http://dx.doi.org/10.1016/j.lfs.2006.09.007] [PMID: 17055538]

[31] Vickers C, Hales P, Kaushik V, *et al.* Hydrolysis of biological peptides by human angiotensin-converting enzyme-related carboxypeptidase. J Biol Chem 2002; 277(17): 14838-43. [http://dx.doi.org/10.1074/jbc.M200581200] [PMID: 11815627]

[32] Zisman LS, Meixell GE, Bristow MR, Canver CC. Angiotensin-(1-7) formation in the intact human heart: *in vivo* dependence on angiotensin II as substrate. Circulation 2003; 108(14): 1679-81. [http://dx.doi.org/10.1161/01.CIR.0000094733.61689.D4] [PMID: 14504185]

[33] Zisman LS, Keller RS, Weaver B, *et al.* Increased angiotensin-(1-7)-forming activity in failing human heart ventricles: evidence for upregulation of the angiotensin-converting enzyme Homologue ACE2. Circulation 2003; 108(14): 1707-12. [http://dx.doi.org/10.1161/01.CIR.0000094734.67990.99] [PMID: 14504186]

[34] Rice GI, Thomas DA, Grant PJ, Turner AJ, Hooper NM. Evaluation of angiotensin-converting enzyme (ACE), its homologue ACE2 and neprilysin in angiotensin peptide metabolism. Biochem J 2004; 383(Pt 1): 45-51. [http://dx.doi.org/10.1042/BJ20040634] [PMID: 15283675]

[35] Stanziola L, Greene LJ, Santos RA. Effect of chronic angiotensin converting enzyme inhibition on angiotensin I and bradykinin metabolism in rats. Am J Hypertens 1999; 12(10 Pt 1): 1021-9. [http://dx.doi.org/10.1016/S0895-7061(99)00090-4] [PMID: 10560789]

[36] Campbell DJ, Zeitz CJ, Esler MD, Horowitz JD. Evidence against a major role for angiotensin converting enzyme-related carboxypeptidase (ACE2) in angiotensin peptide metabolism in the human coronary circulation. J Hypertens 2004; 22(10): 1971-6. [http://dx.doi.org/10.1097/00004872-200410000-00020] [PMID: 15361769]

[37] Ferreira AJ, Moraes PL, Foureaux G, *et al.* The angiotensin-(1-7)/Mas receptor axis is expressed in sinoatrial node cells of rats The journal of histochemistry and cytochemistry : official journal of the Histochemistry Society 2011; 59(8): 761-8.

[38] Santos RA, Brum JM, Brosnihan KB, Ferrario CM. The renin-angiotensin system during acute myocardial ischemia in dogs. Hypertension 1990; 15(2) (Suppl.): I121-7. [http://dx.doi.org/10.1161/01.HYP.15.2_Suppl.I121] [PMID: 2404854]

[39] Averill DB, Ishiyama Y, Chappell MC, Ferrario CM. Cardiac angiotensin-(1-7) in ischemic cardiomyopathy. Circulation 2003; 108(17): 2141-6. [http://dx.doi.org/10.1161/01.CIR.0000092888.63239.54] [PMID: 14517166]

[40] Ferreira AJ, Jacoby BA, Araújo CA, *et al.* The nonpeptide angiotensin-(1-7) receptor Mas agonist AVE-0991 attenuates heart failure induced by myocardial infarction. Am J Physiol Heart Circ Physiol 2007; 292(2): H1113-9. [http://dx.doi.org/10.1152/ajpheart.00828.2006] [PMID: 17056670]

[41] Ferreira AJ, Oliveira TL, Castro MC, *et al.* Isoproterenol-induced impairment of heart function and remodeling are attenuated by the nonpeptide angiotensin-(1-7) analogue AVE 0991. Life Sci 2007; 81(11): 916-23. [http://dx.doi.org/10.1016/j.lfs.2007.07.022] [PMID: 17825326]

[42] Marques FD, Ferreira AJ, Sinisterra RD, *et al.* An oral formulation of angiotensin-(1-7) produces cardioprotective effects in infarcted and isoproterenol-treated rats. Hypertension 2011; 57(3): 477-83.

[http://dx.doi.org/10.1161/HYPERTENSIONAHA.110.167346] [PMID: 21282558]

[43] Neves LA, Almeida AP, Khosla MC, Santos RA. Metabolism of angiotensin I in isolated rat hearts. Effect of angiotensin converting enzyme inhibitors. Biochem Pharmacol 1995; 50(9): 1451-9. [http://dx.doi.org/10.1016/0006-2952(95)02049-7] [PMID: 7503796]

[44] Fraga-Silva RA, Costa-Fraga FP, Murça TM, *et al.* Angiotensin-converting enzyme 2 activation improves endothelial function. Hypertension 2013; 61(6): 1233-8. [http://dx.doi.org/10.1161/HYPERTENSIONAHA.111.00627] [PMID: 23608648]

[45] Fraga-Silva RA, Sorg BS, Wankhede M, *et al.* ACE2 activation promotes antithrombotic activity. Mol Med 2010; 16(5-6): 210-5. [http://dx.doi.org/10.2119/molmed.2009.00160] [PMID: 20111697]

[46] Hernández Prada JA, Ferreira AJ, Katovich MJ, *et al.* Structure-based identification of small-molecule angiotensin-converting enzyme 2 activators as novel antihypertensive agents. Hypertension 2008; 51(5): 1312-7. [http://dx.doi.org/10.1161/HYPERTENSIONAHA.107.108944] [PMID: 18391097]

[47] Shenoy V, Gjymishka A, Jarajapu YP, *et al.* Diminazene attenuates pulmonary hypertension and improves angiogenic progenitor cell functions in experimental models. Am J Respir Crit Care Med 2013; 187(6): 648-57. [http://dx.doi.org/10.1164/rccm.201205-0880OC] [PMID: 23370913]

[48] Walther T, Wessel N, Kang N, *et al.* Altered heart rate and blood pressure variability in mice lacking the Mas protooncogene Brazilian journal of medical and biological research = Revista brasileira de pesquisas medicas e biologicas / Sociedade Brasileira de Biofisica (et al) 2000; 33(1): 1-9. [http://dx.doi.org/10.1590/S0100-879X2000000100001]

[49] Santos RA, Ferreira AJ, Nadu AP, *et al.* Expression of an angiotensin-(1-7)-producing fusion protein produces cardioprotective effects in rats. Physiol Genomics 2004; 17(3): 292-9. [http://dx.doi.org/10.1152/physiolgenomics.00227.2003] [PMID: 15039487]

[50] Martins Lima A, Xavier CH, Ferreira AJ, *et al.* Activation of angiotensin-converting enzyme 2/angiotensin-(1-7)/Mas axis attenuates the cardiac reactivity to acute emotional stress. Am J Physiol Heart Circ Physiol 2013; 305(7): H1057-67. [http://dx.doi.org/10.1152/ajpheart.00433.2013] [PMID: 23873801]

[51] Braga AN, da Silva Lemos M, da Silva JR, Fontes WR, dos Santos RA. Effects of angiotensins on day-night fluctuations and stress-induced changes in blood pressure. Am J Physiol Regul Integr Comp Physiol 2002; 282(6): R1663-71. [http://dx.doi.org/10.1152/ajpregu.00583.2001] [PMID: 12010748]

[52] Liu E, Xu Z, Li J, Yang S, Yang W, Li G. Enalapril, irbesartan, and angiotensin-(1-7) prevent atrial tachycardia-induced ionic remodeling. Int J Cardiol 2011; 146(3): 364-70. [http://dx.doi.org/10.1016/j.ijcard.2009.07.015] [PMID: 19732978]

[53] Dias-Peixoto MF, Santos RA, Gomes ER, *et al.* Molecular mechanisms involved in the angiotensin-(--7)/Mas signaling pathway in cardiomyocytes. Hypertension 2008; 52(3): 542-8. [http://dx.doi.org/10.1161/HYPERTENSIONAHA.108.114280] [PMID: 18695148]

[54] Santos RA, Castro CH, Gava E, *et al.* Impairment of *in vitro* and *in vivo* heart function in angiotensin-

(1-7) receptor MAS knockout mice. Hypertension 2006; 47(5): 996-1002. [http://dx.doi.org/10.1161/01.HYP.0000215289.51180.5c] [PMID: 16567589]

[55] Gironacci MM, Adler-Graschinsky E, Peña C, Enero MA. Effects of angiotensin II and angiotensin-(--7) on the release of [3H]norepinephrine from rat atria. Hypertension 1994; 24(4): 457-60. [http://dx.doi.org/10.1161/01.HYP.24.4.457] [PMID: 8088911]

[56] Byku M, Macarthur H, Westfall TC. Inhibitory effects of angiotensin-(1-7) on the nerve stimulation-induced release of norepinephrine and neuropeptide Y from the mesenteric arterial bed. Am J Physiol Heart Circ Physiol 2010; 298(2): H457-65. [http://dx.doi.org/10.1152/ajpheart.00400.2009] [PMID: 19933420]

[57] Oliveira DR, Santos RA, Santos GF, Khosla M, Campagnole-Santos MJ. Changes in the baroreflex control of heart rate produced by central infusion of selective angiotensin antagonists in hypertensive rats. Hypertension 1996; 27(6): 1284-90. [http://dx.doi.org/10.1161/01.HYP.27.6.1284] [PMID: 8641737]

[58] Chaves GZ, Caligiorne SM, Santos RA, Khosla MC, Campagnole-Santos MJ. Modulation of the baroreflex control of heart rate by angiotensin-(1-7) at the nucleus tractus solitarii of normotensive and spontaneously hypertensive rats. J Hypertens 2000; 18(12): 1841-8. [http://dx.doi.org/10.1097/00004872-200018120-00019] [PMID: 11132609]

[59] Kar S, Gao L, Belatti DA, Curry PL, Zucker IH. Central angiotensin (1-7) enhances baroreflex gain in conscious rabbits with heart failure. Hypertension 2011; 58(4): 627-34. [http://dx.doi.org/10.1161/HYPERTENSIONAHA.111.177600] [PMID: 21844487]

[60] Brosnihan KB, Li P, Ferrario CM. Angiotensin-(1-7) dilates canine coronary arteries through kinins and nitric oxide. Hypertension 1996; 27(3 Pt 2): 523-8. [http://dx.doi.org/10.1161/01.HYP.27.3.523] [PMID: 8613197]

[61] Neves LA, Almeida AP, Khosla MC, *et al.* Effect of angiotensin-(1-7) on reperfusion arrhythmias in isolated rat hearts Brazilian journal of medical and biological research = Revista brasileira de pesquisas medicas e biologicas/Sociedade Brasileira de Biofisica (et al) 1997; 30(6): 801-9.

[62] Kumagai H, Khosla M, Ferrario C, Fouad-Tarazi FM. Biological activity of angiotensin-(1-7) heptapeptide in the hamster heart. Hypertension 1990; 15(2) (Suppl.): I29-33. [http://dx.doi.org/10.1161/01.HYP.15.2_Suppl.I29] [PMID: 2298473]

[63] Fraga-Silva RA, Costa-Fraga FP, De Sousa FB, *et al.* An orally active formulation of angiotensin-(1-7) produces an antithrombotic effect. Clinics (Sao Paulo) 2011; 66(5): 837-41. [http://dx.doi.org/10.1590/S1807-59322011000500021] [PMID: 21789389]

[64] Fraga-Silva RA, Da Silva DG, Montecucco F, *et al.* The angiotensin-converting enzyme 2/angiotensin-(1-7)/Mas receptor axis: a potential target for treating thrombotic diseases. Thromb Haemost 2012; 108(6): 1089-96. [http://dx.doi.org/10.1160/TH12-06-0396] [PMID: 23093373]

[65] da Costa Gonçalves AC, Leite R, Fraga-Silva RA, *et al.* Evidence that the vasodilator angiotensin-(--7)-Mas axis plays an important role in erectile function. Am J Physiol Heart Circ Physiol 2007; 293(4): H2588-96. [http://dx.doi.org/10.1152/ajpheart.00173.2007] [PMID: 17616753]

[66] Pörsti I, Bara AT, Busse R, Hecker M. Release of nitric oxide by angiotensin-(1-7) from porcine coronary endothelium: implications for a novel angiotensin receptor. Br J Pharmacol 1994; 111(3): 652-4.
[http://dx.doi.org/10.1111/j.1476-5381.1994.tb14787.x] [PMID: 8019744]

[67] Almeida AP, Frabregas BC, Madureira MM, *et al.* Angiotensin-(1-7) potentiates the coronary vasodilatory effect of bradykinin in the isolated rat heart Brazilian journal of medical and biological research = Revista brasileira de pesquisas medicas e biologicas / Sociedade Brasileira de Biofisica (et al) 2000; 33(6): 709-13.

[68] Sampaio WO, Souza dos Santos RA, Faria-Silva R, da Mata Machado LT, Schiffrin EL, Touyz RM. Angiotensin-(1-7) through receptor Mas mediates endothelial nitric oxide synthase activation *via* Akt-dependent pathways. Hypertension 2007; 49(1): 185-92.
[http://dx.doi.org/10.1161/01.HYP.0000251865.35728.2f] [PMID: 17116756]

[69] Fernandes L, Fortes ZB, Nigro D, Tostes RC, Santos RA, Catelli De Carvalho MH. Potentiation of bradykinin by angiotensin-(1-7) on arterioles of spontaneously hypertensive rats studied *in vivo.* Hypertension 2001; 37(2 Pt 2): 703-9.
[http://dx.doi.org/10.1161/01.HYP.37.2.703] [PMID: 11230360]

[70] Oliveira MA, Fortes ZB, Santos RA, Kosla MC, De Carvalho MH. Synergistic effect of angiotensin-(1-7) on bradykinin arteriolar dilation *in vivo.* Peptides 1999; 20(10): 1195-201.
[http://dx.doi.org/10.1016/S0196-9781(99)00123-0] [PMID: 10573291]

[71] Carvalho MB, Duarte FV, Faria-Silva R, *et al.* Evidence for Mas-mediated bradykinin potentiation by the angiotensin-(1-7) nonpeptide mimic AVE 0991 in normotensive rats. Hypertension 2007; 50(4): 762-7.
[http://dx.doi.org/10.1161/HYPERTENSIONAHA.107.094987] [PMID: 17664388]

[72] Bader M, Peters J, Baltatu O, Müller DN, Luft FC, Ganten D. Tissue renin-angiotensin systems: new insights from experimental animal models in hypertension research. J Mol Med 2001; 79(2-3): 76-102.
[http://dx.doi.org/10.1007/s001090100210] [PMID: 11357942]

[73] Rosenkranz S. TGF-beta1 and angiotensin networking in cardiac remodeling. Cardiovasc Res 2004; 63(3): 423-32.
[http://dx.doi.org/10.1016/j.cardiores.2004.04.030] [PMID: 15276467]

[74] Santiago NM, Guimarães PS, Sirvente RA, *et al.* Lifetime overproduction of circulating Angiotensin-(1-7) attenuates deoxycorticosterone acetate-salt hypertension-induced cardiac dysfunction and remodeling. Hypertension 2010; 55(4): 889-96.
[http://dx.doi.org/10.1161/HYPERTENSIONAHA.110.149815] [PMID: 20212262]

[75] Nadu AP, Ferreira AJ, Reudelhuber TL, Bader M, Santos RA. Reduced isoproterenol-induced renin-angiotensin changes and extracellular matrix deposition in hearts of TGR(A1-7)3292 rats. J Am Soc Hypertens 2008; 2(5): 341-8.
[http://dx.doi.org/10.1016/j.jash.2008.04.012] [PMID: 20409916]

[76] Trask AJ, Groban L, Westwood BM, *et al.* Inhibition of angiotensin-converting enzyme 2 exacerbates cardiac hypertrophy and fibrosis in Ren-2 hypertensive rats. Am J Hypertens 2010; 23(6): 687-93.
[http://dx.doi.org/10.1038/ajh.2010.51] [PMID: 20300067]

[77] Ferreira AJ, Shenoy V, Qi Y, *et al.* Angiotensin-converting enzyme 2 activation protects against hypertension-induced cardiac fibrosis involving extracellular signal-regulated kinases. Exp Physiol 2011; 96(3): 287-94.
[http://dx.doi.org/10.1113/expphysiol.2010.055277] [PMID: 21148624]

[78] Huentelman MJ, Grobe JL, Vazquez J, *et al.* Protection from angiotensin II-induced cardiac hypertrophy and fibrosis by systemic lentiviral delivery of ACE2 in rats. Exp Physiol 2005; 90(5): 783-90.
[http://dx.doi.org/10.1113/expphysiol.2005.031096] [PMID: 16049057]

[79] Díez-Freire C, Vázquez J, Correa de Adjounian MF, *et al.* ACE2 gene transfer attenuates hypertension-linked pathophysiological changes in the SHR. Physiol Genomics 2006; 27(1): 12-9.
[http://dx.doi.org/10.1152/physiolgenomics.00312.2005] [PMID: 16788004]

[80] Der Sarkissian S, Grobe JL, Yuan L, *et al.* Cardiac overexpression of angiotensin converting enzyme 2 protects the heart from ischemia-induced pathophysiology. Hypertension 2008; 51(3): 712-8.
[http://dx.doi.org/10.1161/HYPERTENSIONAHA.107.100693] [PMID: 18250366]

[81] Zhao YX, Yin HQ, Yu QT, *et al.* ACE2 overexpression ameliorates left ventricular remodeling and dysfunction in a rat model of myocardial infarction. Hum Gene Ther 2010; 21(11): 1545-54.
[http://dx.doi.org/10.1089/hum.2009.160] [PMID: 20507236]

[82] Shenoy V, Ferreira AJ, Qi Y, *et al.* The angiotensin-converting enzyme 2/angiogenesis-(1-7)/Mas axis confers cardiopulmonary protection against lung fibrosis and pulmonary hypertension. Am J Respir Crit Care Med 2010; 182(8): 1065-72.
[http://dx.doi.org/10.1164/rccm.200912-1840OC] [PMID: 20581171]

[83] Grobe JL, Mecca AP, Mao H, Katovich MJ. Chronic angiotensin-(1-7) prevents cardiac fibrosis in DOCA-salt model of hypertension. Am J Physiol Heart Circ Physiol 2006; 290(6): H2417-23.
[http://dx.doi.org/10.1152/ajpheart.01170.2005] [PMID: 16415071]

[84] Iwata M, Cowling RT, Gurantz D, *et al.* Angiotensin-(1-7) binds to specific receptors on cardiac fibroblasts to initiate antifibrotic and antitrophic effects. Am J Physiol Heart Circ Physiol 2005; 289(6): H2356-63.
[http://dx.doi.org/10.1152/ajpheart.00317.2005] [PMID: 16024575]

[85] Pan CH, Wen CH, Lin CS. Interplay of angiotensin II and angiotensin(1-7) in the regulation of matrix metalloproteinases of human cardiocytes. Exp Physiol 2008; 93(5): 599-612.
[http://dx.doi.org/10.1113/expphysiol.2007.041830] [PMID: 18296491]

[86] Giani JF, Gironacci MM, Muñoz MC, Turyn D, Dominici FP. Angiotensin-(1-7) has a dual role on growth-promoting signalling pathways in rat heart *in vivo* by stimulating STAT3 and STAT5a/b phosphorylation and inhibiting angiotensin II-stimulated ERK1/2 and Rho kinase activity. Exp Physiol 2008; 93(5): 570-8.
[PMID: 18448663]

[87] Gomes ER, Lara AA, Almeida PW, *et al.* Angiotensin-(1-7) prevents cardiomyocyte pathological remodeling through a nitric oxide/guanosine 3′,5′-cyclic monophosphate-dependent pathway. Hypertension 2010; 55(1): 153-60.
[http://dx.doi.org/10.1161/HYPERTENSIONAHA.109.143255] [PMID: 19996065]

CHAPTER 6

Essential Roles of Renin-Angiotensin System in the Kidney

Ingrid Kazue Mizuno Watanabe[1,*,#], **Zaira Palomino Jara**[1,#], **Roberto Mesquita Soler**[1,*], **Nestor Schor**[1] and **Flavia F. Jung**[2]

[1] *Nephrology Division, Department of Medicine, Escola Paulista de Medicina, Federal University of São Paulo, São Paulo, Brazil*

[2] *Washington Hospital, Washington DC, USA*

Abstract: The renin angiotensin system (RAS) has crucial action in the kidney; it is able to modulate intrarenal hemodynamics, glomerular filtration, and fluid and electrolytes homeostasis. Currently, six components of this system mediate their action through receptor(s). Four peptides, Ang II, Ang-(1-7), Ang III and Ang IV; and two enzymes, renin and prorenin through the renin and prorenin receptor, respectively. Angiotensin II (Ang II), the main peptide of RAS, through its type 1 receptor (AT1R) alters intrarenal hemodynamics, glomerular filtration, and fluid and electrolytes homeostasis readjusting blood pressure and body fluid balance. In the later functions, direct action of Ang II on the sodium and water transport was observed and related to diuretic/anti-diuretic and natriuretic/anti-natriuretic action depending on Ang II concentration. Angiotensin-(1-7) also influences the glomerular filtration rate but without changing the blood pressure. This heptapeptide showed biphasic direct action on tubular transport of sodium and water, but there is no consensus which receptor translates its tubular effect. Reports showed that Angiotensin III and Angiotensin IV could present natriuretic action; the pressor effect of both peptides is unclear. Direct action on tubular transport via renin and prorenin receptor has not yet been reported.

[*] **Corresponding author Ingrid Kazue Mizuno Watanabe:** Nephrology Division, Department of Medicine, Escola Paulista de Medicina, Federal University of São Paulo, São Paulo, Brazil; Tel: 55 11 5576 4841; Fax: 55 11 5904 1684; E-mails: ingridwatanabe@gmail.com, roberto_soler@hotmail.com

[#] Both authors equally contributed to this chapter.

Dulce Elena Casarini, Danielle Yuri Arita, Tatiana Sousa Cunha & Juliana Almada Colucci (Eds.)

Keywords: Angiotensin II (Ang II), Angiotensin III (Ang III), Angiotensin IV (Ang IV), Angiotensin-(1-7) (Ang-(1-7)), AT1R, AT2R, Blood pressure, Distal tubule, Diuresis, Loop of Henle, Kidney, MAS receptor, Natriuresis, Pro(renin) receptor, Proximal tubule, Renin-angiotensin system.

INTRODUCTION

The kidney is a pivotal organ for regulation of blood pressure and water and electrolytes balance. These functions, regardless of exposure to environment fluctuation, must be maintained in restricted range of variation. Thus, the body orchestrates production and release of humoral factors that interact with the uniquely engineered cells within the kidney adjusting the process to maintain water and electrolyte balance. One of these factors is the renin-angiotensin system (RAS).

The fascinating history of RAS began in 1898 with the discovery of a substance isolated from the kidney, later named renin, capable of increasing blood pressure [1]. Since then, the system has been constantly unraveled by the discovery of other members and the existence of a local RAS in different organs.

Classically, under physiological conditions, angiotensin II (Ang II) formation initiates with the secretion of renin by the juxtaglomerular apparatus stimulated by decrease of blood pressure detected by the baroreceptors. Decrease of sodium levels is sensed by the macula densa, and responds with overactivity of sympathetic nervous system. Since its discovery, the RAS has been characterized in many organs. Despite of that, the action of Ang II is fascinating in the kidney, where the peptide is able to alter intrarenal hemodynamics, glomerular filtration, and fluid and electrolytes homeostasis readjusting blood pressure and body fluid balance. The critical role of RAS in renal physiology is supported by the observation that intrarenal Ang II blockade augmented glomerular filtration rate, sodium and water excretion, and renal plasma flow without any alteration of systemic pressor responses [2]. During many years, Ang II was used as synonym for RAS because it was believed that only Ang II possessed biological action. However, in the present scenario, there are strong physiological evidence supporting that smaller peptides of this system, such as angiotensin III (Ang III), angiotensin IV (Ang IV), and angiotensin-(1-7) (Ang-(1-7)), also modulate their activities through receptor(s). It was observed that in the nephron these peptides participated in the fluid and electrolytes homeostasis by their action on sodium and water transporters.

RAS – Bioactive Angiotensins and Receptors

The RAS has been constantly expanded by the discovery of other member including new enzymes, bioactive peptides and receptors, thus increasing its importance. The current versatile and complex system has six biological active components that translate its activity through receptor(s): four peptides (Ang II, Ang III, Ang IV, and Ang-(1-7)); and enzymes (renin and prorenin).

The mentioned peptides are formed by the action of an array of enzymes. It starts with renin hydrolyzing angiotensinogen (AGT) to form angiotensin I (Ang I) followed by the conversion of Ang I to Ang II by angiotensin-converting enzyme (ACE) [3]. Besides this classical pathway formed by two enzymatic steps, AGT can also be hydrolyzed by cathepsin D to form Ang I and in turn Ang I can be cleaved by chymase to form Ang II [4]. Additionally, Ang II can be produced directly from AGT in one enzymatic step by the following enzymes: either tonin, cathepsin G or chymotrypsin [5 - 7].

Furthermore, Ang I and Ang II can also be substrates to produce Ang-(1-7). Direct and indirect pathways are described to form Ang-(1-7) from Ang I. Direct formation of this heptapeptide occurs by the activity of thimet oligopeptidase (TOP), neprilysin (NEP) or prolyl endopeptidase (POP) on Ang I [8]. Indirect production of this heptapeptide occurs *via* two enzymatic steps: angiotensin-converting enzyme 2 (ACE2) cleaves Ang I to Angiotensin-1-9, and in turn angiotensin-1-9 is hydrolyzed by ACE to produce Ang-(1-7). Ang II can also be hydrolyzed to Ang-(1-7) by ACE2 [9, 10].

Likewise, Ang II can generate Ang III by the action of aminopeptidase A (APA), and Ang III in turn can be hydrolyzed into Ang IV by aminopeptidase N (APN) [11]. Ang II, Ang-(1-7), and Ang IV are further cleaved into smaller inactive fragments.

The biological active RAS components must bind to their angiotensin receptor(s) in order to translate activities. It is well established that Ang II acts through Ang II type I receptor (AT1R) and type 2 receptor (AT2R). In humans only one gene is translate to AT1R, while in rat and mouse two genes are translated into AT1aR and AT1bR [12]. The information available indicates that Ang III also binds to AT1R and AT2R; however, the AT1R binding site preferentially docks to Ang II. Regarding to Ang II and Ang III binding to AT2R, data indicates that this receptor docks individually to these two peptides, and in nanomolar concentration there is not difference in the affinity for AT1R. It has also been discovered the binding site for Ang IV, initially named AT4R, lately also called insulin-regulated aminopeptidase (IRAP) [13, 14] . Extensive literature about Ang-(1-7) has been published. Initially its effects were related to the binding to the AT1R and AT2R, lately, physiologists related its activity through the binding to MAS receptor.

According to the International Unit of Pharmacology (IUPHAR), the AT1R and AT2R fulfill all the criteria to be accepted as angiotensin receptors [15, 16], as well as the IRAP/AT4R for Ang IV. Interestingly, MAS, an orphan GPCR, based on the physiological responses is a strong candidate for mediating the action of Ang-(1-7). However, according to the pharmacological data obtained, up to now, by the scientific community, MAS does not fulfill the requirements to be considered an angiotensin receptor [16].

Finally, as aforementioned two enzymes, one in its inactive form and another in its active form, the pro-renin and renin, respectively, bind to the (pro)renin receptor (PRR), and its signal transduction is distinct from Ang II pathway [17, 18].

RAS Production in the Kidney

All RAS components are expressed in the kidney, however, it is very important to know the local distributions of these components within the kidney, whether or not they coexist in the same target cell. Each organ has unique responses to the biological active angiotensins based on: the concentration and lifetime of these peptides, the existence and density of the receptors, and their binding selectivity for agonists, among other characteristics [16]. Therefore, these features together with unique capability of functions of the different kidney cell types give specific tissue response to the angiotensins.

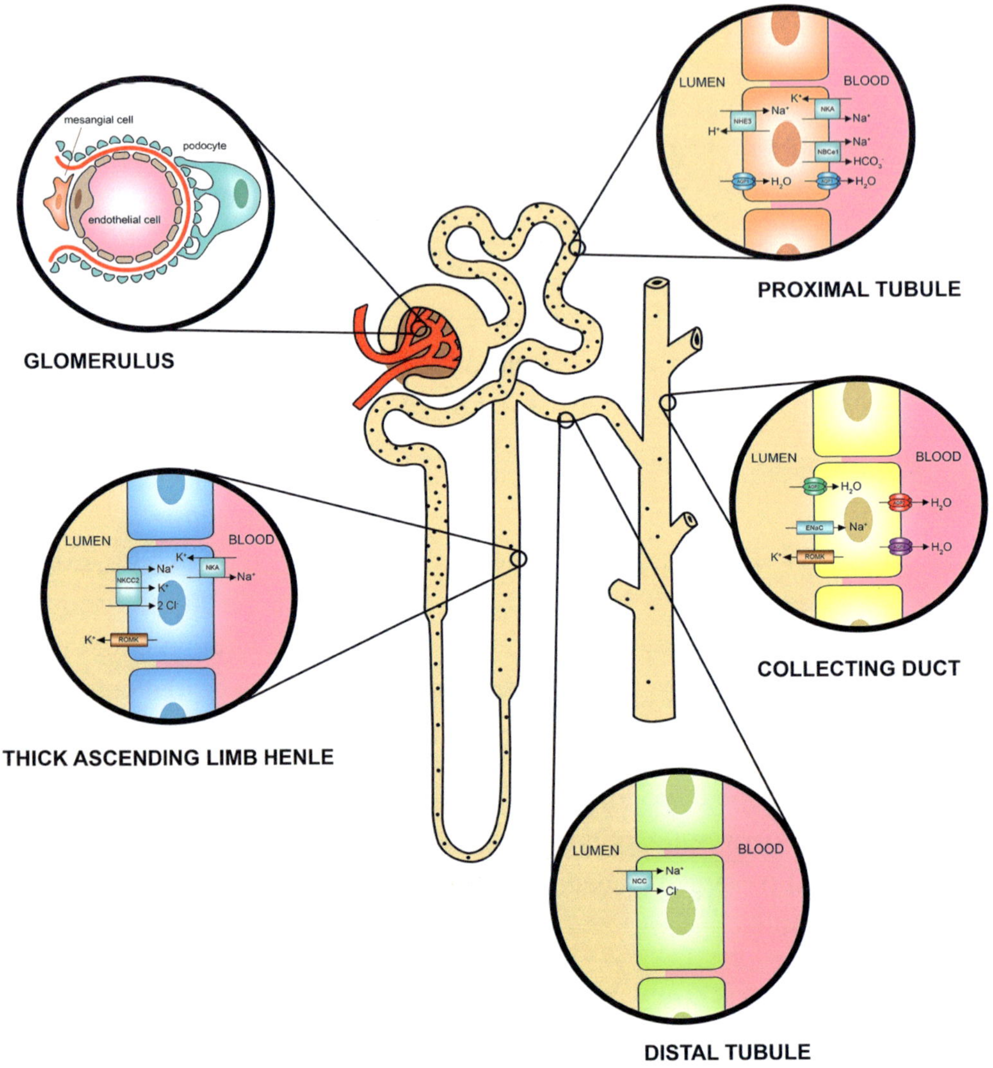

Fig. (1). Nephron, one functional unit depicted showing amplification of its regions. The ultrafiltration barrier located within the glomerulus, and sodium and water transporters along the tubules.

Each kidney has approximately 1 million of nephrons, functional units composed by glomeruli and tubules. The glomerulus, formed by Bowman's capsule and capillary network, performs the blood ultrafiltration. The composition of the filtrate is regulated by interaction of the capillary endothelium fenestration, the endothelial cell, the glomerulus basement membrane (GBM), the podocytes, glycocalyces on the podocyte and the subpodocyte space above the GBM [19, 20]. Once the blood is filtrated, it migrates through the renal tubules lumen. 99% of water, electrolytes and solutes are selectively reabsorbed to the bloodstream through a variety of channels, transporters and exchangers (Table **1** and Fig. (**1**)) located along the proximal tubule (PT), loop of Henle, distal tubule, and collecting tubule [21, 22].

Table 1. Transporters along the nephron tubules.

	Proximal tubule	Reference	Loop of Henle	Reference	Distal tubule	Reference	Collecting duct	Reference
Apical membrane	NHE-3 SGLT2 SLC9A3 NaPi2 AQP-1	[22, 23] [21, 24]	NHE-3 (TAL) NKCC2 AQP-1	[25]	NCC		ENaC AQP2 AQP3 AQP4	[26]
Basolateral membrane	Na^+/K^+-ATPase $Na^+/Ca2^+$ Na^+/HCO_3^- Na^+-ATPase AQP-1 AQP-7	[21, 27] [28] [21] [21 - 29] [30] [24, 31] [32]	Na+/K+-ATPase	[28]	Na+/K+-ATPase	[28]	Na+/K+-ATPase	[28]

NHE-3: sodium-hydrogen exchanger isoform 3; SGLT2: sodium-glucose co-transporter; SLC9A3: sodium amino acid transporters; NaPi2: sodium phosphate co-transporter; AQP-1: aquaporin-1; Na^+/K^+-ATPase: sodium-potassium-adenosine triphosphatase pump; $Na^+/Ca2^+$: sodium-calcium exchanger; Na^+/HCO_3^-: sodium-bicarbonate co-transporter; Na^+-ATPase: sodium-adenosine triphosphatase; NKCC2: sodium-potassium-chloride. co-transporter.

Regarding to specific expression of RAS components in the kidney, it has been published that the circulating AGT can reach the glomerulus by afferent arteriole. Additionally, its expression has been demonstrated locally in the kidney especially in the proximal tubule [33]. It is important to highlight that in physiological conditions AGT cannot pass the glomerulus filtration barrier [34].

The main peptide of the RAS, Ang II, is present in the intraluminal proximal tubule fluid in concentrations between 5 to 10 pmol/L [35], while concentration in urine is 0.5 pmol/L. Concentration in the lumen of other nephron segments has been difficult to quantify [34]. Casarini *et al.* described the presence of ACE activity along the nephron. The authors found highest activity in the proximal portion of the nephron and lower activity in the other portions. Interestingly, higher level was found in the urine compare with the distal nephron [36].

The expression of the Ang-(1-7) was observed in the podocytes and along the nephron. In the podocyte, this heptapeptide seems to be formed preferentially from Ang I as substrate for NEP, although ACE2 imnunostaining colocalizes with the podocyte marker [37, 38]. Along segments of the nephron, positive immunostaining for Ang-(1-7) was reported [35, 39], as well as ACE2 mRNA was expressed in most renal tubules, being the medullary collecting duct and *vasa rectae* the exception . The proximal tubule showed the higher expression of ACE2 colocalized with Ang-(1-7) [40, 41]. In humans, Ang-(1-7) was found in urine [42].

APA activity and immunostaining confirmed the presence of this enzyme along the nephron, however, higher activity was observed in the cortex than in the medulla [43]. Other enzymes, such as, NEP, TOP and POP were also located on renal brush-border membranes. In addition, it is important to highlight that enzymes that further cleave Ang-(1-7) in smaller peptides are present in the proximal tubule [44 - 45].

AT1R is widely found in glomerular, tubular and vascular cells along the nephron. The expression of AT2R is lower and restricted to the renal vasculature and some tubular segments, particularly in proximal tubular cells. The role of AT2R is not fully understood and its activation leads to vasodilation and hypotensive effects observed in conditions of upregulated Ang II/AT1R axis and AT1R blockade, counterbalancing the biological actions of AT1R [46 - 49]. The opposing actions of AT2R are also supported by the observation that AT2R diminishes function and expression of AT1 *via* nitric oxide/cGMP/Sp1 and by the heterodimerization of both receptors in proximal tubule cells [50].

The topographic expression of AT4R and MAS receptor is still less understood. The AT4R presence has been reported in cortex and outer medulla of kidney [51,

52]. And, even though the expression of MAS receptor has been reported in kidney of murine animals [53, 54], the only study published using human proximal cells could not detect any expression of this receptor [55].

Lastly, the (P)RR is located in the collecting duct and distal nephron [56]. Gonzalez *et al.* suggested that its colocalization with H+-ATPase might indicate a functional role in the H+ transport [56, 57].

Ang II

It is well established that Ang II through its main receptor, AT1R, participates in the adjustment of glomerular filtration, sodium and water reabsorption and renal hemodynamics and modulation of blood pressure. Recently, it has been discovered that the presence of AT1R in the kidney is essential for the development of Ang II-dependent hypertension and sodium reabsorption supporting the concept of the central role of this receptor in renal function in physiological and pathophysiological scenarios [58, 59].

Ang II Actions in the Glomerulus

Ang II is a powerful vasoactive peptide, capable of vasoconstricting pre- and postglomerular microvasculature altering the glomerular filtration coefficient [60], and stimulating mesangial cell contraction, and, consequentially, reducing glomerular filtration rate. Ang II also alters the glomerular permeability to macromolecules by its actions on podocytes. It has been thought that this increased permeability would be due to an increase of the glomerular capillary pressure. Nonetheless, growing evidence indicates that structural anomalies in glomerular podocytes are associated to tubulointerstitial injury and glomerular sclerosis. Recent studies have shown that Ang II *via* AT1R induces changes in the cytoskeleton of podocytes, which are capable of altering the glomerular filtration barrier according to the contractile status [61 - 63]. *In vitro* study indicates that Ang II *via* AT1R reduces mRNA expression of nephrin in podocytes, once ARB treatment was able to abolish this effect [64]. Moreover, AT1R blockade abrogates reduction of nephrin and podocin expression in an experimental nephropathy model. This effect was not observed with hydralazine (non-Ang II action-mediated antihypertensive drug). Intrarenal Ang II has also a relevant modulatory effect over the sensitivity of the tubuloglomerular feedback (TGF) [65, 66]. Infusion of exogenous Ang II enhances TGF response *via* AT1R present on vascular muscle cells and macula densa cells, and ACE inhibition and AT1R blockade attenuate TGF responsiveness.

Ang II Actions in the Proximal Tubules

In proximal tubules, which are responsible for the reabsorption of 65% of filtered sodium, Ang II has a biphasic effect on transport. Ang II concentrations lower than 10^{-9} M lead to sodium reabsorption *via* activation of apical NHE-3, basolateral Na^+/HCO_3^- cotransporter type 1 and Na^+/K^+-ATPase [23, 29]. On the other hand, high concentrations of Ang II (nanomolar to micromolar) inhibit the activity of NHE-3, Na^+/HCO_3^-, and Na^+/K^+-ATPase reducing sodium reabsorption.

The importance of RAS in proximal tubules has been highlighted by studies using double transgenic mice expressing human renin and AGT specifically in the kidney [67]. In spite of unaltered plasmatic levels of Ang II, these animals, expressing human AGT only in the proximal tubule cells, are hypertensive indicating that the hypertension in this case is due to modifications of sodium and water transport by the Ang II locally produced in the proximal tubules. Moreover, deletion of AT1R in renal proximal tubule using Cre-Lox technology is able to lower blood pressure without any alteration of vascular properties [68]. Lack of AT1R protects mice against hypertension induced by infusion of Ang II. This protection is apparently due to increased natriuresis indicating that the sodium handling is a key for AT1R actions in blood pressure control. In addition, bicarbonate absorption is also regulated by intrarenal Ang II in a dose-dependent manner. Low dose of Ang II stimulates bicarbonate reabsorption, while high dose reduces it [69]. Candesartan increases bicarbonate reabsorption, while AT2R blockade reduces bicarbonate absorption [70].

Ang II Actions in the Thick Ascending Limbs

Thick ascending limbs (TALs) are responsible for 20% to 30% of sodium reabsorption. Increased sodium reabsorption in this segment has been associated to hypertension [71 - 73]. There are discrepancies in data related to Ang II effects on sodium transport, which seems to depend on the dose, treatment duration and the amplitude of blood pressure alteration. A 2-week infusion of Ang II at a dose of 400 ng/kg/min in mice increased protein expression and phosphorylation of NKCC2 in loop of Henle indicating higher sodium transport activity [74]. On the other hand, a higher dose of 1000 ng/kg/min decreased NKCC2 expression by 25%. The effect of Ang II on NKCC2 abundance and activity seems to depend on the localization of the transporter. After a 2-week of Ang II infusion, NKCC2 protein expression and activity were differentially modulated in cortex and medulla [75]. Ang II increased expression of total NKCC2 in cortex and decreased in medulla, while altered NKCC2 phosphorylation only in cortex. These opposing effects in cortex *versus* medulla may be consequence of an expression of different isoforms of NKCC2. The isoform NKCC2F is mainly found in the medullary TALs, while NKCC2B is mainly expressed in cortical TALs [76]. Under AT1 blockade conditions, Ang II stimulates NO production *via* AT2R in TALs leading to inhibition of NKCC2 and, consequentially, reducing sodium reabsorption [77].

Ang II in the Distal Tubules

Distal tubules absorb 10% to 20% of filtered sodium. Innumerous studies have shown that Ang II regulates sodium handling in the distal nephron. Besides the well-known role of aldosterone, there are growing evidence that Ang II directly regulates sodium transport in distal nephron. Infusion of Ang II in isolated tubules stimulates Na^+/H^+ exchange in the early distal tubule, and AT1 blockade abolishes this effect [78]. Ang II administration also induces the transport of Na^+/Cl^- cotransporter (NCC) to the apical membrane [79], supporting the idea that Ang II stimulates sodium reabsorption in distal tubules. Based on the well-known action of aldosterone over NCC activity, and the fact that Ang II stimulates aldosterone release, NCC activation following Ang II infusion could be *via* aldosterone. Infusion of Ang II in the mouse kidney increases NCC activation, however, aldosterone seems to be the predominant regulator of the phosphorylation cascade involved in the transporter activation [80]. On the other hand, chronic infusion of Ang II in adrenalectomized rats increases total and phosphorylated NCC levels independent of aldosterone [81]. Therefore, Ang II and aldosterone appear to stimulate sodium transport in a separate and additive manner.

Ang II Actions in the Collecting Ducts

Collecting ducts have a minor participation in the renal sodium reabsorption compared to the other nephron segments, but they are responsible for the final adjustment of sodium and water homeostasis. In the last segment of the nephron, the epithelial sodium channel (ENac) mainly performs sodium reabsorption. Ang II delivery at low concentration in isolated cortical collecting duct stimulates apical membrane ENaC activity *via* AT1R [82]. Growing evidence indicates that Ang II regulates ENac expression *via* AT1R. Infusion of Ang II enhances protein expression of alpha ENac, and AT1R blockade downregulated alpha ENac mRNA levels, even under mineralocorticoid receptor blockade, indicating that AT1R regulates directly alpha ENac gene expression [83]. Moreover, Oshawa *et al.* observed that depletion of the angiotensin II type 1 receptor–associated protein (ATRAP), which promotes AT1R internalization, upregulates renal expression of alpha subunit of ENac under chronic infusion with Ang II in an aldosterone-independent manner [84]. Ang II also seems to exert influence over urinary concentration process. Oliverio *et al.* observed that AT1R knockout animals are unable to increase urinary osmolality, despite normal levels of vasopressin [85]. *In vitro* study showed that Ang II augments vasopressin-stimulated facilitated urea transport in the collecting duct cells [86].

Ang II and Water Balance

Aquaporins are membrane proteins specialized in water transport in several cells and tissues. In particularly, they are critical elements in the control of water excretion in the kidney. Aquaporin 1 (AQP1) is remarkably expressed in the proximal tubules and thin descending limb of Henle, which are segments highly permeable to water [87]. Nephron segments with low water permeability do not seem to express aquaporins. The connecting tubules and collecting ducts present a fluctuating water permeability controlled by vasopressin. In this terminal part of the nephron, aquaporin 2 (AQP2) is found in the apical cell membrane [88] and aquaporin 3 and 4 are present in the basolateral cell membrane [89, 90]. AQP2, abundantly expressed in the principal cells of collecting ducts, is the target for vasopressin actions playing a key role in urine concentration and water balance [91, 92]. Most forms of nephrogenic diabetes insipidus (DI) are observed in patients with mutations in the vasopressin type 2 receptor (V2R) gene and 10% have mutations in AQP2 gene. These mutations are associated with polyuria in these patients [93], leading to a severe impaired urinary concentrating defect [94].

Proximal tubule and thin descending limb Henle, where AQP1 is highly expressed, are responsible for 80% of intratubular fluid reabsorption. The importance of AQP1 in water reabsorption is highlighted by the observation of urine concentration defect in AQP1 null mice [95, 96]. Growing indirect evidence indicates that Ang II can regulate AQP1 expression. Infusion of Ang I stimulates AQP1 gene expression in sheep fetal kidney [97], and RAS blockade inhibits expression of AQP1 in the rat peritoneum [98]. Recent study demonstrated that, in fact, Ang II stimulates AQP1 expression *in vivo* and *in vitro* [99]. Higher levels of AQP1 mRNA were detected in proximal tubule cells incubated with Ang II. This effect was blunted by the presence of losartan indicating that Ang II influences AQP1 gene expression *via* AT1R. Moreover, Ang II increased AQP1 protein expression and stimulated the AQP1 translocation to apical and basolateral plasma membrane. *In vivo* experiments showed that Ang II infusion increased immunostaining for AQP1 in proximal tubule segments 1 and 2 and thick descending limb Henle, which was abolished by AT1R blockade, indicating that Ang II regulates AQP1 redistribution in these nephron segments through AT1R.

Experimental studies have supported the idea of a potential relationship between Ang II and vasopressin. Simultaneous treatment with Ang II and vasopressin potentiated the production of cAMP *via* vasopressin V2 receptor in cells transfected with AT1 and V2 receptors [100]. Ang II also stimulates the gene expression of V2 receptor in collecting ducts, and AT1 blockade diminishes water reabsorption induced by vasopressin, expression, phosphorylation, and trafficking of AQP2 [101, 102]. Growing evidence has shown that Ang II can upregulate AQP2 expression in the absence of vasopressin [102] suggesting that RAS is able to regulate water reabsorption in collecting ducts. Ang II actions on AQP2 appears to be mediated by AT1R. The lack of AT1A receptors in collecting ducts decreases AQP2 expression in the medulla of knockout mice and the ability of urine concentration after water deprivation or vasopressin treatment [103].

Ang-(1-7)

Santos and Baracho in 1992 reported that Ang-(1-7) administrated peripherally into intraperitoneal-water-load male Wistar rat had antidiuretic action. When compared to vasopressin at same molar range, Ang-(1-7) is slightly less potent and when administrated simultaneously it seems to demonstrate an additive effect [104]. Up to this point, there were scientific reports indicating the central effects of both vasopressin and Ang-(1-7). The possibility of tissue specific expression and effect of Ang-(1-7) start to open fields to study this heptapeptide.

In 1993 it was published one of the first evidences that Ang-(1-7) affects the kidney. In isolated rat kidney, the heptapeptide had increased dose-dependent response on glomerular filtration rate as well as increased water and electrolyte excretion without changing the renal vascular resistance [105]. In this report Dellipizzi *et al.* hypothesized that the observed action may be through either by activation of both peptides, Ang II and Ang-(1-7), or by the activation solely of Ang-(1-7). In the last case, Ang II conversion to Ang-(1-7) probably had happened prior to receptor activation. This work gave the initiation of an array of studies about possible actions of Ang-(1-7) on the proximal and distal tubules.

Ang-(1-7) Actions in Proximal Tubule

The first study reporting the effect of Ang-(1-7) on proximal tubule was in 1994 by Garcia *et al.* In isolated rat proximal straight tubule, they observed a biphasic effect of this heptapeptide: concentrations of 10^{-12} M and 10^{-8} M increased and decreased fluid absorption, respectively, and AT1R antagonist blocked both effects. Thus, Ang-(1-7) could have biphasic effect on tubular transport in the proximal nephron [106].

Studies of Ang-(1-7) effect on the proximal nephron continued and were extended to other transporters. Special attention was payed to sodium reabsorption. Thus, Na^+/K^+-ATPase and Na^+-ATPase, two active transporters, placed on the basolateral membrane were the focus of study. In 1996, Handa *et al.* reported that in the proximal tubule Ang-(1-7) can inhibit Na^+/K^+-ATPase , and suggested that the major receptor to translate this inhibition was not either AT1R or AT2R, although the minor receptor to modulate this effect was AT1R [107].

Later, in 1998, study using the whole kidney showed also a biphasic effect of Ang-(1-7) on Na^+/K^+-ATPase activity. Concentrations of 10^{-6} M to 10^{-10} M of Ang-(1-7) decreased between 40 to 70% the activity of pump, while concentration of 10^{-12} M increased in 22% Na^+/K^+-ATPase pump [108]. In disagreement with this study, Caruso-Neves *et al.* 1999 reported that concentrations of 10^{-11} M to 10^{-5} M of Ang-(1-7) did not regulate the Na^+/K^+-ATPase activity present in the kidney cortex and in proximal tubule-basolateral-preparation from pig kidney [109].

In basolateral membrane of proximal tubule, Ang-(1-7) has also affected Na^+-ATPase, whether this peptide affects the Na^+-ATPase in biphasic manner is open field for new studies. Data published showed that Ang-(1-7) stimulates this pump. The highest increase observed, 68%, was observed with 10^{-9} M concentration. AT1R antagonist reverted the observed stimulation [30, 110]. Additionally, De Souza *et al.* reported inhibition of Na^+-ATPase in the range from 10^{-11} M to 10^{-5} M, being the highest inhibition at 10^{-7} M. Only AT2R antagonist completely blocked this inhibition, and not by losartan or A779, AT1R and Ang-(1-7) receptor antagonists, respectively [111, 112].

In the proximal tubule, NH3 is found in the apical membrane, this exchanger is involved in the sodium and bicarbonate reabsorption. In 1994, Garcia *et al.* also reported increased of bicarbonate absorption together with fluid absorption at physiological concentration. Only in 2013, Castelo Branco *et al.* published data showing the direct effect of the heptapeptide on bicarbonate reabsorption. *In vivo* luminal microperfusion of the proximal tubules in rat with Ang-(1-7) decreased and increased bicarbonate reabsorption in 10^{-9} M and 10^{-6} M, respectively. A779, antagonist of Ang-(1-7) receptor, blocked both effects, thus MAS receptor mediates the biphasic effects [113]. Taken together, it is possible to conclude that the Ang-(1-7) may have diuretic and antidiuretic effects depending on the concentration.

Ang-(1-7) Actions in the Distal Tubule

The role of Ang-(1-7) on Na^+/K^+-ATPase in the distal tubule was studied using MDCK cells. Dose-dependent inhibition was observed within the range of 10^{-12} to 10^{-7} M, and the highest inhibitory action was with 10^{-8} M. This inhibition seems to be mediated by AT1R, since and AT1R antagonist blocked this effect [114]. Because the effects in the proximal nephron may be biphasic, further studies are needed in the later segment of the nephron to verify whether Ang-(1-7) behaves in the same manner as in the early nephron.

Ang-(1-7) and Water Balance

At the beginning of the boom of studies regarding to Ang-(1-7), this heptapeptide was reported to cause antidiuresis. Later, studies showed that this heptapeptide could also have diuretic effect. Diuresis was observed after Ang-(1-7) infusion *via* intrarenal artery, and neither AT1R nor AT2R antagonist completely abolished this effect [115]. In the proximal nephron, study from our group using immortalized proximal tubule cells observed downregulation of AQP-1 mRNA and protein at 10^{-7} M concentration [116].

In 2008, Joyner *et al.* using animals in two physiological states, virgins and pregnant rats, observed reduction and increase of urine volume, respectively. Diuresis was associated with increased levels of Ang-(1-7) in the kidney and urine of pregnant rat. The antinatriuretic effect was associated with upregulation of AQP-1 [117].

Ang III Actions in the Kidney

Padia *et al.* suggested that systemic infusion of Ang III in rat previously treated with an antagonist of AT1R, candesartan, could cause natriuresis *via* Ang III binding to AT2R [118]. In fact, AT2R antagonism abolished this increase in sodium excretion [119, 120]. This sodium excretion probably took place in the proximal tubule cell [121]. Further experiments of the same group showed data indicating that rat infused with Ang III that were previously pre-treated with inhibitor of aminopeptidase N, enzyme that cleaves Ang III to Ang IV, increased natriuresis.

Ang IV Actions in the Kidney

Contrasting data indicate that the role of Ang IV in the kidney is unclear. Infusion of Ang IV in renal artery led to an increase in cortical flow in dose-dependent manner. Increased natriuresis was also observed without changing systemic blood pressure, glomerular filtration rate and urine volume. Only a specific antagonist of AT4R was able to block these effects [52, 122].

On the other hand, systemic infusion of Ang IV demonstrated dose-dependent increase of blood pressure and decrease in renal cortical blood flow, effects blocked by AT1R antagonist [123]. Interestingly, Handa observed both effects vasoconstriction and vasodilation caused by Ang IV, the first effect lasted second and the second minutes. When studied the receptor, neither AT4R or AT2R antagonists blocked these effect, only AT1R antagonist reduced both vasoactive responses [124]. Studies using transgenic mice models, AT1a, AT1b, AT2R and IRAP knockout animals demonstrated that the vasoconstriction caused by Ang IV in the wild type was *via* AT1R. This conclusion was based on the lack of vasoconstriction in AT1a and AT2 knockout animals, and in the similar pressor effect of Ang IV in wild type, AT1b and IRAP knockout mice [125].

In this scenario, only one study has related the reported natriuretic effect of Ang IV to direct action on the proximal tubule [126]. Treatment of proximal tubule cells with Ang IV increased Na^+/K^+-ATPase activity and expression, which were not observed with siRNA knockdown of either APN or AT4R [127].

CONCLUSION

The actual understanding of the physiological role of RAS in the kidney is the result of enormous effort in the field. Ang II is a powerful vasoactive peptide, capable of modulating glomerular filtration through alterations in the microvasculature status, mesangial cell contraction, and changes in the cytoskeleton of podocytes. In addition to that, Ang II alters sodium reabsorption in a concentration and transporter-localization manner. In proximal tubules, Ang II activates or inhibits sodium channels, such as NHE-3 and Na^+/HCO_3^- cotransporter, depending on its concentration, *via* AT1R. In thick ascending limbs, Ang II increased expression of total NKCC2 in cortex and decreased in medulla. Water balance is also modulated by Ang II, which is able to stimulate gene and protein expression of AQP1 and its translocation to apical membrane. The sum of all Ang II actions aims to orchestrate glomerular filtration, sodium and water reabsorption, renal hemodynamics and, ultimately, blood pressure.

Ang-(1-7) effect on renal hemodynamics seem not as potent as Ang II, however the direct effect on modulation of sodium transporters water channel in the proximal nephron: NH^{-}_{3}, Na^{+}/HCO^{-}_{3}, Na^{+}/K^{+}-ATPase, Na^{+}-ATPase, and AQP-1 affect the final net result of natriuresis and diuresis. The mechanism that this heptapeptide uses to modulate these transporters is quite a conundrum; some studies showed the heptapeptide effects through AT1R other through AT2R and more recently studies through Mas receptor. Few studies showed Ang-(1-7) on sodium transport of the distal nephron. In the present there is not enough information about Ang-(1-7) action on the other tubules segments. Ang III and Ang IV can cause natriuresis, however little is known about their side of action along the nephron.

CONFLICT OF INTEREST

The authors confirm that they have no conflict of interest to declare for this publication.

ACKNOWLEDGEMENTS

We acknowledge Dr. Roberto Mesquita Soler for designing the Figure.

REFERENCES

[1] Tigerstedt R, Bergman P. Niere und Kreislauf. Skand Arch Physiol 1898; 8: 223-71. [http://dx.doi.org/10.1111/j.1748-1716.1898.tb00272.x]

[2] Kimbrough HM Jr, Vaughan ED Jr, Carey RM, Ayers CR. Effect of intrarenal angiotensin II blockade on renal function in conscious dogs. Circ Res 1977; 40(2): 174-8. [http://dx.doi.org/10.1161/01.RES.40.2.174] [PMID: 191213]

[3] Ng KK, Vane JR. Conversion of angiotensin I to angiotensin II. Nature 1967; 216(5117): 762-6. [http://dx.doi.org/10.1038/216762a0] [PMID: 4294626]

[4] Wasse H, Naqvi N, Husain A. Impact of Mast Cell Chymase on Renal Disease Progression. Curr Hypertens Rev 2012; 8(1): 15-23. [http://dx.doi.org/10.2174/157340212800505007] [PMID: 23503162]

[5] Kramkowski K, Mogielnicki A, Buczko W. The physiological significance of the alternative pathways of angiotensin II production. J Physiol Pharmacol 2006; 57(4): 529-39. [PMID: 17229979]

[6] Kokkonen JO, Saarinen J, Kovanen PT. Angiotensin II formation in the human heart: an ACE or non-ACE-mediated pathway? Ann Med 1998; 30 (Suppl. 1): 9-13. [PMID: 9800878]

[7] Kumar R, Boim MA. Diversity of pathways for intracellular angiotensin II synthesis. Curr Opin Nephrol Hypertens 2009; 18(1): 33-9. [http://dx.doi.org/10.1097/MNH.0b013e32831a9e20] [PMID: 19077687]

[8] Alzayadneh EM, Chappell MC. Nuclear expression of renin-angiotensin system components in NRK-52E renal epithelial cells. J Renin Angiotensin Aldosterone Syst 2014. [PMID: 24961503]

[9] Donoghue M, Hsieh F, Baronas E, *et al.* A novel angiotensin-converting enzyme-related carboxypeptidase (ACE2) converts angiotensin I to angiotensin 1-9. Circ Res 2000; 87(5): E1-9. [http://dx.doi.org/10.1161/01.RES.87.5.e1] [PMID: 10969042]

[10] Tipnis SR, Hooper NM, Hyde R, Karran E, Christie G, Turner AJ. A human homolog of angiotensin-converting enzyme. Cloning and functional expression as a captopril-insensitive carboxypeptidase. J Biol Chem 2000; 275(43): 33238-43. [http://dx.doi.org/10.1074/jbc.M002615200] [PMID: 10924499]

[11] Ardaillou R. Active fragments of angiotensin II: enzymatic pathways of synthesis and biological effects. Curr Opin Nephrol Hypertens 1997; 6(1): 28-34. [http://dx.doi.org/10.1097/00041552-199701000-00006] [PMID: 9051351]

[12] de Gasparo M. New basic science initiatives with the angiotensin II receptor blocker valsartan. J Renin Angiotensin Aldosterone Syst 2000; 1(2) (Suppl.): S3-5. [http://dx.doi.org/10.3317/jraas.2000.052] [PMID: 17199210]

[13] de Gasparo M, Catt KJ, Inagami T, Wright JW, Unger T. International union of pharmacology. XXIII. The angiotensin II receptors. Pharmacol Rev 2000; 52(3): 415-72. [PMID: 10977869]

[14] Teerlink JR. Neurohumoral mechanisms in heart failure: a central role for the renin-angiotensin system. J Cardiovasc Pharmacol 1996; 27 (Suppl. 2): S1-8. [http://dx.doi.org/10.1097/00005344-199600002-00002] [PMID: 8723392]

[15] Humphrey PP, Barnard EA. International Union of Pharmacology. XIX. The IUPHAR receptor code: a proposal for an alphanumeric classification system. Pharmacol Rev 1998; 50(2): 271-7. [PMID: 9647868]

[16] Karnik SS, Unal H, Kemp JR, *et al.* International Union of Basic and Clinical Pharmacology. XCIX. Angiotensin Receptors: Interpreters of Pathophysiological Angiotensinergic Stimuli [corrected]. Pharmacol Rev 2015; 67(4): 754-819. [http://dx.doi.org/10.1124/pr.114.010454] [PMID: 26315714]

[17] Nguyen G. Renin/prorenin receptors. Kidney Int 2006; 69(9): 1503-6. [http://dx.doi.org/10.1038/sj.ki.5000265] [PMID: 16672920]

[18] Schefe JH, Menk M, Reinemund J, *et al.* A novel signal transduction cascade involving direct physical interaction of the renin/prorenin receptor with the transcription factor promyelocytic zinc finger protein. Circ Res 2006; 99(12): 1355-66. [http://dx.doi.org/10.1161/01.RES.0000251700.00994.0d] [PMID: 17082479]

[19] Deen WM, Lazzara MJ, Myers BD. Structural determinants of glomerular permeability. Am J Physiol Renal Physiol 2001; 281(4): F579-96.

[PMID: 11553505]

[20] Neal CR, Muston PR, Njegovan D, *et al.* Glomerular filtration into the subpodocyte space is highly restricted under physiological perfusion conditions. Am J Physiol Renal Physiol 2007; 293(6): F1787-98.
[http://dx.doi.org/10.1152/ajprenal.00157.2007] [PMID: 17715264]

[21] Li XC, Zhuo JL. Proximal tubule-dominant transfer of AT(1a) receptors induces blood pressure responses to intracellular angiotensin II in AT(1a) receptor-deficient mice. Am J Physiol Regul Integr Comp Physiol 2013; 304(8): R588-98.
[http://dx.doi.org/10.1152/ajpregu.00338.2012] [PMID: 23427083]

[22] Hall G. Tratado de Fisiologia Médica. In: Editora E, Ed.

[23] Houillier P, Chambrey R, Achard JM, Froissart M, Poggioli J, Paillard M. Signaling pathways in the biphasic effect of angiotensin II on apical Na/H antiport activity in proximal tubule. Kidney Int 1996; 50(5): 1496-505.
[http://dx.doi.org/10.1038/ki.1996.464] [PMID: 8914015]

[24] Verkman AS, Shi LB, Frigeri A, *et al.* Structure and function of kidney water channels. Kidney Int 1995; 48(4): 1069-81.
[http://dx.doi.org/10.1038/ki.1995.390] [PMID: 8569068]

[25] Umenishi F, Schrier RW. Hypertonicity-induced aquaporin-1 (AQP1) expression is mediated by the activation of MAPK pathways and hypertonicity-responsive element in the AQP1 gene. J Biol Chem 2003; 278(18): 15765-70.
[http://dx.doi.org/10.1074/jbc.M209980200] [PMID: 12600999]

[26] Nielsen S, Frøkiaer J, Marples D, Kwon TH, Agre P, Knepper MA. Aquaporins in the kidney: from molecules to medicine. Physiol Rev 2002; 82(1): 205-44.
[http://dx.doi.org/10.1152/physrev.00024.2001] [PMID: 11773613]

[27] Clapp WL, Bowman P, Shaw GS, Patel P, Kone BC. Segmental localization of mRNAs encoding Na(+)-K(+)-ATPase alpha- and beta-subunit isoforms in rat kidney using RT-PCR. Kidney Int 1994; 46(3): 627-38.
[http://dx.doi.org/10.1038/ki.1994.315] [PMID: 7996786]

[28] Féraille E, Doucet A. Sodium-potassium-adenosinetriphosphatase-dependent sodium transport in the kidney: hormonal control. Physiol Rev 2001; 81(1): 345-418.
[PMID: 11152761]

[29] Horita S, Zheng Y, Hara C, *et al.* Biphasic regulation of Na+-HCO3- cotransporter by angiotensin II type 1A receptor. Hypertension 2002; 40(5): 707-12.
[http://dx.doi.org/10.1161/01.HYP.0000036449.70110.DE] [PMID: 12411466]

[30] Caruso-Neves C, Lara LS, Rangel LB, Grossi AL, Lopes AG. Angiotensin-(1-7) modulates the ouabain-insensitive Na+-ATPase activity from basolateral membrane of the proximal tubule. Biochim Biophys Acta 2000; 1467(1): 189-97.
[http://dx.doi.org/10.1016/S0005-2736(00)00219-4] [PMID: 10930521]

[31] Maunsbach AB, Marples D, Chin E, *et al.* Aquaporin-1 water channel expression in human kidney. J Am Soc Nephrol 1997; 8(1): 1-14.

[PMID: 9013443]

[32] Sohara E, Rai T, Miyazaki J, Verkman AS, Sasaki S, Uchida S. Defective water and glycerol transport in the proximal tubules of AQP7 knockout mice. Am J Physiol Renal Physiol 2005; 289(6): F1195-200.
[http://dx.doi.org/10.1152/ajprenal.00133.2005] [PMID: 15998844]

[33] Ingelfinger JR, Zuo WM, Fon EA, Ellison KE, Dzau VJ. *In situ* hybridization evidence for angiotensinogen messenger RNA in the rat proximal tubule. An hypothesis for the intrarenal renin angiotensin system. J Clin Invest 1990; 85(2): 417-23.
[http://dx.doi.org/10.1172/JCI114454] [PMID: 2298917]

[34] Navar LG, Prieto MC, Satou R, Kobori H. Intrarenal angiotensin II and its contribution to the genesis of chronic hypertension. Curr Opin Pharmacol 2011; 11(2): 180-6.
[http://dx.doi.org/10.1016/j.coph.2011.01.009] [PMID: 21339086]

[35] Nishiyama A, Seth DM, Navar LG. Renal interstitial fluid concentrations of angiotensins I and II in anesthetized rats. Hypertension 2002; 39(1): 129-34.
[http://dx.doi.org/10.1161/hy0102.100536] [PMID: 11799091]

[36] Casarini DE, Boim MA, Stella RC, Krieger-Azzolini MH, Krieger JE, Schor N. Angiotensin I-converting enzyme activity in tubular fluid along the rat nephron. Am J Physiol 1997; 272(3 Pt 2): F405-9.
[PMID: 9087685]

[37] Ye M, Wysocki J, William J, Soler MJ, Cokic I, Batlle D. Glomerular localization and expression of Angiotensin-converting enzyme 2 and Angiotensin-converting enzyme: implications for albuminuria in diabetes. J Am Soc Nephrol 2006; 17(11): 3067-75.
[http://dx.doi.org/10.1681/ASN.2006050423] [PMID: 17021266]

[38] Velez JC, Bland AM, Arthur JM, Raymond JR, Janech MG. Characterization of renin-angiotensin system enzyme activities in cultured mouse podocytes. Am J Physiol Renal Physiol 2007; 293(1): F398-407.
[http://dx.doi.org/10.1152/ajprenal.00050.2007] [PMID: 17429035]

[39] Navar LG, Imig JD, Zou L, Wang CT. Intrarenal production of angiotensin II. Semin Nephrol 1997; 17(5): 412-22.
[PMID: 9316209]

[40] Brosnihan KB, Neves LA, Joyner J, *et al.* Enhanced renal immunocytochemical expression of ANG-(1-7) and ACE2 during pregnancy. Hypertension 2003; 42(4): 749-53.
[http://dx.doi.org/10.1161/01.HYP.0000085220.53285.11] [PMID: 12874086]

[41] Li N, Zimpelmann J, Cheng K, Wilkins JA, Burns KD. The role of angiotensin converting enzyme 2 in the generation of angiotensin 1-7 by rat proximal tubules. Am J Physiol Renal Physiol 2005; 288(2): F353-62.
[http://dx.doi.org/10.1152/ajprenal.00144.2004] [PMID: 15467007]

[42] Ferrario CM, Martell N, Yunis C, *et al.* Characterization of angiotensin-(1-7) in the urine of normal and essential hypertensive subjects. Am J Hypertens 1998; 11(2): 137-46.
[http://dx.doi.org/10.1016/S0895-7061(97)00400-7] [PMID: 9524041]

[43] Hus-Citharel A, Gasc JM, Zini S, *et al.* Aminopeptidase A activity and angiotensin III effects on [Ca2+]i along the rat nephron. Kidney Int 1999; 56(3): 850-9. [http://dx.doi.org/10.1046/j.1523-1755.1999.00634.x] [PMID: 10469354]

[44] Ward PE, Erdös EG, Gedney CD, Dowben RM, Reynolds RC. Isolation of membrane-bound renal enzymes that metabolize kinins and angiotensins. Biochem J 1976; 157(3): 643-50. [http://dx.doi.org/10.1042/bj1570643] [PMID: 186028]

[45] Ward PE, Sheridan MS. Converting enzyme, kininase and angiotensinase of renal and intestinal brush border 1983.

[46] Schießl IM, Castrop H. Angiotensin II AT2 receptor activation attenuates AT1 receptor-induced increases in the glomerular filtration of albumin: a multiphoton microscopy study. Am J Physiol Renal Physiol 2013; 305(8): F1189-200. [http://dx.doi.org/10.1152/ajprenal.00377.2013] [PMID: 23946289]

[47] Carey RM, Howell NL, Jin XH, Siragy HM. Angiotensin type 2 receptor-mediated hypotension in angiotensin type-1 receptor-blocked rats. Hypertension 2001; 38(6): 1272-7. [http://dx.doi.org/10.1161/hy1201.096576] [PMID: 11751702]

[48] Li XC, Widdop RE. AT2 receptor-mediated vasodilatation is unmasked by AT1 receptor blockade in conscious SHR. Br J Pharmacol 2004; 142(5): 821-30. [http://dx.doi.org/10.1038/sj.bjp.0705838] [PMID: 15197103]

[49] Singh RR, Lankadeva YR, Denton KM, Moritz KM. Improvement in renal hemodynamics following combined angiotensin II infusion and AT1R blockade in aged female sheep following fetal unilateral nephrectomy. PLoS One 2013; 8(7): e68036. [http://dx.doi.org/10.1371/journal.pone.0068036] [PMID: 23840884]

[50] Yang J, Chen C, Ren H, *et al.* Angiotensin II AT(2) receptor decreases AT(1) receptor expression and function *via* nitric oxide/cGMP/Sp1 in renal proximal tubule cells from Wistar-Kyoto rats. J Hypertens 2012; 30(6): 1176-84. [http://dx.doi.org/10.1097/HJH.0b013e3283532099] [PMID: 22504846]

[51] Wright JW, Krebs LT, Stobb JW, Harding JW. The angiotensin IV system: functional implications. Front Neuroendocrinol 1995; 16(1): 23-52. [http://dx.doi.org/10.1006/frne.1995.1002] [PMID: 7768321]

[52] Coleman JK, Krebs LT, Hamilton TA, *et al.* Autoradiographic identification of kidney angiotensin IV binding sites and angiotensin IV-induced renal cortical blood flow changes in rats. Peptides 1998; 19(2): 269-77. [http://dx.doi.org/10.1016/S0196-9781(97)00291-X] [PMID: 9493859]

[53] Santos RA, Haibara AS, Campagnole-Santos MJ, *et al.* Characterization of a new selective antagonist for angiotensin-(1-7), D-pro7-angiotensin-(1-7). Hypertension 2003; 41(3 Pt 2): 737-43. [http://dx.doi.org/10.1161/01.HYP.0000052947.60363.24] [PMID: 12623989]

[54] Pinheiro SV, Simões e Silva AC, Sampaio WO, *et al.* Nonpeptide AVE 0991 is an angiotensin-(1-7) receptor Mas agonist in the mouse kidney. Hypertension 2004; 44(4): 490-6. [http://dx.doi.org/10.1161/01.HYP.0000141438.64887.42] [PMID: 15326087]

[55] Shalamanova L, Wilkinson MC, McArdle F, Jackson MJ, Rustom R. Characterisation of the

expression of the Renin-Angiotensin system in primary and immortalised human renal proximal tubular cells. Nephron, Exp Nephrol 2010; 116(3): e53-61.
[http://dx.doi.org/10.1159/000318176] [PMID: 20616569]

[56] Gonzalez AA, Prieto MC. Renin and the (pro)renin receptor in the renal collecting duct: Role in the pathogenesis of hypertension. Clin Exp Pharmacol Physiol 2015; 42(1): 14-21.
[http://dx.doi.org/10.1111/1440-1681.12319] [PMID: 25371190]

[57] Advani A, Kelly DJ, Cox AJ, *et al.* The (Pro)renin receptor: site-specific and functional linkage to the vacuolar H+-ATPase in the kidney. Hypertension 2009; 54(2): 261-9.
[http://dx.doi.org/10.1161/HYPERTENSIONAHA.109.128645] [PMID: 19546380]

[58] Crowley SD, Gurley SB, Herrera MJ, *et al.* Angiotensin II causes hypertension and cardiac hypertrophy through its receptors in the kidney. Proc Natl Acad Sci USA 2006; 103(47): 17985-90.
[http://dx.doi.org/10.1073/pnas.0605545103] [PMID: 17090678]

[59] Crowley SD, Zhang J, Herrera M, Griffiths R, Ruiz P, Coffman TM. Role of AT□ receptor-mediated salt retention in angiotensin II-dependent hypertension. Am J Physiol Renal Physiol 2011; 301(5): F1124-30.
[http://dx.doi.org/10.1152/ajprenal.00305.2011] [PMID: 21849491]

[60] Yamamoto T, Hayashi K, Matsuda H, *et al.* *In vivo* visualization of angiotensin II- and tubuloglomerular feedback-mediated renal vasoconstriction. Kidney Int 2001; 60(1): 364-9.
[http://dx.doi.org/10.1046/j.1523-1755.2001.00808.x] [PMID: 11422773]

[61] Hsu HH, Hoffmann S, Endlich N, *et al.* Mechanisms of angiotensin II signaling on cytoskeleton of podocytes. J Mol Med 2008; 86(12): 1379-94.
[http://dx.doi.org/10.1007/s00109-008-0399-y] [PMID: 18773185]

[62] Saleem MA, Zavadil J, Bailly M, *et al.* The molecular and functional phenotype of glomerular podocytes reveals key features of contractile smooth muscle cells. Am J Physiol Renal Physiol 2008; 295(4): F959-70.
[http://dx.doi.org/10.1152/ajprenal.00559.2007] [PMID: 18684887]

[63] Axelsson J, Rippe A, Oberg CM, Rippe B. Rapid, dynamic changes in glomerular permeability to macromolecules during systemic angiotensin II (ANG II) infusion in rats. Am J Physiol Renal Physiol 2012; 303(6): F790-9.
[http://dx.doi.org/10.1152/ajprenal.00153.2012] [PMID: 22718887]

[64] Suzuki K, Han GD, Miyauchi N, *et al.* Angiotensin II type 1 and type 2 receptors play opposite roles in regulating the barrier function of kidney glomerular capillary wall. Am J Pathol 2007; 170(6): 1841-53.
[http://dx.doi.org/10.2353/ajpath.2007.060484] [PMID: 17525253]

[65] Navar LG. Tuma RF, Duran WN, Ley K. The renal microcirculation. Handbook of physiology: microcirculation. 2nd ed. Academic Press 2008; pp. 550-683.
[http://dx.doi.org/10.1016/B978-0-12-374530-9.00015-2]

[66] Persson AE, Lai EY, Gao X, Carlström M, Patzak A. Interactions between adenosine, angiotensin II and nitric oxide on the afferent arteriole influence sensitivity of the tubuloglomerular feedback. Front Physiol 2013; 4: 187.
[http://dx.doi.org/10.3389/fphys.2013.00187] [PMID: 23882224]

[67] Davisson RL, Ding Y, Stec DE, Catterall JF, Sigmund CD. Novel mechanism of hypertension revealed by cell-specific targeting of human angiotensinogen in transgenic mice. Physiol Genomics 1999; 1(1): 3-9.
[PMID: 11015555]

[68] Gurley SB, Riquier-Brison AD, Schnermann J, *et al.* AT1A angiotensin receptors in the renal proximal tubule regulate blood pressure. Cell Metab 2011; 13(4): 469-75.
[http://dx.doi.org/10.1016/j.cmet.2011.03.001] [PMID: 21459331]

[69] Boron WF. Acid-base transport by the renal proximal tubule. J Am Soc Nephrol 2006; 17(9): 2368-82.
[http://dx.doi.org/10.1681/ASN.2006060620] [PMID: 16914536]

[70] Haithcock D, Jiao H, Cui XL, Hopfer U, Douglas JG. Renal proximal tubular AT2 receptor: signaling and transport. J Am Soc Nephrol 1999; 10 (Suppl. 11): S69-74.
[PMID: 9892143]

[71] Haque MZ, Ares GR, Caceres PS, Ortiz PA. High salt differentially regulates surface NKCC2 expression in thick ascending limbs of Dahl salt-sensitive and salt-resistant rats. Am J Physiol Renal Physiol 2011; 300(5): F1096-104.
[http://dx.doi.org/10.1152/ajprenal.00600.2010] [PMID: 21307126]

[72] Good DW, Caflisch CR, George T. Prostaglandin E2 regulation of ion transport is absent in medullary thick ascending limbs from SHR. Am J Physiol 1995; 269(1 Pt 2): F47-54.
[PMID: 7631831]

[73] O'Connor PM, Lu L, Liang M, Cowley AW Jr. A novel amiloride-sensitive h+ transport pathway mediates enhanced superoxide production in thick ascending limb of salt-sensitive rats, not na+/h+ exchange. Hypertension 2009; 54(2): 248-54.
[http://dx.doi.org/10.1161/HYPERTENSIONAHA.109.134692] [PMID: 19564541]

[74] Gonzalez-Villalobos RA, Janjoulia T, Fletcher NK, *et al.* The absence of intrarenal ACE protects against hypertension. J Clin Invest 2013; 123(5): 2011-23.
[http://dx.doi.org/10.1172/JCI65460] [PMID: 23619363]

[75] Nguyen MT, Lee DH, Delpire E, McDonough AA. Differential regulation of Na+ transporters along nephron during ANG II-dependent hypertension: distal stimulation counteracted by proximal inhibition. Am J Physiol Renal Physiol 2013; 305(4): F510-9.
[http://dx.doi.org/10.1152/ajprenal.00183.2013] [PMID: 23720346]

[76] Castrop H, Schnermann J. Isoforms of renal Na-K-2Cl cotransporter NKCC2: expression and functional significance. Am J Physiol Renal Physiol 2008; 295(4): F859-66.
[http://dx.doi.org/10.1152/ajprenal.00106.2008] [PMID: 18495801]

[77] Hong NJ, Garvin JL. Angiotensin II type 2 receptor-mediated inhibition of NaCl absorption is blunted in thick ascending limbs from Dahl salt-sensitive rats. Hypertension 2012; 60(3): 765-9.
[http://dx.doi.org/10.1161/HYPERTENSIONAHA.112.199216] [PMID: 22777935]

[78] Wang T, Giebisch G. Effects of angiotensin II on electrolyte transport in the early and late distal tubule in rat kidney. Am J Physiol 1996; 271(1 Pt 2): F143-9.
[PMID: 8760255]

[79] Sandberg MB, Riquier AD, Pihakaski-Maunsbach K, McDonough AA, Maunsbach AB. ANG II

provokes acute trafficking of distal tubule Na+-Cl(-) cotransporter to apical membrane. Am J Physiol Renal Physiol 2007; 293(3): F662-9. [http://dx.doi.org/10.1152/ajprenal.00064.2007] [PMID: 17507603]

[80] Talati G, Ohta A, Rai T, *et al.* Effect of angiotensin II on the WNK-OSR1/SPAK-NCC phosphorylation cascade in cultured mpkDCT cells and *in vivo* mouse kidney. Biochem Biophys Res Commun 2010; 393(4): 844-8. [http://dx.doi.org/10.1016/j.bbrc.2010.02.096] [PMID: 20175999]

[81] van der Lubbe N, Lim CH, Fenton RA, *et al.* Angiotensin II induces phosphorylation of the thiazide-sensitive sodium chloride cotransporter independent of aldosterone. Kidney Int 2011; 79(1): 66-76. [http://dx.doi.org/10.1038/ki.2010.290] [PMID: 20720527]

[82] Peti-Peterdi J, Warnock DG, Bell PD. Angiotensin II directly stimulates ENaC activity in the cortical collecting duct *via* AT(1) receptors. J Am Soc Nephrol 2002; 13(5): 1131-5. [http://dx.doi.org/10.1097/01.ASN.0000013292.78621.FD] [PMID: 11960999]

[83] Beutler KT, Masilamani S, Turban S, *et al.* Long-term regulation of ENaC expression in kidney by angiotensin II. Hypertension 2003; 41(5): 1143-50. [http://dx.doi.org/10.1161/01.HYP.0000066129.12106.E2] [PMID: 12682079]

[84] Ohsawa M, Tamura K, Wakui H, *et al.* Deletion of the angiotensin II type 1 receptor-associated protein enhances renal sodium reabsorption and exacerbates angiotensin II-mediated hypertension. Kidney Int 2014; 86(3): 570-81. [http://dx.doi.org/10.1038/ki.2014.95] [PMID: 24694992]

[85] Oliverio MI, Delnomdedieu M, Best CF, *et al.* Abnormal water metabolism in mice lacking the type 1A receptor for ANG II. Am J Physiol Renal Physiol 2000; 278(1): F75-82. [PMID: 10644657]

[86] Kato A, Klein JD, Zhang C, Sands JM. Angiotensin II increases vasopressin-stimulated facilitated urea permeability in rat terminal IMCDs. Am J Physiol Renal Physiol 2000; 279(5): F835-40. [PMID: 11053043]

[87] Nielsen S, Smith BL, Christensen EI, Knepper MA, Agre P. CHIP28 water channels are localized in constitutively water-permeable segments of the nephron. J Cell Biol 1993; 120(2): 371-83. [http://dx.doi.org/10.1083/jcb.120.2.371] [PMID: 7678419]

[88] Fushimi K, Uchida S, Hara Y, Hirata Y, Marumo F, Sasaki S. Cloning and expression of apical membrane water channel of rat kidney collecting tubule. Nature 1993; 361(6412): 549-52. [http://dx.doi.org/10.1038/361549a0] [PMID: 8429910]

[89] Ecelbarger CA, Terris J, Frindt G, *et al.* Aquaporin-3 water channel localization and regulation in rat kidney. Am J Physiol 1995; 269(5 Pt 2): F663-72. [PMID: 7503232]

[90] Terris J, Ecelbarger CA, Marples D, Knepper MA, Nielsen S. Distribution of aquaporin-4 water channel expression within rat kidney. Am J Physiol 1995; 269(6 Pt 2): F775-85. [PMID: 8594871]

[91] Nielsen S, Chou CL, Marples D, Christensen EI, Kishore BK, Knepper MA. Vasopressin increases water permeability of kidney collecting duct by inducing translocation of aquaporin-CD water

channels to plasma membrane. Proceedings of the National Academy of Sciences of the United States of America. 1013-7.
[http://dx.doi.org/10.1073/pnas.92.4.1013]

[92] Yamamoto T, Sasaki S, Fushimi K, *et al.* Vasopressin increases AQP-CD water channel in apical membrane of collecting duct cells in Brattleboro rats. Am J Physiol 1995; 268(6 Pt 1): C1546-51.
[PMID: 7541941]

[93] Loonen AJ, Knoers NV, van Os CH, Deen PM. Aquaporin 2 mutations in nephrogenic diabetes insipidus. Semin Nephrol 2008; 28(3): 252-65.
[http://dx.doi.org/10.1016/j.semnephrol.2008.03.006] [PMID: 18519086]

[94] Rojek A, Füchtbauer EM, Kwon TH, Frøkiaer J, Nielsen S. Severe urinary concentrating defect in renal collecting duct-selective AQP2 conditional-knockout mice. Proc Natl Acad Sci USA 2006; 103(15): 6037-42.
[http://dx.doi.org/10.1073/pnas.0511324103] [PMID: 16581908]

[95] Schnermann J, Chou CL, Ma T, Traynor T, Knepper MA, Verkman AS. Defective proximal tubular fluid reabsorption in transgenic aquaporin-1 null mice. Proceedings of the National Academy of Sciences of the United States of America. 9660-4.
[http://dx.doi.org/10.1073/pnas.95.16.9660]

[96] Yang B, Ma T, Dong JY, Verkman AS. Partial correction of the urinary concentrating defect in aquaporin-1 null mice by adenovirus-mediated gene delivery. Hum Gene Ther 2000; 11(4): 567-75.
[http://dx.doi.org/10.1089/10430340050015752] [PMID: 10724035]

[97] Wintour EM, Earnest L, Alcorn D, Butkus A, Shandley L, Jeyaseelan K. Ovine AQP1: cDNA cloning, ontogeny, and control of renal gene expression. Pediatr Nephrol 1998; 12(7): 545-53.
[http://dx.doi.org/10.1007/s004670050502] [PMID: 9761352]

[98] Imai H, Nakamoto H, Ishida Y, *et al.* Renin-angiotensin system plays an important role in the regulation of water transport in the peritoneum. Adv Perit Dial 2001; 17: 20-4.
[PMID: 11510275]

[99] Bouley R, Palomino Z, Tang SS, *et al.* Angiotensin II and hypertonicity modulate proximal tubular aquaporin 1 expression. Am J Physiol Renal Physiol 2009; 297(6): F1575-86.
[http://dx.doi.org/10.1152/ajprenal.90762.2008] [PMID: 19776169]

[100] Klingler C, Ancellin N, Barrault MB, Morel A, Corman B. Potentiation of receptor-mediated cAMP production: role in the cross-talk between vasopressin V1a and V2 receptor transduction pathways. Biochem J 1998; 330(Pt 2): 1023-8.
[http://dx.doi.org/10.1042/bj3301023] [PMID: 9480925]

[101] Kwon TH, Nielsen J, Knepper MA, Frøkiaer J, Nielsen S. Angiotensin II AT1 receptor blockade decreases vasopressin-induced water reabsorption and AQP2 levels in NaCl-restricted rats. Am J Physiol Renal Physiol 2005; 288(4): F673-84.
[http://dx.doi.org/10.1152/ajprenal.00304.2004] [PMID: 15585668]

[102] Wang W, Li C, Summer S, Falk S, Schrier RW. Interaction between vasopressin and angiotensin II *in vivo* and *in vitro*: effect on aquaporins and urine concentration. Am J Physiol Renal Physiol 2010; 299(3): F577-84.
[http://dx.doi.org/10.1152/ajprenal.00168.2010] [PMID: 20576679]

[103] Stegbauer J, Gurley SB, Sparks MA, *et al.* AT1 receptors in the collecting duct directly modulate the concentration of urine. J Am Soc Nephrol 2011; 22(12): 2237-46.
[http://dx.doi.org/10.1681/ASN.2010101095] [PMID: 22052052]

[104] Santos RA, Baracho NC. Angiotensin-(1-7) is a potent antidiuretic peptide in rats. Braz J Med Biol Res 1992; 25(6): 651-4.
[PMID: 1342241]

[105] DelliPizzi AM, Hilchey SD, Bell-Quilley CP. Natriuretic action of angiotensin(1-7). Br J Pharmacol 1994; 111(1): 1-3.
[http://dx.doi.org/10.1111/j.1476-5381.1994.tb14014.x] [PMID: 8012686]

[106] Garcia NH, Garvin JL. Angiotensin 1-7 has a biphasic effect on fluid absorption in the proximal straight tubule. J Am Soc Nephrol 1994; 5(4): 1133-8.
[PMID: 7849254]

[107] Handa RK, Ferrario CM, Strandhoy JW. Renal actions of angiotensin-(1-7): *in vivo* and *in vitro* studies. Am J Physiol 1996; 270(1 Pt 2): F141-7.
[PMID: 8769832]

[108] López Ordieres MG, Gironacci M, Rodríguez de Lores Arnaiz G, Peña C. Effect of angiotensin-(1-7) on ATPase activities in several tissues. Regul Pept 1998; 77(1-3): 135-9.
[http://dx.doi.org/10.1016/S0167-0115(98)00113-X] [PMID: 9809807]

[109] Caruso-Neves C, Siqueira AS, Iso-Cohen G, Lopes AG. Bradykinin modulates the ouabain-insensitive Na+-ATPase activity from basolateral membrane of the proximal tubule. Biochim Biophys Acta 1999; 1431(2): 483-91.
[http://dx.doi.org/10.1016/S0167-4838(99)00080-1] [PMID: 10350623]

[110] Lara LS, Correa JS, Lavelle AB, Lopes AG, Caruso-Neves C. The angiotensin receptor type 1-Gq protein-phosphatidyl inositol phospholipase Cbeta-protein kinase C pathway is involved in activation of proximal tubule Na+-ATPase activity by angiotensin(1-7) in pig kidneys. Exp Physiol 2008; 93(5): 639-47.
[http://dx.doi.org/10.1113/expphysiol.2007.040584] [PMID: 18245203]

[111] De Souza AM, Lopes AG, Pizzino CP, *et al.* Angiotensin II and angiotensin-(1-7) inhibit the inner cortex Na+ -ATPase activity through AT2 receptor. Regul Pept 2004; 120(1-3): 167-75.
[http://dx.doi.org/10.1016/j.regpep.2004.03.005] [PMID: 15177935]

[112] Lara LdaS, Cavalcante F, Axelband F, De Souza AM, Lopes AG, Caruso-Neves C. Involvement of the Gi/o/cGMP/PKG pathway in the AT2-mediated inhibition of outer cortex proximal tubule Na+-ATPase by Ang-(1-7). Biochem J 2006; 395(1): 183-90.
[http://dx.doi.org/10.1042/BJ20051455] [PMID: 16390332]

[113] Castelo-Branco RC, Leite-Delova DC, de Mello-Aires M. Dose-dependent effects of angiotensin-(1-7) on the NHE3 exchanger and [Ca(2+)](i) in *in vivo* proximal tubules. Am J Physiol Renal Physiol 2013; 304(10): F1258-65.
[http://dx.doi.org/10.1152/ajprenal.00401.2012] [PMID: 23515716]

[114] Lara LS, De Carvalho T, Leão-Ferreira LR, Lopes AG, Caruso-Neves C. Modulation of the (Na(+)+K+)ATPase activity by Angiotensin-(1-7) in MDCK cells. Regul Pept 2005; 129(1-3): 221-6.

[http://dx.doi.org/10.1016/j.regpep.2005.02.014] [PMID: 15927719]

[115] Heller J, Kramer HJ, Malý J, Cervenka L, Horácek V. Effect of intrarenal infusion of angiotensin-(1-7) in the dog. Kidney Blood Press Res 2000; 23(2): 89-94.
[http://dx.doi.org/10.1159/000025959] [PMID: 10765110]

[116] Zaira PJ, Elena CD, Flavia JF. Angiotensin (1-7) donwregulation of AQP-1 in rat proximal cell is mediated by ACE and ACE2 balance Experimental Biology (EB) Meeting. New Orleans -USA 2009.

[117] Joyner J, Neves LA, Stovall K, Ferrario CM, Brosnihan KB. Angiotensin-(1-7) serves as an aquaretic by increasing water intake and diuresis in association with downregulation of aquaporin-1 during pregnancy in rats. Am J Physiol Regul Integr Comp Physiol 2008; 294(3): R1073-80.
[http://dx.doi.org/10.1152/ajpregu.00572.2007] [PMID: 18184763]

[118] Padia SH, Howell NL, Siragy HM, Carey RM. Renal angiotensin type 2 receptors mediate natriuresis *via* angiotensin III in the angiotensin II type 1 receptor-blocked rat. Hypertension 2006; 47(3): 537-44.
[http://dx.doi.org/10.1161/01.HYP.0000196950.48596.21] [PMID: 16380540]

[119] Padia SH, Kemp BA, Howell NL, *et al.* Intrarenal aminopeptidase N inhibition augments natriuretic responses to angiotensin III in angiotensin type 1 receptor-blocked rats. Hypertension 2007; 49(3): 625-30.
[http://dx.doi.org/10.1161/01.HYP.0000254833.85106.4d] [PMID: 17190872]

[120] Padia SH, Kemp BA, Howell NL, Fournie-Zaluski MC, Roques BP, Carey RM. Conversion of renal angiotensin II to angiotensin III is critical for AT2 receptor-mediated natriuresis in rats. Hypertension 2008; 51(2): 460-5.
[http://dx.doi.org/10.1161/HYPERTENSIONAHA.107.103242] [PMID: 18158338]

[121] Kemp BA, Bell JF, Rottkamp DM, *et al.* Intrarenal angiotensin III is the predominant agonist for proximal tubule angiotensin type 2 receptors. Hypertension 2012; 60(2): 387-95.
[http://dx.doi.org/10.1161/HYPERTENSIONAHA.112.191403] [PMID: 22689743]

[122] Hamilton TA, Handa RK, Harding JW, Wright JW. A role for the angiotensin IV/AT4 system in mediating natriuresis in the rat. Peptides 2001; 22(6): 935-44.
[http://dx.doi.org/10.1016/S0196-9781(01)00405-3] [PMID: 11390024]

[123] Li XC, Campbell DJ, Ohishi M, Yuan S, Zhuo JL. AT1 receptor-activated signaling mediates angiotensin IV-induced renal cortical vasoconstriction in rats. Am J Physiol Renal Physiol 2006; 290(5): F1024-33.
[http://dx.doi.org/10.1152/ajprenal.00221.2005] [PMID: 16380463]

[124] Handa RK. Biphasic actions of angiotensin IV on renal blood flow in the rat. Regul Pept 2006; 136(1-3): 23-9.
[http://dx.doi.org/10.1016/j.regpep.2006.04.008] [PMID: 16780972]

[125] Yang R, Walther T, Gembardt F, *et al.* Renal vasoconstrictor and pressor responses to angiotensin IV in mice are AT1a-receptor mediated. J Hypertens 2010; 28(3): 487-94.
[http://dx.doi.org/10.1097/HJH.0b013e3283343250] [PMID: 19907343]

[126] Chai SY, Fernando R, Peck G, *et al.* The angiotensin IV/AT4 receptor. Cell Mol Life Sci 2004; 61(21): 2728-37.
[http://dx.doi.org/10.1007/s00018-004-4246-1] [PMID: 15549174]

[127] Kotlo K, Shukla S, Tawar U, Skidgel RA, Danziger RS. Aminopeptidase N reduces basolateral Na+ -K+ -ATPase in proximal tubule cells. Am J Physiol Renal Physiol 2007; 293(4): F1047-53. [http://dx.doi.org/10.1152/ajprenal.00074.2007] [PMID: 17634404]

CHAPTER 7

Renin-Angiotensin System Along the Nephron and its Role in Hypertension

Alexis A. Gonzalez[1,2], **L. Gabriel Navar**[2,3] and **Minolfa C. Prieto**[2,3,*]

[1] *Instituto de Química, Pontificia Universidad Católica de Valparaíso, Chile*

[2] *Department of Physiology Tulane University, School of Medicine, New Orleans, LA, 70112, USA*

[3] *Tulane Hypertension and Renal Center, Tulane University, School of Medicine, New Orleans, LA, 70112, USA*

Abstract: There is increasing evidence regarding the pivotal role of the intrarenal renin angiotensin system (RAS) in the pathogenesis of hypertension and its independent role in the regulation of interstitial and intratubular fluids. The presence of high intrarenal angiotensin II (Ang II) levels and the localization of Ang II type 1 receptor (AT1R) in proximal and distal nephron segments suggested a physiological role for this receptor. In the collecting duct, luminal AT1R activation directly stimulates the activity of epithelial sodium channel (ENaC), contributing to enhance sodium reabsorption. Several reports have demonstrated the expression of angiotensinogen (AGT) and prorenin/renin in proximal tubules and collecting ducts, respectively. Both, tubular AGT and prorenin/renin are upregulated during Ang II-dependent hypertension despite the suppression of renin in juxtaglomerular cells. The (pro)renin receptor (PRR) is a new member of the RAS. PRR by binding renin or prorenin, enhances renin activity and activates the non active enzyme prorenin. The PRR and its soluble form are increased in the renal tissue and urine of Ang II hypertensive rats; however, the contribution of PRR to enhance renin activity in the distal nephron remains unclear. The presence of angiotensin converting enzyme (ACE), the enzyme that converts Ang I into Ang II in the nephron, along with the augmentation of intratubular AGT, renin and PRR may contribute to additional production of Ang II in the tubular lumen, which enhances sodium reabsorption and high blood pressure.

* **Corresponding author Minolfa C. Prieto:** Department of Physiology, Tulane University Health Sciences Center, 1430 Tulane Avenue, SL39, New Orleans, LA 70112, USA; Tel: 504-988-2445; Fax: 504-988-2675; E-mail: mprieto@tulane.edu.

Dulce Elena Casarini, Danielle Yuri Arita, Tatiana Sousa Cunha & Juliana Almada Colucci (Eds.)

Keywords: Angiotensin, Angiotensinogen, Angiotensin converting enzyme, Blood pressure, Collecting duct, Cyclic AMP, Cyclooxygenase-2, Hypertension, Intracellular pathways, Kidney, Prorenin, Protein kinase C, Renal medulla, Renin, Sodium, Transport, Urine.

INTRODUCTION

The renin-angiotensin system (RAS) plays crucial role in controlling blood pressure and body volume. Beside the systemic RAS, which is mainly controlled by the production and release of renin from the kidneys into the circulation, locally acting RAS in abnormal or sustained activated conditions has been related to the pathogenesis and development of hypertension. A change in the paradigm occurred when it was discovered that proximal intratubular concentrations of Ang II were greater than plasma [1 - 3]. The presence of angiotensin (Ang) type 1 receptors (AT1R) along the luminal membrane of the proximal and distal nephron [4] also suggested a physiological role for the AT1R, despite the abundant expression of degrading enzymes in the proximal tubules. Evidence demonstrating the increased expression and secretion of AGT by the proximal tubule cells [5, 6] and prorenin and renin in the collecting duct in Ang II-dependent hypertension [7 - 10], further support the increased generation of local intratubular Ang II during intrarenal RAS activation [11, 12]. ACE is another key enzyme of the RAS that is also present in collecting duct cells [13]. This enzyme is augmented in Ang II-dependent hypertension [14, 15] and other models of kidney injury [16]. These findings, along with the demonstration of the PRR expression in the collecting ducts establish the basis for a physiologically important role of the tubular RAS.

Intratubular Ang II and AT1R Along the Nephron

Ang I and Ang II concentrations in the proximal tubule are around 5-10 pmol/ml [17]. Which is similar to what have been found in interstitial fluid [18, 19]. these concentrations are elevated in Ang II-dependent hypertensive rats [20], 2K1C Goldblatt hypertensive rats [21] and TGR(mRen2) rats [22]. The AT1aR are essential for in the regulation of blood pressure and the increase in blood pressure in response to Ang II [23]. Furthermore, AT1aR knockout mice fail to develop hypertension in response to unilateral renal arterial constriction [24]. There is evidence that Ang II concentrations are about 0.5 pmol/ml; this value increases during chronic Ang II infusions in mice [25, 26]. These responses can be blocked by AT1R antagonists in rats [27]. Ang II concentrations are sufficiently high to influence distal transport [28, 29]. AT1R are responsible for internalizing Ang II in proximal tubules, since AT1R blockade prevents this effect [30]. Internalized Ang II can migrate to the nucleus and exert transcriptional effects [31], including the activation of several profibrotic and proliferative genes [32]. Thus, intrarenal and intratubular Ang II may contribute to sustained de novo Ang II formation and profibrotic responses in the kidney.

Increased Expression of AGT in Proximal Tubules in Hypertension

Angiotensinogen (AGT) mRNA has been found in proximal tubules [5, 33, 34]. This observation generated interest about its function. The augmentation of AGT mRNA and AGT protein in the urine during chronic Ang II infusion (Fig. **1**) [5, 6, 35, 36] are mediated by AT1R, since AT1R blockers prevented AGT upregulation [18]. The same phenomenon occurs *in vitro* using proximal tubule cell [36]. Also, augmentation of AGT in proximal tubules requires the presence of inflammatory factors like IL-6, and oxidative stress [37 - 39].

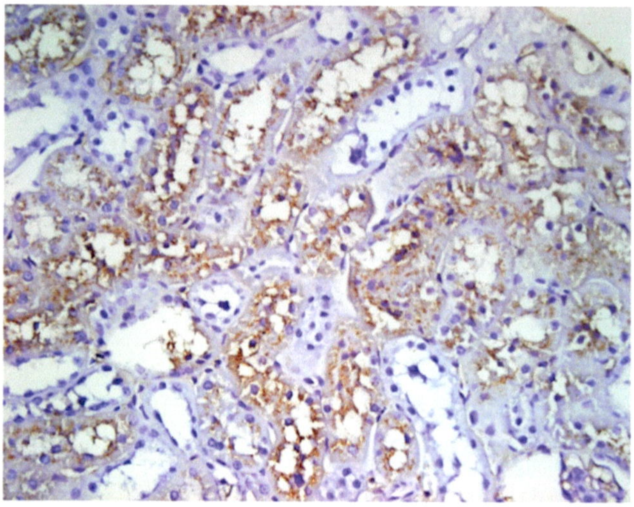

Fig. (1). Angiotensinogen (AGT) specific immunostaining in the proximal tubules of an Angiotensin II-infused rat kidney section (5 μm). Sheep anti-AGT antibody was used at a dilution of 1:60,000.

The role of AGT has been established using genetic models that lead to overexpression of AGT and hypertension [40]. Therefore, AGT has been used as a marker, since it reflects the intratubular RAS status [18, 41]. Because of its potential importance in identifying Ang II-dependent hypertension in human subjects, direct methods to measure urinary AGT using AGT enzyme-link immunosorbent assay (ELISA), were recently reported [42 - 44]. Urinary AGT excretion might provide information of the status of intrarenal RAS in patients with kidney disease [18, 45], diabetes mellitus [46], and hypertension [18, 47, 48].

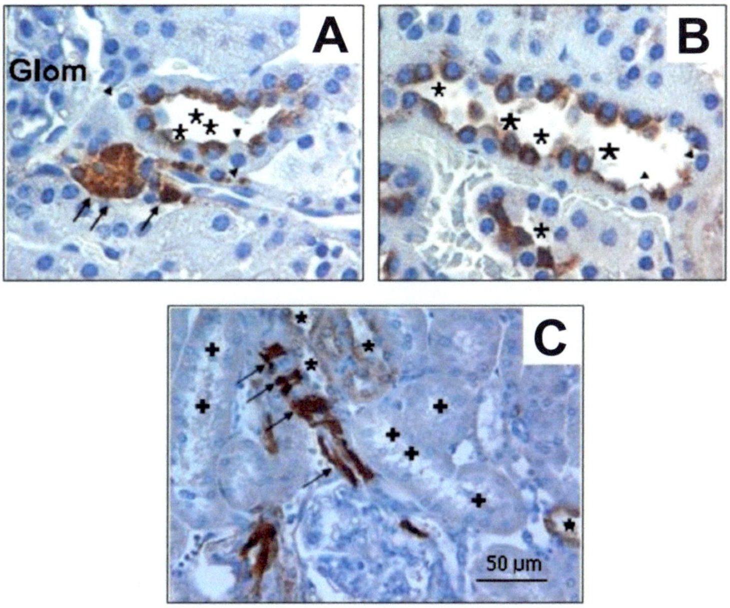

Fig. (2). Renin immunostaining in rat kidney sections showing specific localization in juxtaglomerular cells (arrows) of the glomerulus (Glom; A and C) and collecting ducts (asterisks; A-C) in paraffin embedded rat kidney sections (5 µm). Proximal tubules show no specific renin immunostaining. A rabbit anti-renin antibody was used at a dilution of 1:4,000 (antibody generously provided as a gift by Dr. Tadashi Inagami, Vanderbilt University).

Renin in the Collecting Duct

Renin is synthesized mostly by the juxtaglomerular cells (JG), however there is evidence about the presence of renin mRNA and protein in renal tubular segments, including the proximal tubules, connecting tubules and collecting ducts (Fig. **2A-C**) [7, 8, 49, 50]. In contrast to the effect of Ang II on JG renin expression, renin synthesis is increased in the collecting ducts of chronic Ang II-infused rats and mice (Fig. **3C-E**), Cyp1a1Ren2 transgenic rats, and both kidneys of Goldblatt hypertensive rats [7, 8, 51, 52].

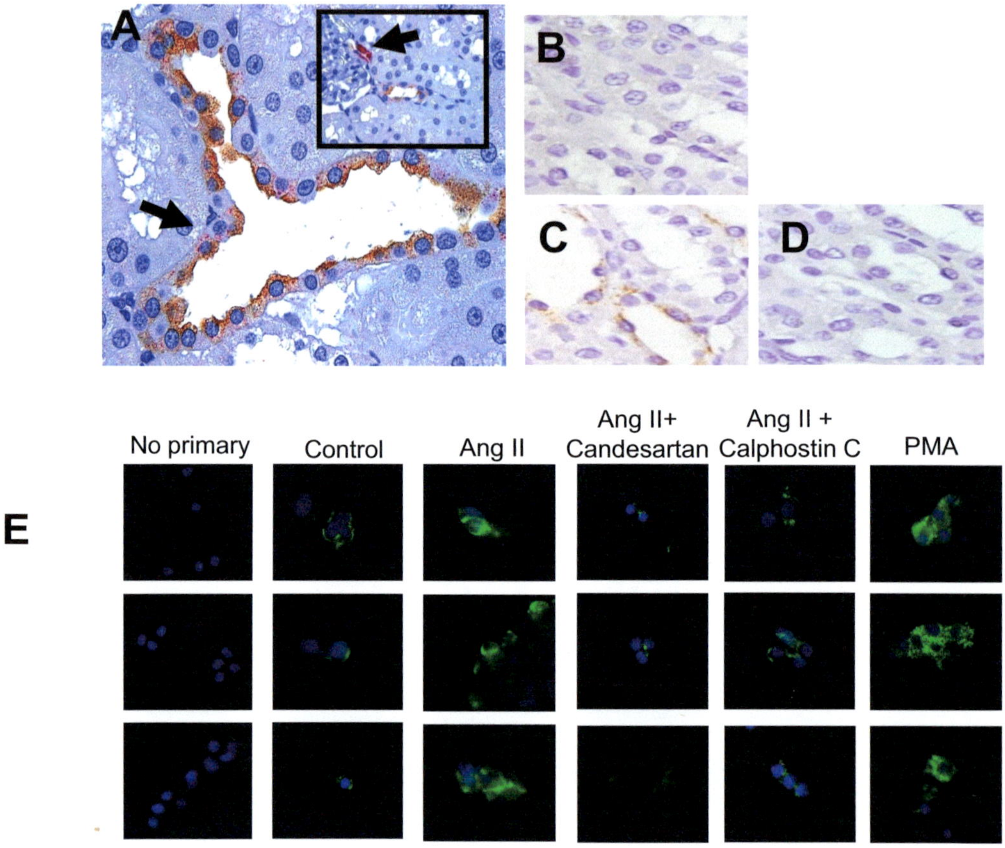

Fig. (3). A. Renin expression in juxtaglomerular cells (insert in red and arrow) and in collecting ducts (red). Brown chromogen indicates aquaporin-2 immunostaining, which is a specific marker for principal cells of the collecting duct. **B.** Renin immunolabeling in collecting ducts of a control rat; **C.** Renin is augmented in collecting ducts of Ang II infused rats, and this effect was suppressed in Ang II infused rats treated with AT1 receptor blocker **D.** (Modified from Prieto-Carrasquero *et al.*, 2005). **E.** Effect of Ang II (10^{-7} M), Ang II plus PKC inhibition with Calphostin C (Cal C) and PKC activator Phorbol 12-myristate 13-acetate (PMA) on renin expression in freshly isolated rat inner medullary collecting ducts (modified from Gonzalez *et al.*, 2011).

Ang II stimulates renin in collecting duct cells *via* AT1R and independent of blood pressure [7, 8]. On the other hand, activation of AT1R suppresses renin synthesis in JG cells *via* protein kinase C (PKC) and Ca^{+2} [53 - 55].

We have shown that renin is increased in rat inner medullary collecting duct cells and that this effect is mediated by AT1R *via* PKC [9]. Using a PKC activator, PMA (Phorbol 12-myristate 13-acetate) renin levels were higher than control and PKC inhibition with Calphostin C prevented the stimulatory effect of Ang II (Fig. **3E**).

The (Pro) Renin Receptor

The (pro)renin receptor (PRR) is a new discovered receptor for renin and for the inactive prorenin. The discovery of this protein has opened the possibility of a role in regulating intrarenal RAS. PRR was described as an associated protein of the V-ATPase (vacuolar H+-ATPase, ATP6AP2). Ang II may activates H+-ATPase, which causes the addition of H+ into the urine suggesting that PRR is involved in H+ transport through Ang II stimulation. PRR is expressed predominantly in glomeruli and renal arteries [56]. Other studies demonstrated that PRR is expressed particularly in podocytes, and intercalated type-A cells of distal nephron segments [57 - 59]. We demonstrated that the full length PRR (37 kDa) is decreased in the renal medulla of Ang II-infused rats [60]. In Fig. (**4A**), we show a co-immunostaining for renin (in red, representing principal cells) and PRR (in green, representing intercalated cells) in a mouse collecting duct cell line. The PRR binds renin and prorenin with affinity in the nanomolar range [61], increasing the catalytic activity of renin and activating prorenin by exposing its active site [62, 63]. Binding of prorenin to PRR increases renin enzymatic activity and also triggers the intracellular phosphorylation of mitogen activated protein kinases (MAPK) ERK1/2 [56, 64]. Activation of MAPK/ERK1/2 upregulates cyclooxygenase-2 (COX-2) in heart [65] and kidney [66]. Transgenic rats over-expressing PRR have increased expression of COX-2 and phosphorylated-ERK1/2 (p-ERK1/2) in the renal cortex with normal renal Ang II content, suggesting that PRR-mediated COX-2 upregulation may be independent of Ang II [67 - 69]. In Ang II-infused rats, augmentation of COX-2 expression and activity in isolated glomeruli is associated with the activation of MAPK/ERK1/2 pathways [70, 71]. We recently reported the expression of PRR not only in intercalated but also in renal interstitial cells [69], and that, Ang II and PRR, both stimulate COX-

2 in these cells *via* activation of ERK 1/2 pathway (Fig. **4B**).

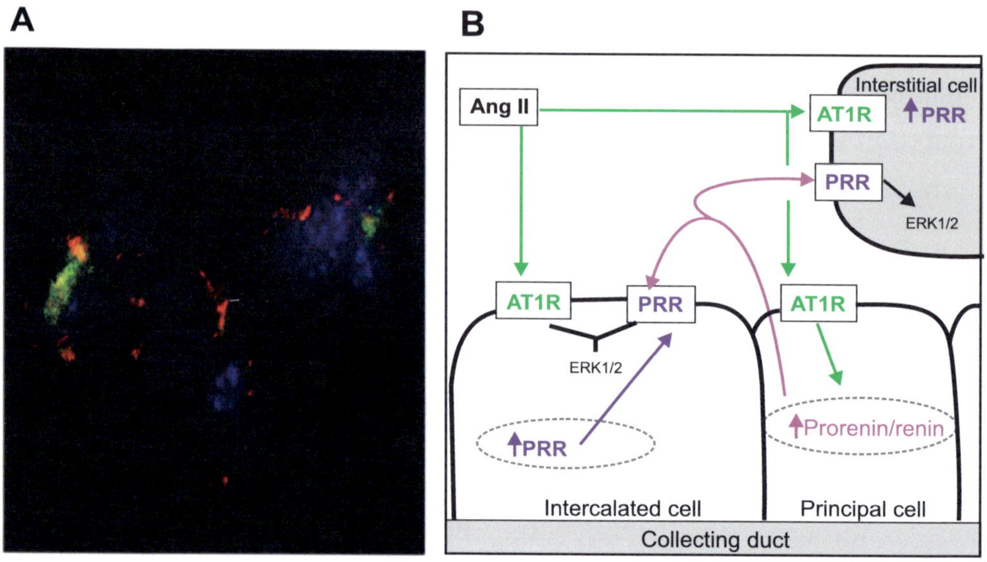

Fig. (4). A. Immunocolocalization of renin in principal cells (red) and PRR (green) in M-1 cells. Blue, nuclei (DAPI; 4',6-diamidino-2-phenylindole). **B.** Hypothetic role of PRR. Ang II increases renin in principal cells as well as PRR expression in intercalated cells. PRR activates ERK 1/2 pathways stimulating COX-2 expression, but also membrane located PRR in interstitial cells can be stimulated by the increased prorenin/renin secreted by principal cells in response to AT1R activation. The PRR and renin immunofluorescence were performed using a rabbit anti-PRR antibody (1:400 dilution; Cat HPA003156; Sigma, Co, LLC) and mouse anti-renin B-12 (1:400; Cat 133145; Santa Cruz, Inc), respectively.

The actions of the PRR have been associated to diabetic nephropathy [72]. Despite low f plasma renin in patients with diabetic nephropathy, prorenin is high in the plasma, and is associated to microalbuminuria and retinopathy [73, 74]. Blockade of prorenin binding to PRR prevents and even reverses diabetic nephropathy [75]. Prorenin is augmented in the collecting ducts in diabetes, which may lead to activation of PRR promoting tissue injury [76]. This is relevant in view of the fact that plasma prorenin are not correlated with plasma renin [77]. Interestingly, activation of PRR induces a four-fold increase in the catalytic efficiency of Ang I formation from AGT [78, 79]. This may provide an alternative pathway for Ang I generation on the cell surface.

Renin and PRR Upregulation During Angiotensin II-Dependent Hypertension.

Chronic Ang II infusion for 14 days in male Sprague-Dawley rats show increases in renal PRR transcript in renal medulla, and the soluble form of PRR (sPRR) [60]. Urines, from Ang II infused rats show high Ang I formation [60]. These *in vivo* observations are of relevance in light of the demonstration that renin is augmented in the collecting ducts of Ang II hypertensive rats [7 - 9, 51, 52]. Augmentation of renin in the principal cells could stimulate the membrane bound PRR in the intercalated cells or bind the sPRR in the intratubular space, leading to Ang I formation. *In vitro* studies have shown that furin (a protease) cleaves the full-length form of PRR [80]. Taking together, this evidence supports the notion that in Ang II-dependent hypertension, the PRR contribute to increase intratubular Ang II content by enhancing renin activity *via* two mechanisms: First, by binding renin secreted by the principal cell [8, 51, 76, 81] at its location in the apical side of the intercalated cells. And second, by binding renin in the lumen [60], which contribute even further to enhance the intraluminal Ang I, and Ang II since ACE is also present in the collecting ducts [82]. Thus, the renin and PRR in the collecting ducts are new candidates to study RAS dysregulation.

CONCLUSION

Collectively this evidence indicates that the distal nephron segments contain the machinery necessary to generate intratubular Ang II. Augmented intrarenal Ang II levels elicit an increase in AGT, prorenin/renin and PRR, along with the sustained activation of ACE, thus leading to increase further the de novo Ang II formation. Increased content of Ang II in the tubular lumen augments sodium reabsorption *via* AT1R-mediated stimulation of proximal and distal nephron transporters, including ENaC. Ang II also increases the expression of apical PRR in intercalated cells of the collecting ducts allowing for a greater interaction between this receptor and prorenin/renin secreted by the principal cells, thus resulting in further Ang I formation. This positive augmentation of intrarenal Ang II by itself appears to be counter-intuitive to normal feedback regulation but is a self-limiting process [83, 84]. The upregulation of these RAS elements in the proximal and distal nephron segments suggest that inappropriate stimulation of the intratubular

RAS is an key factor to the development and progression of hypertension and associated renal injury [85].

CONFLICT OF INTEREST

The authors Alexis A. Gonzalez, Minolfa C. Prieto and L. Gabriel Navar declare no conflicts of interest in preparing this chapter.

ACKNOWLEDGEMENTS

We want to thank Camille R. Bourgeois, MS and Dale M. Seth, MS, for their excellent technical assistance.

SOURCES OF FOUNDING

Research reported in this publication was supported by the National Institute of General Medical Sciences of the National Institutes of Health-Institutional Developmental Award Program of the National Center for Research Resources, under the awards P20RR-017659 and P30GM103337. The content is solely the responsibility of the authors and does not necessarily represent the official views of the National Institutes of Health. In addition, funds were provided to M.C.P by the American Heart Association (09BGIA2280440) and the Eunice Kennedy Shriver National Institute of Child Health & Human Development (K12HD043451) and to A.A.G., by FONDECYT (11121217).

DISCLOSURE

Part of this chapter has been previously published in Clinical and Experimental Pharmacology and Physiology.Volume 42, Issue 1, pages 14–21, January 2015 DOI: 10.1111/1440-1681.12319

REFERENCES

[1] Navar LG, Harrison-Bernard LM, Wang C-T, Cervenka L, Mitchell KD. Concentrations and actions of intraluminal angiotensin II. J Am Soc Nephrol 1999; 10 (Suppl. 11): S189-95. [PMID: 9892162]

[2] Seikaly MG, Arant BS Jr, Seney FD Jr. Endogenous angiotensin concentrations in specific intrarenal fluid compartments of the rat. J Clin Invest 1990; 86(4): 1352-7. [http://dx.doi.org/10.1172/JCI114846] [PMID: 2212017]

[3] Braam B, Mitchell KD, Fox J, Navar LG. Proximal tubular secretion of angiotensin II in rats. Am J Physiol 1993; 264(5 Pt 2): F891-8.
[PMID: 8388654]

[4] Douglas JG, Hopfer U. Novel aspect of angiotensin receptors and signal transduction in the kidney. Annu Rev Physiol 1994; 56: 649-69.
[http://dx.doi.org/10.1146/annurev.ph.56.030194.003245] [PMID: 8010754]

[5] Schunkert H, Ingelfinger JR, Jacob H, Jackson B, Bouyounes B, Dzau VJ. Reciprocal feedback regulation of kidney angiotensinogen and renin mRNA expressions by angiotensin II. Am J Physiol 1992; 263(5 Pt 1): E863-9.
[PMID: 1443118]

[6] Kobori H, Harrison-Bernard LM, Navar LG. Enhancement of angiotensinogen expression in angiotensin II-dependent hypertension. Hypertension 2001; 37(5): 1329-35.
[http://dx.doi.org/10.1161/01.HYP.37.5.1329] [PMID: 11358949]

[7] Prieto-Carrasquero MC, Harrison-Bernard LM, Kobori H, *et al.* Enhancement of collecting duct renin in angiotensin II-dependent hypertensive rats. Hypertension 2004; 44(2): 223-9.
[http://dx.doi.org/10.1161/01.HYP.0000135678.20725.54] [PMID: 15226276]

[8] Prieto-Carrasquero MC, Kobori H, Ozawa Y, Gutiérrez A, Seth D, Navar LG. AT1 receptor-mediated enhancement of collecting duct renin in angiotensin II-dependent hypertensive rats. Am J Physiol Renal Physiol 2005; 289(3): F632-7.
[http://dx.doi.org/10.1152/ajprenal.00462.2004] [PMID: 15870381]

[9] Gonzalez AA, Liu L, Lara LS, *et al.* Angiotensin II stimulates renin in inner medullary collecting duct cells via protein kinase C and independent of epithelial sodium channel and mineralocorticoid receptor activity. Hypertension 2011; 57(3): 594-9.
[http://dx.doi.org/10.1161/HYPERTENSIONAHA.110.165902] [PMID: 21282553]

[10] Liu L, Gonzalez AA, McCormack M, *et al.* Increased renin excretion is associated with augmented urinary angiotensin II levels in chronic angiotensin II-infused hypertensive rats. Am J Physiol Renal Physiol 2011; 301(6): F1195-201.
[http://dx.doi.org/10.1152/ajprenal.00339.2011] [PMID: 21865264]

[11] Shao W, Seth DM, Navar LG. Augmentation of endogenous intrarenal angiotensin II levels in Val5-ANG II-infused rats. Am J Physiol Renal Physiol 2009; 296(5): F1067-71.
[http://dx.doi.org/10.1152/ajprenal.90596.2008] [PMID: 19244403]

[12] Shao W, Seth DM, Navar LG. Angiotensin II type 1 receptor-mediated augmentation of urinary excretion of endogenous angiotensin II in Val5-angiotensin II-infused rats. Hypertension 2010; 56(3): 378-83.
[http://dx.doi.org/10.1161/HYPERTENSIONAHA.110.153106] [PMID: 20625079]

[13] Casarini DE, Boim MA, Stella RC, Krieger-Azzolini MH, Krieger JE, Schor N. Angiotensin I-converting enzyme activity in tubular fluid along the rat nephron. Am J Physiol 1997; 272(3 Pt 2): F405-9.
[PMID: 9087685]

[14] Harrison-Bernard LM, Zhuo J, Kobori H, Ohishi M, Navar LG. Intrarenal AT(1) receptor and ACE

binding in ANG II-induced hypertensive rats. Am J Physiol Renal Physiol 2002; 282(1): F19-25. [http://dx.doi.org/10.1152/ajprenal.0335.2000] [PMID: 11739108]

[15] Gonzalez-Villalobos RA, Satou R, Ohashi N, *et al.* Intrarenal mouse renin-angiotensin system during ANG II-induced hypertension and ACE inhibition. Am J Physiol Renal Physiol 2010; 298(1): F150-7. [http://dx.doi.org/10.1152/ajprenal.00477.2009] [PMID: 19846570]

[16] Vío CP, Jeanneret VA. Local induction of angiotensin-converting enzyme in the kidney as a mechanism of progressive renal diseases. Kidney Int Suppl 2003; (86): S57-63. [http://dx.doi.org/10.1046/j.1523-1755.64.s86.11.x] [PMID: 12969129]

[17] Navar LG, Harrison-Bernard LM, Nishiyama A, Kobori H. Regulation of intrarenal angiotensin II in hypertension. Hypertension 2002; 39(2 Pt 2): 316-22. [http://dx.doi.org/10.1161/hy0202.103821] [PMID: 11882566]

[18] Kobori H, Nishiyama A, Harrison-Bernard LM, Navar LG. Urinary angiotensinogen as an indicator of intrarenal Angiotensin status in hypertension. Hypertension 2003; 41(1): 42-9. [http://dx.doi.org/10.1161/01.HYP.0000050102.90932.CF] [PMID: 12511528]

[19] Nishiyama A, Seth DM, Navar LG. Angiotensin II type 1 receptor-mediated augmentation of renal interstitial fluid angiotensin II in angiotensin II-induced hypertension. J Hypertens 2003; 21(10): 1897-903. [http://dx.doi.org/10.1097/00004872-200310000-00017] [PMID: 14508196]

[20] Wang C-T, Navar LG, Mitchell KD. Proximal tubular fluid angiotensin II levels in angiotensin II-induced hypertensive rats. J Hypertens 2003; 21(2): 353-60. [http://dx.doi.org/10.1097/00004872-200302000-00027] [PMID: 12569266]

[21] Cervenka L, Wang C-T, Mitchell KD, Navar LG. Proximal tubular angiotensin II levels and renal functional responses to AT1 receptor blockade in nonclipped kidneys of Goldblatt hypertensive rats. Hypertension 1999; 33(1): 102-7. [http://dx.doi.org/10.1161/01.HYP.33.1.102] [PMID: 9931089]

[22] Mitchell KD, Jacinto SM, Mullins JJ. Proximal tubular fluid, kidney, and plasma levels of angiotensin II in hypertensive ren-2 transgenic rats. Am J Physiol 1997; 273(2 Pt 2): F246-53. [PMID: 9277585]

[23] Crowley SD, Gurley SB, Herrera MJ, *et al.* Angiotensin II causes hypertension and cardiac hypertrophy through its receptors in the kidney. Proc Natl Acad Sci USA 2006; 103(47): 17985-90. [http://dx.doi.org/10.1073/pnas.0605545103] [PMID: 17090678]

[24] Cervenka L, Horácek V, Vanecková I, *et al.* Essential role of AT1A receptor in the development of 2K1C hypertension. Hypertension 2002; 40(5): 735-41. [http://dx.doi.org/10.1161/01.HYP.0000036452.28493.74] [PMID: 12411470]

[25] Zhao D, Navar LG. Acute angiotensin II infusions elicit pressure natriuresis in mice and reduce distal fractional sodium reabsorption. Hypertension 2008; 52(1): 137-42. [http://dx.doi.org/10.1161/HYPERTENSIONAHA.108.111435] [PMID: 18504321]

[26] Zhao D, Seth DM, Navar LG. Enhanced distal nephron sodium reabsorption in chronic angiotensin II-infused mice. Hypertension 2009; 54(1): 120-6. [http://dx.doi.org/10.1161/HYPERTENSIONAHA.109.133785] [PMID: 19487583]

[27] Shao W, Seth DM, Prieto MC, Kobori H, Navar LG. Activation of the renin-angiotensin system by a low-salt diet does not augment intratubular angiotensinogen and angiotensin II in rats. Am J Physiol Renal Physiol 2013; 304(5): F505-14.
[http://dx.doi.org/10.1152/ajprenal.00587.2012] [PMID: 23303412]

[28] Peti-Peterdi J, Warnock DG, Bell PD. Angiotensin II directly stimulates ENaC activity in the cortical collecting duct *via* AT(1) receptors. J Am Soc Nephrol 2002; 13(5): 1131-5.
[http://dx.doi.org/10.1097/01.ASN.0000013292.78621.FD] [PMID: 11960999]

[29] Komlosi P, Fuson AL, Fintha A, *et al.* Angiotensin I conversion to angiotensin II stimulates cortical collecting duct sodium transport. Hypertension 2003; 42(2): 195-9.
[http://dx.doi.org/10.1161/01.HYP.0000081221.36703.01] [PMID: 12835330]

[30] Zhuo JL, Imig JD, Hammond TG, Orengo S, Benes E, Navar LG. Ang II accumulation in rat renal endosomes during Ang II-induced hypertension: role of AT(1) receptor. Hypertension 2002; 39(1): 116-21.
[http://dx.doi.org/10.1161/hy0102.100780] [PMID: 11799089]

[31] Pendergrass KD, Averill DB, Ferrario CM, Diz DI, Chappell MC. Differential expression of nuclear AT1 receptors and angiotensin II within the kidney of the male congenic mRen2. Lewis rat. Am J Physiol Renal Physiol 2006; 290(6): F1497-506.
[http://dx.doi.org/10.1152/ajprenal.00317.2005] [PMID: 16403834]

[32] Cook JL, Zhang Z, Re RN. *In vitro* evidence for an intracellular site of angiotensin action. Circ Res 2001; 89(12): 1138-46.
[http://dx.doi.org/10.1161/hh2401.101270] [PMID: 11739278]

[33] Yanagawa N. Angiotensin II and proximal tubule sodium transport. Ren Physiol Biochem 1991; 14(4-5): 208-15.
[PMID: 1708907]

[34] Darby IA, Sernia C. *In situ* hybridization and immunohistochemistry of renal angiotensinogen in neonatal and adult rat kidneys. Cell Tissue Res 1995; 281(2): 197-206.
[http://dx.doi.org/10.1007/BF00583388] [PMID: 7648615]

[35] Kobori H, Harrison-Bernard LM, Navar LG. Expression of angiotensinogen mRNA and protein in angiotensin II-dependent hypertension. J Am Soc Nephrol 2001; 12(3): 431-9.
[PMID: 11181790]

[36] Ingelfinger JR, Jung F, Diamant D, *et al.* Rat proximal tubule cell line transformed with origin-defective SV40 DNA: autocrine ANG II feedback. Am J Physiol 1999; 276(2 Pt 2): F218-27.
[PMID: 9950952]

[37] Satou R, Gonzalez-Villalobos RA, Miyata K, *et al.* Costimulation with angiotensin II and interleukin 6 augments angiotensinogen expression in cultured human renal proximal tubular cells. Am J Physiol Renal Physiol 2008; 295(1): F283-9.
[http://dx.doi.org/10.1152/ajprenal.00047.2008] [PMID: 18463317]

[38] Satou R, Gonzalez-Villalobos RA, Miyata K, *et al.* IL-6 augments angiotensinogen in primary cultured renal proximal tubular cells. Mol Cell Endocrinol 2009; 311(1-2): 24-31.
[http://dx.doi.org/10.1016/j.mce.2009.06.013] [PMID: 19583994]

[39] Satou R, Miyata K, Gonzalez-Villalobos RA, Ingelfinger JR, Navar LG, Kobori H. Interferon-γ biphasically regulates angiotensinogen expression via a JAK-STAT pathway and suppressor of cytokine signaling 1 (SOCS1) in renal proximal tubular cells. FASEB J 2012; 26(5): 1821-30. [http://dx.doi.org/10.1096/fj.11-195198] [PMID: 22302831]

[40] Kim H-S, Krege JH, Kluckman KD, *et al.* Genetic control of blood pressure and the angiotensinogen locus. Proc Natl Acad Sci USA 1995; 92(7): 2735-9. [http://dx.doi.org/10.1073/pnas.92.7.2735] [PMID: 7708716]

[41] Kobori H, Harrison-Bernard LM, Navar LG. Urinary excretion of angiotensinogen reflects intrarenal angiotensinogen production. Kidney Int 2002; 61(2): 579-85. [http://dx.doi.org/10.1046/j.1523-1755.2002.00155.x] [PMID: 11849399]

[42] Suzaki Y, Ozawa Y, Kobori H. Quantification of human angiotensinogen by a novel sandwich ELISA. Peptides 2006; 27(11): 3000-2. [http://dx.doi.org/10.1016/j.peptides.2006.05.006] [PMID: 16793172]

[43] Katsurada A, Hagiwara Y, Miyashita K, *et al.* Novel sandwich ELISA for human angiotensinogen. Am J Physiol Renal Physiol 2007; 293(3): F956-60. [http://dx.doi.org/10.1152/ajprenal.00090.2007] [PMID: 17553939]

[44] Kobori H, Katsurada A, Miyata K, *et al.* Determination of plasma and urinary angiotensinogen levels in rodents by newly developed ELISA. Am J Physiol Renal Physiol 2008; 294(5): F1257-63. [http://dx.doi.org/10.1152/ajprenal.00588.2007] [PMID: 18353869]

[45] Yamamoto T, Nakagawa T, Suzuki H, *et al.* Urinary angiotensinogen as a marker of intrarenal angiotensin II activity associated with deterioration of renal function in patients with chronic kidney disease. J Am Soc Nephrol 2007; 18(5): 1558-65. [http://dx.doi.org/10.1681/ASN.2006060554] [PMID: 17409316]

[46] Ogawa S, Kobori H, Ohashi N, *et al.* Angiotensin II Type 1 Receptor Blockers Reduce Urinary Angiotensinogen Excretion and the Levels of Urinary Markers of Oxidative Stress and Inflammation in Patients with Type 2 Diabetic Nephropathy. Biomark Insights 2009; 4: 97-102. [PMID: 19652765]

[47] Lantelme P, Rohrwasser A, Vincent M, *et al.* Significance of urinary angiotensinogen in essential hypertension as a function of plasma renin and aldosterone status. J Hypertens 2005; 23(4): 785-92. [http://dx.doi.org/10.1097/01.hjh.0000163147.20330.f5] [PMID: 15775783]

[48] Kobori H, Urushihara M, Xu JH, Berenson GS, Navar LG. Urinary angiotensinogen is correlated with blood pressure in men (Bogalusa Heart Study). J Hypertens 2010; 28(7): 1422-8. [http://dx.doi.org/10.1097/HJH.0b013e3283392673] [PMID: 20375906]

[49] Rohrwasser A, Morgan T, Dillon HF, *et al.* Elements of a paracrine tubular renin-angiotensin system along the entire nephron. Hypertension 1999; 34(6): 1265-74. [http://dx.doi.org/10.1161/01.HYP.34.6.1265] [PMID: 10601129]

[50] Rohrwasser A, Ishigami T, Gociman B, *et al.* Renin and kallikrein in connecting tubule of mouse. Kidney Int 2003; 64(6): 2155-62. [http://dx.doi.org/10.1046/j.1523-1755.2003.00302.x] [PMID: 14633138]

[51] Prieto-Carrasquero MC, Botros FT, Pagan J, *et al.* Collecting duct renin is upregulated in both kidneys

of 2-kidney, 1-clip goldblatt hypertensive rats. Hypertension 2008; 51(6): 1590-6. [http://dx.doi.org/10.1161/HYPERTENSIONAHA.108.110916] [PMID: 18426992]

[52] Prieto-Carrasquero MC, Botros FT, Kobori H, Navar LG. Collecting Duct Renin: A major player in Angiotensin II-dependent Hypertension. J Am Soc Hypertens 2009; 3(2): 96-104. [http://dx.doi.org/10.1016/j.jash.2008.11.003] [PMID: 20046983]

[53] Kurtz A. Cellular control of renin secretion. Rev Physiol Biochem Pharmacol 1989; 113: 1-40. [http://dx.doi.org/10.1007/BFb0032674] [PMID: 2697067]

[54] Kurtz A, Wagner C. Cellular control of renin secretion. J Exp Biol 1999; 202(Pt 3): 219-25. [PMID: 9882634]

[55] Müller MW, Todorov V, Krämer BK, Kurtz A. Angiotensin II inhibits renin gene transcription *via* the protein kinase C pathway. Pflugers Arch 2002; 444(4): 499-505. [http://dx.doi.org/10.1007/s00424-002-0835-8] [PMID: 12136269]

[56] Nguyen G, Contrepas A. Physiology and pharmacology of the (pro)renin receptor. Curr Opin Pharmacol 2008; 8(2): 127-32. [http://dx.doi.org/10.1016/j.coph.2007.12.009] [PMID: 18243793]

[57] Nguyen G, Delarue F, Berrou J, Rondeau E, Sraer JD. Specific receptor binding of renin on human mesangial cells in culture increases plasminogen activator inhibitor-1 antigen. Kidney Int 1996; 50(6): 1897-903. [http://dx.doi.org/10.1038/ki.1996.511] [PMID: 8943472]

[58] Nguyen G, Danser AH. The (pro)renin receptor: therapeutic consequences. Expert Opin Investig Drugs 2006; 15(10): 1131-5. [http://dx.doi.org/10.1517/13543784.15.10.1131] [PMID: 16989589]

[59] Ichihara A, Sakoda M, Kurauchi-Mito A, Kaneshiro Y, Itoh H. Involvement of (pro)renin receptor in the glomerular filtration barrier. J Mol Med 2008; 86(6): 629-35. [http://dx.doi.org/10.1007/s00109-008-0327-1] [PMID: 18335185]

[60] Gonzalez AA, Lara LS, Luffman C, Seth DM, Prieto MC. Soluble form of the (pro)renin receptor is augmented in the collecting duct and urine of chronic angiotensin II-dependent hypertensive rats. Hypertension 2011; 57(4): 859-64. [http://dx.doi.org/10.1161/HYPERTENSIONAHA.110.167957] [PMID: 21321306]

[61] Nabi AH, Biswas KB, Nakagawa T, Ichihara A, Inagami T, Suzuki F. Prorenin has high affinity multiple binding sites for (pro)renin receptor. Biochim Biophys Acta 2009; 1794(12): 1838-47. [http://dx.doi.org/10.1016/j.bbapap.2009.08.024] [PMID: 19733264]

[62] Nguyen G, Burcklé CA, Sraer JD. Renin/prorenin-receptor biochemistry and functional significance. Curr Hypertens Rep 2004; 6(2): 129-32. [http://dx.doi.org/10.1007/s11906-004-0088-3] [PMID: 15010017]

[63] Nguyen G, Muller DN. The biology of the (pro)renin receptor. J Am Soc Nephrol 2010; 21(1): 18-23. [http://dx.doi.org/10.1681/ASN.2009030300] [PMID: 19917780]

[64] Nguyen G. Renin and prorenin receptor in hypertension: what's new? Curr Hypertens Rep 2011; 13(1): 79-85. [http://dx.doi.org/10.1007/s11906-010-0172-9] [PMID: 21125352]

[65] Adderley SR, Fitzgerald DJ. Oxidative damage of cardiomyocytes is limited by extracellular regulated kinases 1/2-mediated induction of cyclooxygenase-2. J Biol Chem 1999; 274(8): 5038-46. [http://dx.doi.org/10.1074/jbc.274.8.5038] [PMID: 9988750]

[66] Rodríguez-Barbero A, Dorado F, Velasco S, Pandiella A, Banas B, López-Novoa JM. TGF-beta1 induces COX-2 expression and PGE2 synthesis through MAPK and PI3K pathways in human mesangial cells. Kidney Int 2006; 70(5): 901-9. [http://dx.doi.org/10.1038/sj.ki.5001626] [PMID: 16820791]

[67] Kaneshiro Y, Ichihara A, Takemitsu T, *et al.* Increased expression of cyclooxygenase-2 in the renal cortex of human prorenin receptor gene-transgenic rats. Kidney Int 2006; 70(4): 641-6. [http://dx.doi.org/10.1038/sj.ki.5001627] [PMID: 16807542]

[68] Kaneshiro Y, Ichihara A, Sakoda M, *et al.* Slowly progressive, angiotensin II-independent glomerulosclerosis in human (pro)renin receptor-transgenic rats. J Am Soc Nephrol 2007; 18(6): 1789-95. [http://dx.doi.org/10.1681/ASN.2006091062] [PMID: 17494887]

[69] Gonzalez AA, Luffman C, Bourgeois CR, Vio CP, Prieto MC. Angiotensin II-independent upregulation of cyclooxygenase-2 by activation of the (Pro)renin receptor in rat renal inner medullary cells. Hypertension 2013; 61(2): 443-9. [http://dx.doi.org/10.1161/HYPERTENSIONAHA.112.196303] [PMID: 23184385]

[70] Jaimes EA, Tian RX, Pearse D, Raij L. Up-regulation of glomerular COX-2 by angiotensin II: role of reactive oxygen species. Kidney Int 2005; 68(5): 2143-53. [http://dx.doi.org/10.1111/j.1523-1755.2005.00670.x] [PMID: 16221213]

[71] Jaimes EA, Zhou MS, Pearse DD, Puzis L, Raij L. Upregulation of cortical COX-2 in salt-sensitive hypertension: role of angiotensin II and reactive oxygen species. Am J Physiol Renal Physiol 2008; 294(2): F385-92. [http://dx.doi.org/10.1152/ajprenal.00302.2007] [PMID: 18094033]

[72] Satofuka S, Ichihara A, Nagai N, *et al.* (Pro)renin receptor-mediated signal transduction and tissue renin-angiotensin system contribute to diabetes-induced retinal inflammation. Diabetes 2009; 58(7): 1625-33. [http://dx.doi.org/10.2337/db08-0254] [PMID: 19389828]

[73] Bryer-Ash M, Ammon RA, Luetscher JA. Increased inactive renin in diabetes mellitus without evidence of nephropathy. J Clin Endocrinol Metab 1983; 56(3): 557-61. [http://dx.doi.org/10.1210/jcem-56-3-557] [PMID: 6337180]

[74] Luetscher JA, Kraemer FB, Wilson DM. Prorenin and vascular complications of diabetes. Am J Hypertens 1989; 2(5 Pt 1): 382-6. [PMID: 2655663]

[75] Ichihara A, Hayashi M, Kaneshiro Y, *et al.* Inhibition of diabetic nephropathy by a decoy peptide corresponding to the "handle" region for nonproteolytic activation of prorenin. J Clin Invest 2004; 114(8): 1128-35. [http://dx.doi.org/10.1172/JCI21398] [PMID: 15489960]

[76] Kang JJ, Toma I, Sipos A, Meer EJ, Vargas SL, Peti-Peterdi J. The collecting duct is the major source

of prorenin in diabetes. Hypertension 2008; 51(6): 1597-604.
[http://dx.doi.org/10.1161/HYPERTENSIONAHA.107.107268] [PMID: 18413493]

[77] Deinum J, Rønn B, Mathiesen E, Derkx FH, Hop WC, Schalekamp MA. Increase in serum prorenin precedes onset of microalbuminuria in patients with insulin-dependent diabetes mellitus. Diabetologia 1999; 42(8): 1006-10.
[http://dx.doi.org/10.1007/s001250051260] [PMID: 10491762]

[78] Nguyen G, Delarue F, Burcklé C, Bouzhir L, Giller T, Sraer JD. Pivotal role of the renin/prorenin receptor in angiotensin II production and cellular responses to renin. J Clin Invest 2002; 109(11): 1417-27.
[http://dx.doi.org/10.1172/JCI0214276] [PMID: 12045255]

[79] Nguyen G. The (pro)renin receptor: biochemistry and potential significance. J Renin Angiotensin Aldosterone Syst 2005; 6(3): 166-7.
[http://dx.doi.org/10.3317/jraas.2005.026] [PMID: 16532574]

[80] Cousin C, Bracquart D, Contrepas A, Corvol P, Muller L, Nguyen G. Soluble form of the (pro)renin receptor generated by intracellular cleavage by furin is secreted in plasma. Hypertension 2009; 53(6): 1077-82.
[http://dx.doi.org/10.1161/HYPERTENSIONAHA.108.127258] [PMID: 19380613]

[81] Prieto-Carrasquero MC, Navar LG. Role of the intrarenal renin-angiotensin system in hypertension. 2006.

[82] Casarini DE, Plavinik FL, Zanella MT, *et al.* Angiotensin converting enzymes from human urine of mild hypertensive untreated patients resemble the N-terminal fragment of human angiotensin I-converting enzyme. Int J Biochem Cell Biol 2001; 33(1): 75-85.
[http://dx.doi.org/10.1016/S1357-2725(00)00072-8] [PMID: 11167134]

[83] Navar LG, Satou R, Gonzalez-Villalobos RA. The increasing complexity of the intratubular Renin-Angiotensin system. J Am Soc Nephrol 2012; 23(7): 1130-2.
[http://dx.doi.org/10.1681/ASN.2012050493] [PMID: 22677556]

[84] Satou R, Miyata K, Gonzalez-Villalobos RA, Ingelfinger JR, Navar LG, Kobori H. Interferon-γ biphasically regulates angiotensinogen expression *via* a JAK-STAT pathway and suppressor of cytokine signaling 1 (SOCS1) in renal proximal tubular cells. FASEB J 2012; 26(5): 1821-30.
[http://dx.doi.org/10.1096/fj.11-195198] [PMID: 22302831]

[85] Polichnowski AJ, Jin C, Yang C, Cowley AW Jr. Role of renal perfusion pressure *versus* angiotensin II on renal oxidative stress in angiotensin II-induced hypertensive rats. Hypertension 2010; 55(6): 1425-30.
[http://dx.doi.org/10.1161/HYPERTENSIONAHA.110.151332] [PMID: 20404214]

CHAPTER 8

Tonin: An Overview and Functional Analysis

Fernanda Rezende[1], **Amanda Aparecida Ribeiro**[2], **Zaira Palomino Jara**[2], **Valéria Alves Fernades**[3], **Mercia de Paula Lima**[3], **Dulce Elena Casarini**[2] and **Jorge Luiz Pesquero**[3,*]

[1] *Universidade de Mogi das Cruzes, Sao Paulo, Brazil*

[2] *Department of Medicine, Nephrology Division, Universidade Federal de São Paulo, Sao Paulo, Brazil*

[3] *Departmentof Physiology and Biophysics, Universidade Federal de São Paulo, Brazil*

Abstract: Tonin, a serinoproteinase, is capable of releasing angiotensin II by the hydrolysis of Phe[8]-His[9] bond in the angiotensinogen, angiotensin I and synthetic peptides corresponding to the N-terminal portion of angiotensinogen. Tonin is able to hydrolyze beta-lipotropic hormone releasing an opiate-like segment. It is capable of degrading adrenocorticotropic hormone, substance P but not bradykinin. Hydrolysis of Phe.His bond depends on a minimum sequence involving residues Ile.His.Pro.Phe.His.Leu. Tonin activity is present in human and rat tissues. In the rat, tonin is present in various tissues including kidney, brain and heart, and the activity levels vary according to age and sex being higher in males. Tonin is released into bloodstream and saliva after beta-adrenergic stimulation. There is evidence that tonin is involved in blood pressure control and participates in the hydromineral balance. Intracerebroventricular injection of tonin induces salt appetite and water intake and increases urinary volume and blood pressure. TGM(rTon), a transgenic mouse that expresses rat tonin, presents increased blood pressure. The levels of angiotensin II in the plasma are increased in TGM(rTon) and the AT1 receptors desensitized when compared to the wild type. A significant increase in the plasmatic and a decrease in urinary sodium were observed in TGM(rTon), suggesting alterations in the renal function. Induction of cardiac hypertrophy by isoproterenol injection in rats showed that tonin may be involved in this process. TGM(rTon) presents resistance to develop isoproterenol-induced hypertrophy. The molecular basis for the hypertrophy resistance

* **Corresponding author Jorge Luiz Pesquero:** Departamento de Fisiologia e Biofísica, ICB-UFMG, Av. Antonio Carlos, 6627 31270-901, Belo Horizonte, Minas Gerais, Brasil; Tel: +55-31-34092942; Fax: +55-31-34092924; E-mail: jlpesq@icb.ufmg.br.

Dulce Elena Casarini, Danielle Yuri Arita, Tatiana Sousa Cunha & Juliana Almada Colucci (Eds.)

is to be determined. These results lead us to conclude that tonin, an angiotensin II liberating enzyme may represent an alternative pathway with effects on the renal and cardiovascular systems.

Keywords: Angiotensin I, Angiotensin II, Angiotensinogen, Antinociceptive effect, Blood pressure, Converting enzyme, Heart, Hypertension, Hypertrophy resistance, Isoproterenol, Renin, Serine proteinase, Tonin, Transgenic mouse, Water intake.

HISTORICAL REVIEW

The first citation of tonin was in the 70s, when a group of researchers, coordinated by Jacques Genest from the Clinical Research Institute of Montreal, Canada, described the presence of this enzyme in large amounts in the submandibular gland (SMG) of the rat. It was described as a new angiotensin-converting enzyme (ACE) and named as ß- converting enzyme [1]. Due to several differences in the properties of this enzyme, compared to renin and ACE, as specificity, catalytic activity, factors of activation and inhibition it was renamed as tonin.

While ACE is able to release angiotensin II (Ang II) by hydrolysis of the Phe^{8}-His^{9} bond of angiotensin I (Ang I), tonin is also capable of releasing Ang II by hydrolysis of the Phe^{8}-His^{9} bond from angiotensinogen (AG) [2] and from synthetic substrates homologues to the tetradecapeptide, a synthetic substrate corresponding to the 14 residues of N-terminal portion of angiotensinogen (AG(1-14)) [3, 4] as shown in the Fig. (**1**).

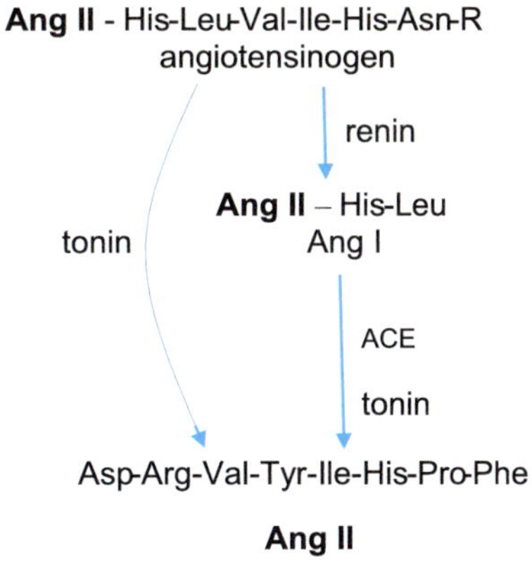

Fig. (1). Tonin-angiotensin II system.

Tonin activity was observed in various rat tissues such as the testes, liver, renal cortex and medulla, spleen, brain, lung, parotid, prostate, pancreas and submandibular gland where it is present at higher levels [3, 5 - 8]. Tonin, in the rat SMG, represents around 8% of the protein content. Woodley-Miller *et al.* (1987) [8] found that the levels of immunoreactive tonin in the SMG are approximately 10% of the protein content (105.27 ± 2.71 μg/mg protein) [8]. A similar result was found by Johansen *et al.* (1987) [7] who observed that the levels are of the order of 69 μg/mg of protein [7]. Tonin activity in this tissue varies according to age and sex being higher in males. The difference in sex becomes more evident after 60-80 days of age [9].

Orstavik and colleagues (1982) [10] investigated the cellular localization of tonin in the rat salivary glands by indirect immunofluorescence and observed that the enzyme is abundantly present in the granular tubular cells. In the striated duct cells tonin-specific staining was detected only as a thin luminal rim and no signal in any other structure of the gland [10]. Ledoux and collaborators (1982) [11] determined, by the indirect immunofluorescence and by the unlabeled antibody technique, the localization of tonin in salivary glands and kidney. The results were identical with both techniques. Immunoreactive tonin was localized in the cytoplasm of granular convoluted tubular cells and on the apical surface of striated duct cells and collecting duct cells. In the parotid and sublingual glands tonin was only found on the apical surface of striated duct and collecting duct cells. In the kidney, immunoreactive tonin was found associated with cells of the distal convoluted tubules [11]. Zacharatos *et al.* (1983) [12] also determined the levels of tonin in the rat SMG and tonin release. Their results show that a tonin-like substance appears, in the ducts, late, during gestation, where it is present at high levels in the adult. They also found that tonin amount in females increases during lactation; the granules are discharged during stimulation and are rapidly replaced [12]. Lis and collaborators (1977) [9] verified that hypophysectomy led to a sharp drop of tonin activity, whereas adrenalectomy, thyroidectomy, and gonadectomy have little effect. Treatment of hypophysectomized male rats with growth hormone and testosterone restored tonin activity. Treatment with prolactin, alone or in combination with testosterone had no effect in hypophysectomized animals [9]. Shih and collaborators (1986) [13] found that levels of immunoreactive tonin in rat SMG decrease after castration and was restored after treatment with testosterone. These data show that tonin is an androgen-dependent enzyme [13].

Data obtained by Garcia *et al.* (1983) [14] show that tonin is released into the bloodstream and saliva after beta-adrenergic stimulation. The results of these authors showed that synthesis and release of tonin in SMG increase by beta-adrenergic stimulation, and that these effects are mediated by cAMP [14]. On the other hand, Hirata and collaborators, in 1986 [15], determined the *in vitro* secretion of immunoreactive tonin from dispersed rat submandibular gland cells and observed that tonin release is stimulated by norepinephrine, epinephrine, and phenylephrine. They observed also that phentolamine, but not propranolol, inhibited this effect. Isoproterenol, carbachol, histamine, and serotonin do not stimulate tonin release. A very interesting result obtained by these authors is that removal of Ca^{2+} from the medium or addition of selective calcium channel blockers inhibited the stimulatory effect elicited by alpha- adrenergic agonists. Tonin release was stimulated by the cation ionophore A23187, in the presence of Ca^{2+}, but not Mg^{2+}. They concluded that the *in vitro* secretion of tonin from rat SMG is initiated by activation of alpha-adrenergic receptors and apparently involves a mechanism dependent not on cyclic adenosine 3',5'-monophosphate, but on the influx of extracellular Ca^{2+} [15].

The presence of tonin in rat brain was first described by Woodley-Miller *et al.* (1987) [8]. These authors determined, by direct radioimmunoassay, the levels of the enzyme in some tissues including the brain. They found that the levels of brain immunoreactive tonin are approximately 0.12 ng/mg of protein, in the order of 106-times lower than that found in the SMG [8]. In a study developed by Lopes *et al.* (1997) [16], it was found that tonin is expressed in various brain regions of the rat. Tonin activity is present in the adenohypophysis, neurohypophysis, cerebellum, hypothalamus, medulla, pons, and midbrain. The highest values of specific tonin activity were found in the neurohypophysis and in the archicerebellum. The highest level of total tonin activity was observed in the archicerebellum which retained 97% of total tonin activity of whole cerebellum [16]. More recently, it was determined the expression levels of tonin in rat brain regions. The tonin mRNA was detected in the anterior pituitary, diencephalon rostral, pons astrocytes and medulla [17].

The determination of tonin activity in plasma is difficult due the fact the enzyme is bound to a strong inhibitor. This inhibitor is a protein which was isolated from rat plasma by Tremblay *et al.* (1981) [18], who reported its molecular mass of approximately 360 kDa, and characterized as a α1-macroglobulin, the major circulating proteinase inhibitor of the rat. An assay to determine the levels of tonin in plasma and various tissue homogenates was described by Johansen and collaborators, in 1987 [7]. Using tonin specific antibody, these authors showed that the levels of immunoreactive tonin in normal blood plasma from adult male rat is 0.90 ± 0.53 ng/mL, which decrease after removal of SMG. They also observed that tonin in the plasma is bound to one inhibitor with a molecular mass around 650,000-750,000 Da [7]. Probably the difference in molecular mass of the inhibitor observed by these authors and that observed by Tremblay *et al.* (1981) [18] is due the fact that alpha-macroglobulins are able to form dimers. The enzymatic activity of tonin-α1-macroglobulin complex was studied *in vitro* and *in vivo* by Ikeda *et al.* (1988) [19]. The complex can quantitatively hydrolyze angiotensin I and the synthetic tridecapeptide renin substrate to form angiotensin II. These results suggest that tonin bound to α1-macroglobulin in the plasma keeps the active site intact and therefore may be linked to some forms of hypertension through angiotensin II formation [19].

Using 125I-labeled tonin, Morris and Cheng (1982) [20] determined the clearance and metabolism of tonin in the rat. They verified that radio iodinated tonin immediately bound to α1-macroglobulin. The clearing of tonin-α1-macroglobulin complex was in a biexponential manner being 1.8 ± 0.1 min the t1/2 of the fast component and 84 ± 10 min for the slow component. So, it seems that tonin circulates as a complex with α1-macroglobulin, which is quickly eliminated from the bloodstream by tissue uptake and metabolism [20].

Biophysics of Tonin

Tonin has been purified from rat SMG and human tissue by conventional methods [3, 5, 18, 21], affinity chromatography [22, 23] and by isoelectric focusing chromatography [24]. In rat tissue, tonin is present as a single polypeptide chain containing 272 amino acids. The molecular mass of tonin, determined by electrophoresis on polyacrylamide gel is of the order of 27 kDa. It has an optimum pH for activity around 6.8 for both Ang I and for AG(1-14) as substrates. Its activity is not dependent on chloride ions, is not affected by pepstatin A, angiotensin-converting enzyme inhibitors, as ethylenediamine tetraacetic acid (EDTA) and dipyridyl, but is inhibited by serine proteinase inhibitors. Although it is inhibited by serine proteinase inhibitors, tonin presents some resistance to inhibition by diisopropylfluorophosphate (DFP) [6]. Tonin presents high homology with other enzymes of the serine proteinases family as γ-subunit of the epidermal growth factor binding protein (EGF-BPs), prostate specific antigen (PSA) and kallikrein enzyme in which presents around 80% homology [25]. This led to the hypothesis that tonin may not be as specific as observed by some authors, although it is more resistant to inhibition by DFP as compared to other serine proteinases. In addition to release Ang II, tonin also showed able to cleave beta-lipotropin (LPH) into beta-LPH (l-50), l-51, 51-60, 52-60, 61-78 and 79-91 fragments, to selectively release the segment beta-LPH 61-78 with opiate-like activity [26]. In a similar way it acts upon adrenocorticotropic hormone (ACTH), releasing ACTH(l-8), l-7, 3-8, 3-7 and 9-39 fragments [26]. It is also able to degrade substance P hydrolyzing Arg-Xxx and Phe-Xxx bonds presenting trypsin-chymotrypsin-like activity [3, 27]. Investigating the substrate specificity of tonin, Moreau and collaborators, in 1995 [28], using synthetic peptides which reproduce the region of the activation site of rat pro-atrial natriuretic peptide (ANP), as substrates verified that tonin is able to cleave pro-ANP to generate ANP.

Tonin is an esteroproteinase. It hydrolyzes benzoyl-arginine ethyl ester, benzoyl-arginine methyl ester, tosyl-arginine methyl ester, benzoyl-arginine p-nitroanilide and other small synthetic substrates at an optimum pH of 9.0 [29]. Although capable of hydrolyzing different bonds involving residues Phe or Arg, tonin seems to be more specific than chymotrypsin and trypsin, since the hydrolysis of the above mentioned bonds appears to involve conformational factors as observed by Pesquero *et al.* (1982) [3]. These authors verified that bradykinin is not inactivated by tonin and that the hydrolysis of Phe. His bond of angiotensin I and from synthetic substrates homologues to the tetradecapeptide depends on a minimum sequence around the scissile bond.

The mechanism of action of serine proteinases is explained by the presence of histidine, aspartic acid and serine residues in the active center, forming a catalytic pocket, which is also present in the active center of tonin [30, 31]. According to these authors, although tonin presents tryptic-chymotryptic activity, its specificity is quite different, because it seems to act on peptide bonds involving the carboxyl residues of phenylalanine, arginine, lysine, tyrosine and tryptophan specifically located, in agreement with the results of Pesquero *et al.* (1982) [3]. The X-ray crystallographic structure of tonin, at 1.8 A, resolution was reported by Fuginaga and James in 1987 [32]. The initial phases were obtained using the structure of bovine trypsin as the search model. The structure of the enzyme that was determined is not in its active conformation, but one perturbed by the binding with Zn^{2+} in the active site. Tonin presents tertiary structural homology with kallikrein. These authors observed that the differences in the structures of the two enzymes are concentrated in several loop regions and these structural differences are probably responsible for the differences in their reactivity and specificity [32].

In the pure form, and having Ang I as substrate, tonin is capable to release Ang II at a rate of 14.1 micromole per minute and milligram of protein [3]. Tonin cleaves Ang II from the human plasma AG at an optimum pH of 5.0-5.5, and 1 nanomole of the enzyme is able to release Ang II at a rate of 26 nmol/hour, while 1 nanomole of renin, at optimum pH, is able to cleave the human angiotensinogen to liberate Ang I at the rate of 1320 nanomole per hour [2]. Kinetic studies with rat renin and tonin upon AG and AG(1-14) as substrates were performed by Gutkowska *et al.* (1984) [33]. The Km for renin, determined at the optimum pH, was 2.8 +/- 0.03 μM for AG and 28.8 +/- 2.69 μM for AG(1-14). The Km for tonin was 0.66 +/- 0.18 μM for AG and 2.33 +/- 0.42 μM for AG(1-14). Tonin shows higher affinity to AG and AG(1-14), however the turnover number of AG observed with renin (0.87 s^{-1}) is more than 3700 times higher than that of tonin (2.3 x 10^{-4} s^{-1}). The turnover number of AG(1-14) for renin and tonin were similar (2.8 and 10.0 s^{-1}, respectively) [33].

Araújo *et al.* (1991) [5] purified two enzymes with tonin-simile activity from rat SMG. These enzymes were named rSMT3 and rSMT4. The physicochemical properties of rSMT4 match to that encoded by the gene rKLK2, or the tonin described by Boucher *et al.* in 1972 [1]. The amino acid sequence of the N-terminal portion of rSMT3 is identical in 38 of 39 residues of rSMT4. The only change noted was the insertion of a serine residue at position 27 of the rSMT3 (Fig. **2**) [5]. rSMT3 differs from rSMT4 in molecular mass, specific activity, pH optimum, sensitivity to serine proteinase inhibitors and it presents a potent oxytocic effect on the isolated rat uterus, which was blocked by bradykinin B2 receptor antagonist. It was verified that under optimal conditions, rSMT3 liberates kinin at a rate 19-fold greater than it releases angiotensin II [34].

rSMT4 (tonin): I-V-G-G-Y^{5}-K-C-E-K-N^{10}-S-Q-P-W-Q^{15}-V-A-V-I-N^{20}-E-Y-L-C-G^{25}-G-V-L-I-D^{30}-P-S-W-V-I^{35}-T-A-A-H...

rSMT3: I-V-G-G-Y^{5}-K-C-E-K-N^{10}-S-Q-P-W-Q^{15}-V-A-V-I-N^{20}-E-Y-L-C-G^{25}-G-S-V-L-I^{30}-D-P-S-W-V^{35}-I-T-A-A...

Fig. (2). **N-terminal sequence of rSMT3 [Araujo *et al.* 1991] and rSMT4 [tonin, Lazure *et al.*, 1987]. The amino acid serine inserted at position 27 of the rSMT3 is underlined.**

Gualberto and colleagues published, in 1992 [35], results of purification of an enzyme with tonin activity from human submandibular gland. The enzyme presents molecular mass of 110 kDa, is inhibited by phenylmethanesulfonyl fluoride (PMSF) but not by EDTA or enalaprilat. The pH optima for angiotensin II liberation using angiotensin I as substrate is 4.0, 7.0 for AG(1-14) and 8.0 for angiotensinogen. The total amount of angiotensin II generating activity in the human submandibular gland, measured at optimum conditions for tonin activity is 5,000-times smaller than that in the rat gland [35]. In a study conducted by our group, one enzyme presenting tonin activity and molecular mass of 51 kDa was purified from human placenta. Two hypothetical proteins from human genome data presented identical N-terminal sequence and molecular mass of that purified by our group. The complete amino acid sequence of these hypothetical proteins showed to belong to the serine proteinases family, since the amino acids which form the catalytic triad, typical of these enzymes, are present in positions similar to those found in other components of the family (unpublished data).

There is no in the literature, so far, any study of substrate specificity presented by human tonin. On the other hand, for rat tonin, in a study conducted by Pesquero and collaborators, and published in 1982 [3], it was found that, under similar conditions, the enzyme is able to hydrolyze the AG(1-14) at a rate three times higher than that angiotensin I, presenting greater affinity for AG(1-14) (Km = 6.7 x 10^{-6} M and 5.3 x 10^{-5} M for AG(1-14) and Ang I, respectively), showing that the chain elongation in the C-terminal direction causes the substrate to be better in terms of specificity, affecting much more the mechanism of hydrolysis than the interaction with the substrate. Moreover, shortening of the polypeptide chain from the N-terminal showed that the removal of Asp^1 residue makes better the substrate for tonin through an increase in the affinity (reduction in Km), so that the resulting peptide corresponding to portion 2-14 of angiotensinogen showed to be the best substrate for tonin [3]. On the other hand, in a study by Schiller *et al.* (1976) [4] it was found that the N-terminal portion of the substrate Asp^1-Arg^2-Val^3 is an important recognition site for binding of Ang I to tonin. In this sequence, the positively charged arginine residue is considered essential for a high rate of hydrolysis and enzyme-substrate interaction, perhaps by promoting an ionic interaction with the negatively charged site of the enzyme or by forming hydrogen bonds, or yet, by stabilizing a particular conformation of the peptide, making it a good substrate. These authors also found that the peptide des-Asp^1-angiotensin I is so good as the substrate Ang I, and that tonin is not able to hydrolyse the peptide homologous to the C-terminus of Ang I which contains in the sequence at least eight amino acid residues. They further suggested that the presence of the residue Val^3 is important in the proposed recognition site [4]. Taking into account the importance of C-terminus of Ang I for hydrolysis by tonin, the nonapeptide (des-Leu^{10})-Ang I is not substrate [1]. Combining data from Pesquero *et al.* (1982) [3], Schiller *et al.* (1976) [4] and from Boucher *et al.* (1972) [1], it can be concluded that the minimal sequence to be hydrolyzed by tonin would be the portion 5-10 of Ang I, presenting the sequence Ile-His-P-o-Phe-His-Leu [1, 3, 4]. Pesquero *et al.* (1982) [3] proposed that this would be the minimum sequence to maintain a favorable structure for tonin substrate and that this structure would be a beta-turn involving residues 6 to 9 [3].

To determine the tonin activity in glandular tissue and other tissues it has been employed the radioimmunoassay (RIA) of angiotensin II, as described by

Gualberto *et al.* (1992) [35]. For this purpose, previously the sample from the tissue supernatant is incubated in the presence of one of the substrates AG, Ang I or AG(1-14) according to the protocol established by Araujo *et al.* (1991) [5]. The pH of the buffer is always around 6.8 and this buffer should contain inhibitors of ACE and other peptidases and the amount of Ang II released during the incubation period determined by RIA [35].

Functiona Analysis of Tonin

Tonin was described as an Ang II releasing enzyme, therefore, since its discovery tonin has been studied in order to verify its participation in hypertensive process. Some studies have shown that tonin may actually be involved in the genesis and maintenance of hypertension. The first studies presenting results relating tonin with hypertensive process were published the Genest and collaborators [36 - 38]. In this paper the authors show that: a) the levels of tonin activity in the plasma are increased in humans with essential and renovascular hypertension, b) infusion of tonin intravenously in mice does not alter blood pressure, however, in indomethacin salt- treated rats a marked increase in arterial blood pressure was observed c) a single intravenous administration of rabbit anti-tonin antiserum into one-kidney one-clip hypertensive rats restored blood pressure to normal. These authors suggest that tonin is important in the maintenance of high blood pressure, however, other factors, possibly prostaglandins and sodium, have to be modified in order to activate the tonin-angiotensin II system.

In 1980, Kondo and collaborators [39] determined the effects of intracerebro-ventricular administration of tonin on water intake and blood pressure in the rat. They verified that injection of tonin in the brain stimulated water intake and increased blood pressure. These responses were not affected by an ACE inhibitor but abolished by administration of an Ang II antagonist. They concluded that tonin may participate in the regulation of water balance and blood pressure through local and direct generation of Ang II in the central nervous system [39]. Similar results were obtained by Araujo *et al.* (2002) [17] who also injected purified tonin into rat brain. These authors observed that central microinjection of tonin produced elevation of blood pressure, heart rate, water and saline intake, urinary volume and salt excretion, effects partially blocked by losartan, indicating that tonin induced a central Ang II formation. These results suggest that tonin may be a pathway to Ang II generation in the rat brain and may participate in the physiological effects exerted by Ang II.

In a very important work, Schiffrin and collaborators (1981) [40] injected tonin intravenously in anephric rats and verified that after bilateral nephrectomy tonin produced a pressor effect in these animals. The effect was abolished by [Sar^1-Ala^8]-Ang II, an antagonist of angiotensin II. The levels of Ang II in the plasma increased after tonin injection and decreased biexponentially with a half-life of less than 1 min for the fast component and 9 min for the slow component and correlated with blood pressure. These authors verified that incubating tonin with plasma as substrate, *in vitro*, the initial rate of Ang II generation increased after addition of renin substrate. In nephrectomized rabbits, a pressor effect was produced by tonin, which was not observed in intact rabbits. These data demonstrate the *in vivo* production of Ang II by tonin. Schiffrin and collaborators concluded that these results suggest a role for substrate concentration for tonin activity *in vivo* [40].

Other studies which show that tonin may produce the vasoconstrictor peptide Ang II *in vivo*, and the relationship between aldosterone and tonin, was published by Schiffrin and colleagues (1981, 1983) [41, 42]. These researchers infused tonin intravenously over 2 hours at a rate of 12 μg/kg/min in conscious rats, and found that the levels of secretion of both aldosterone and corticosterone were increased while plasma renin activity significantly reduced in this group. Another observation from these studies is that tonin infusion induces ACTH secretion which contributes to the adrenal response. In chronically hypophysectomized rats, the concentration of aldosterone in the plasma remained unchanged after tonin infusion. The authors concluded that the failure of tonin to stimulate aldosterone in hypophysectomized animals indicates the participation of a pituitary hormone, probably ACTH, in the effect of tonin on adrenal secretion [39, 40]. Lis and collaborators (1977) [9] verified a marked increase in tonin activity in animals bearing MtT-F4 transplantable tumors, known to produce ACTH [9].

The direct effect of tonin was demonstrated by Garcia and collaborators in 1981 [43]. They showed that tonin is able to potentiate the contraction induced by norephinefrine in mesenteric and aortic strips from hypertensive and normotensive rats and rabbits and that saralasin did not inhibit such effect which suggests that Ang II is not the mediator. Indomethacin and alpha- or beta-adrenergic blockers were not able to change the direct contraction or the potentiation of contraction which was blocked by Db-cAMP and theophylline. Ca^{2+}-free medium, La^{3+}, and verapamil inhibited the direct tonin-induced contraction by 75%. Garcia and collaborators suggest that the vasoactive effect of tonin may be mediated by the release of intracellular-bound calcium, an effect dependent on a proteolytic action of tonin, and by increasing the cellular permeability to calcium [43].

In order to clarify the importance of tonin for the cardiovascular system, Cardoso *et al.* (2010) [44], generated a transgenic mice which express rat tonin, the TGM(rTon). These mice present high levels of tonin mRNA and activity specifically in the brain. Plasma Ang II is increased in TGM(rTon) as compared to the wild type. TGM(rTon) presents increased blood pressure and water intake. Lisinopril, an ACE inhibitor, is less hypotensive for TGM(rTon) than for control animals. Candesartan, an AT1 receptor antagonist, equally lowers blood pressure in TGM(rTon) and in control mice. Cardoso and collaborators concluded that tonin may represent, in the brain, an alternative pathway to generate Ang II with effects on the cardiovascular system [44].

Ang II and its metabolite Ang-(1-7) produce antinociception in pain animal models. Recently, Pacheco *et al.* (2013) [45] investigated the nociceptive behavior of TGM(rTon). Nociception was evaluated using the thermal tail-flick and chemical acetic acid writhing tests, and the drugs were administered by intracerebroventricular and subcutaneous pathways, respectively. The results demonstrated that TGM(rTon) presents an antinociceptive effect. Losartan, an AT1 receptor antagonist and A-779 [D-Ala7-Ang-(1-7)], a Mas receptor antagonist attenuated the antinociceptive behavior. These data suggest that the *in vivo* produced Ang II induces antinociception.

Tonin and Cardiac Hypertrophy

Borges and collaborators, in 2003 [46], investigated the possible involvement of tonin on cardiac hypertrophy. Tonin, renin, ACE and AG expression and activity in the heart rat with isoproterenol-induced hypertrophy were determined in the whole heart, atria (left + right) and ventricles. In this study Wistar rats were treated with isoproterenol (ISO) during seven days (5 mg/kg/day – sc). After ISO treatment the levels of tonin specific activity increased 2-fold in the atria but not in the ventricles. Renin expression was not detectable in these structures and ACE expression levels did not change by treatment. Angiotensinogen expression was detected in the left ventricle at very low levels when compared to the atria and increased significantly only in the hypertrophied atria (1.8-fold). Tonin mRNA was not detected in the ventricle but was found at low levels in the atria which increased after isoproterenol treatment. With these results the authors conclude that tonin may play a role on the process of heart hypertrophy in the rat [46].

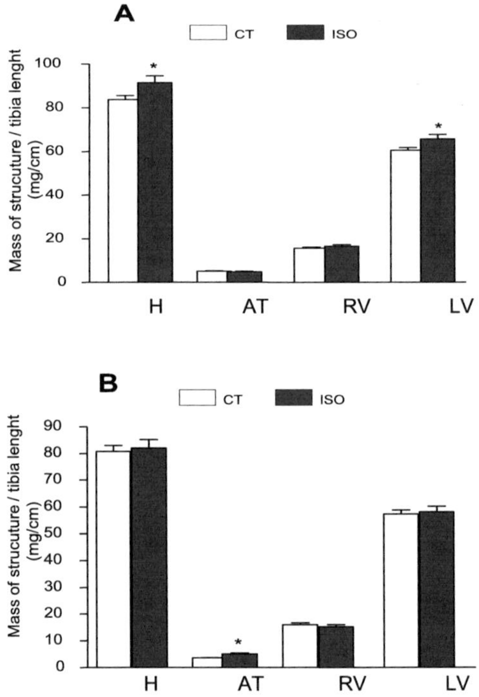

Fig. (3). Specific mass of heart structures, expressed in milligrams/centimeter, after treatment of WT [A] and TGM[rTon] [B] with isoproterenol [ISO] or oil [CT]. H = whole heart, AT = atria, RV = right ventricle and LV = left ventricle. Data are expressed as mean ± SEM. *p < 0.05 *vs.* oil.

Very recently we verified that tonin is able to generate the vasoconstrictor peptide Ang II in the rat isolated heart. The cardiovascular response induced by tonin in the rat heart was completely blocked by candesartan, an indication that the action of Ang II on AT1 receptors is the major mechanism of the heart effects [47].

The generation of the transgenic model TGM(rTon) gave us excellent opportunity to reinforce the importance of tonin on the cardiac hypertrophy. Therefore, the TGM(rTon) was treated with ISO or mineral oil (control) and the parameters body mass, heart mass and the specific heart mass were determined. The hypertrophy was monitored by cardiac index (heart mass/tibia length) and by atrium natriuretic peptide (ANP) expression on the left ventricle of animals. We used the length of the tibia of animals as a control parameter for determining the specific mass of the various structures of the heart [48]. The results in terms of specific mass for different structures (structure mass/tibia length) are shown in Table **1** and were utilized in the construction of Fig. (**3**), where it is possible to verify in which structure(s) hypertrophy is present. From Table **1** we can observe that the length of the tibia for the animals treated with ISO were 1.55 ± 0.01 cm and 1.56 ± 0.01 cm for TGM(rTon) and wild type (WT), respectively. The values observed when the animals were treated with oil are 1.60 ± 0.02 cm and 1.62 ± 0.01 cm, respectively, for TGM(rTon) and WT. After treatment with ISO the specific cardiac mass of transgenic group was significantly lower than that observed for the WT (82 ± 3.2 *vs.* 91.5 ± 5.3 $mg.cm^{-1}$ for the TGM(rTon) and WT, respectively). For the WT animals, we observed a larger difference in the specific mass of different cardiac structures between treated and control groups which increased 7.7 $mg.cm^{-1}$ for the heart, as compared with the increase of 1.3 $mg.cm^{-1}$ verified for TGM(rTon) group. It means that, apparently the animal TGM(rTon) presents greater resistance to develop hypertrophy when compared to WT. With respect to the atria, it is interesting to note that the specific mass for the WT group is not different considering the treatments, but for the transgenic group the values obtained for the treatment with ISO is significantly higher (3.61 ± 0.14 *vs.* 5.07 ± 0.40 $mg.cm^{-1}$, oil *vs.* ISO, respectively). Another interesting fact is related to the values of specific mass observed for the LV. While in the WT group, the treatment with ISO has led to a significant increase in the specific mass of LV (60.54 ± 1.28 $mg.cm^{-1}$ *vs* 65.7 ± 1.97 $mg.cm^{-1}$, oil *vs.* ISO, respectively), in transgenic animal, the data again show protection against hypertrophy, being the values 57.27 ± 1.53 $mg.cm^{-1}$ *vs.* 58.03 ± 2.07 $mg.cm^{-1}$, oil *vs.* ISO, respectively.

Table 1. Mass and specific mass of cardiac structures after treatment of WT or TGM(rTon) with isoproterenol (ISO) or oil.

GROUP	Mass and specific mass																	
	Oil									ISO								
	Tibia	H	Hs	AT	Ats	RV	Rvs	LV	Lvs	Tibia	H	Hs	AT	ATs	RV	RVs	LV	LVs
WT	1.62	135	83.8	8.18	5.07	25.1	15.56	97.74	60.54	1.56	140	91.5*	7.32	4.82	25.27	16.60	100.6	65.7*
	±0.01	±3.0	±1.8	±0.30	±0.20	±0.92	±0.57	±2.11	±1.28	±0.01	±4.6	±3.05	±0.34	±0.24	±1.07	±0.71	±2.90	±1.97
TGM(rTon)	1.60	130	80.7	5.86	3.61	25.55	15.9	92.16	57.27	1.55	130	82.0	8.00	5.07*	23.98	15.16	90.45	58.03
	±0.02	±3.2	±2.28	±0.24	±0.14	±1.04	±0.76	±2.47	±1.53	±0.01	±5.9	±3.2	±0.62	±0.40	±1.34	±0.79	±3.51	±2.07

Values of mass expressed in milligrams and specific mass in milligrams/centimeter. H=whole heart, AT = atria, RV = right ventricle and LV = left ventricle. Hs, Ats, Rvs and Lvs indicate the respective specific mass. Data are expressed as mean ± SEM. *p<0.05 *vs* oil.

FINAL REMARKS

Worldwide, the highest rates of morbidity and mortality result from cardiovascular diseases such as hypertension, myocardial infarction, heart and kidney failure, as well as cerebrovascular diseases. Because of this, extensive studies have been conducted for the development of effective drugs, focused on the renin-angiotensin system, from which the peptide Ang II is the active component. It is not known yet the relative importance of each Ang II forming pathway present in different tissues, however, strong evidences clearly indicate a role for other enzymes in the generation of Ang II in addition to ACE and renin. This is the case of some neurons in the brain, where most of Ang II may be formed by other enzymes. Although it has been demonstrated the presence of all components of the RAS in the brain, yet it was not possible to demonstrate their co-location in the same brain region. The levels of renin and Ang I into the cerebrospinal fluid (CEF) are very low in contrast to the high levels of angiotensinogen, whose concentration is of the order of thousand times higher than Ang I. Some authors suggest that the AG in the brain is of glial origin. These authors observed that astrocytes are the major source of AG in the brain [49, 50]. Another intriguing factor is the expression of renin in the brain. Renin is present in the cortex and brainstem and the renin mRNA is weakly detectable in these regions. The putative areas for expression of angiotensinogen mRNA are the hypothalamus, basal ganglia, septum, amygdala, cortex, nucleus of the solitary tract (NTS) and preoptic area. The levels of renin mRNA in these areas are very low, indicating that the renin may not be involved in the synthesis of angiotensin II in the brain. Another possibility which confirms the previous one is that the Ang I levels in the brain are lower than in plasma [51].

It has been shown that in human heart tissues ACE inhibitors block only 10 to 20% of Ang I conversion and the remaining activity is blocked by serine proteinase inhibitors. ACE inhibitors only partially reduce vessel wall Ang II production, while chymostatin, a strong inhibitor of many proteinases, including chymotrypsin and chymotrypsin-like serine proteinases, is able to completely block the conversion of Ang I to Ang II in human arteries. Wolny *et al.* (1997) [52] verified an incomplete ACE inhibition in human heart tissue after chronic ACE inhibitor therapy. They verified also that ACE contributes only to a small portion of the total Ang I conversion being a serine proteinase responsible for the majority of Ang II production in both the membrane preparation and Ang I–induced contractions of isolated coronary arteries. These authors conclude that, in humans, a serine proteinase pathway is likely to play an important role in cardiac Ang II formation [52]. Combination therapy of ACE inhibition and AT1 receptor blockade has provide greater renoprotection than ACE inhibitor alone in human diabetic nephropathy, which suggest that blockade of formation of Ang II by ACE-independent pathways are of major significance in disease progression [53].

It is known that tonin can act *in vitro* upon other molecules of biological importance such as ANP, beta-LPH and ACTH. Does this action happens in the biological system and if so what would be the role of tonin in these biological pathways? What is the role of tonin in saliva? The animal TGM(rTon) can help us answer these questions.

CONFLICT OF INTEREST

The authors confirm that they have no conflict of interest to declare for this publication.

AKNOWLEDGEMENTS

CNPq [Conselho Nacional de Pesquisa], Fapemig [Fundação de Amparo a Pesquisa do Estado de Minas Gerais] and Fapesp [Fundação de Amparo a Pesquisa do Estado de Sao Paulo].

REFERENCES

[1] Boucher RS, Genest J. A new Angiotensin I converting enzyme system. In: Genest J, Koiw E, Eds. Hypertension 72. Springer-Verlag 1972; pp. 521-3.

[2] Grisé C, Boucher R, Thibault G, Genest J. Formation of angiotensin II by tonin from partially purified human angiotensinogen. Can J Biochem 1981; 59(4): 250-5. [http://dx.doi.org/10.1139/o81-034] [PMID: 6265047]

[3] Pesquero JL, Boschcov P, Oliveira MC, Paiva AC. Effect of substrate size on tonin activity. Biochem Biophys Res Commun 1982; 108(4): 1441-6. [http://dx.doi.org/10.1016/S0006-291X(82)80068-5] [PMID: 6295383]

[4] Schiller PW, Demassieux S, Boucher R. Substrate specificity of tonin from rat submaxillary gland. Circ Res 1976; 39(5): 629-32. [http://dx.doi.org/10.1161/01.RES.39.5.629] [PMID: 184974]

[5] Araujo GW, Pesquero JB, Lindsey CJ, Paiva AC, Pesquero JL. Identification of serine proteinases with tonin-like activity in the rat submandibular and prostate glands. Biochim Biophys Acta 1991; 1074(1): 167-71. [http://dx.doi.org/10.1016/0304-4165(91)90056-M] [PMID: 1646031]

[6] Boucher R, Asselin J, Genest J. A new enzyme leading to the direct formation of angiotensin II. Circ Res 1974; 34/35: I-203-12.

[7] Johansen L, Berg T, Bergundhaugen H, Nustad K, Scicli AG, Carretero OA. Excess antibody immunoassay for the measurement of tonin in rat tissues and plasma. J Immunol Methods 1987; 98(2): 257-65. [http://dx.doi.org/10.1016/0022-1759(87)90013-5] [PMID: 3033082]

[8] Woodley-Miller C, Chao J, Chao L. Identification of tonin in brain and exocrine tissues and in the cell-free translation products encoded by the mRNA of these tissues. Biochem J 1987; 248(2): 477-81. [http://dx.doi.org/10.1042/bj2480477] [PMID: 2829829]

[9] Lis M, Boucher R, Chrétien M, Genest J. Dependence of tonin activity in rat submaxillary gland on growth hormone and testosterone. Am J Physiol 1977; 232(5): E522-5. [PMID: 193408]

[10] Orstavik TB, Carretero OA, Hayashi H, Scicli GA, Johansen L. Immunohistochemical localization of tonin and its relation to kallikrein in rat salivary glands. J Histochem Cytochem 1982; 30(11): 1123-9. [http://dx.doi.org/10.1177/30.11.6292285] [PMID: 6292285]

[11] Ledoux S, Gutkowska J, Garcia R, Thibault G, Cantin M, Genest J. Immunohistochemical localization of tonin in rat salivary glands and kidney. Histochemistry 1982; 76(3): 329-39. [http://dx.doi.org/10.1007/BF00543955] [PMID: 6186645]

[12] Zacharatos DT, Vasak EZ, Cheng ES, van Lennep EW, Morris BJ. Immunohistochemistry of tonin in rat submandibular gland during development, lactation and secretion. Histochemistry 1983; 79(3): 433-42.
[http://dx.doi.org/10.1007/BF00491778] [PMID: 6317619]

[13] Shih HC, Chao L, Chao J. Age and hormonal dependence of tonin levels in rat submandibular gland as determined by a new direct radioimmunoassay. Biochem J 1986; 238(1): 145-9. [eng.].
[http://dx.doi.org/10.1042/bj2380145] [PMID: 3026337]

[14] Garcia R, Thibault G, Gutkowska J, Genest J. Release of tonin and of kallikrein by perfused rat submaxillary gland. Am J Physiol 1983; 244(2): R228-34.
[PMID: 6297317]

[15] Hirata Y, Tomita M, Fujita T, Ikeda M. *In vitro* secretion of immunoreactive tonin from dispersed rat submandibular gland cells. Hypertension 1986; 8(10): 883-9.
[http://dx.doi.org/10.1161/01.HYP.8.10.883] [PMID: 3019887]

[16] Lopes ES, Sumitani M, Juliano L, Beraldo WT, Pesquero JL. Distribution of tonin- and kallikrein-like activities in rat brain. Brain Res 1997; 769(1): 152-7.
[http://dx.doi.org/10.1016/S0006-8993(97)00785-3] [PMID: 9374283]

[17] Araujo RC, Lima MP, Lomez ES, *et al.* Tonin expression in the rat brain and tonin-mediated central production of angiotensin II. Physiol Behav 2002; 76(2): 327-33.
[http://dx.doi.org/10.1016/S0031-9384(02)00720-5] [PMID: 12044607]

[18] Tremblay J, Thibault G, Gutkowska J, Boucher R, Genest J. Purification and partial characterization of a plasma inhibitor of tonin. Can J Biochem 1981; 59(4): 256-61.
[http://dx.doi.org/10.1139/o81-035] [PMID: 6265048]

[19] Ikeda M, Sasaguri M, Maruta H, Arakawa K. Formation of angiotensin II by tonin-inhibitor complex. Hypertension 1988; 11(1): 63-70.
[http://dx.doi.org/10.1161/01.HYP.11.1.63] [PMID: 2448241]

[20] Morris BJ, Cheng ES. Clearance and metabolism of 125I-labeled tonin in the rat. Endocrinology 1982; 111(5): 1462-8.
[http://dx.doi.org/10.1210/endo-111-5-1462] [PMID: 6181985]

[21] Demassieux S, Boucher R, Crise C, Genest J. Purification and characterization of tonin. Can J Biochem 1976; 54(9): 788-95.
[http://dx.doi.org/10.1139/o76-113] [PMID: 9189]

[22] Ikeda M, Arakawa K. Purification of tonin by chromatography using soybean trypsin inhibitor coupled CH-sepharose 4B. Jpn Circ J 1981; 45(9): 1083-9.
[http://dx.doi.org/10.1253/jcj.45.1083] [PMID: 6271996]

[23] Ikeda M, Gutkowska J, Thibault G, Boucher R, Genest J. Purification of tonin by affinity chromatography. Hypertension 1981; 3(1): 81-6.
[http://dx.doi.org/10.1161/01.HYP.3.1.81] [PMID: 6259060]

[24] Cheng ES, Morris BJ. A simple method of isolating tonin using chromatofocusing. Anal Biochem 1982; 126(2): 295-300.
[http://dx.doi.org/10.1016/0003-2697(82)90518-8] [PMID: 6760739]

[25] Seidah NG, Routhier R, Caron M, *et al.* N-Terminal amino acid sequence of rat tonin: homology with serine proteases. Can J Biochem 1978; 56(9): 920-5. [http://dx.doi.org/10.1139/o78-142] [PMID: 215293]

[26] Seidah NG, Chan JS, Mardini G, *et al.* Specific cleavage of beta-LPH and ACTH by tonin: release of an opiate-like peptide beta-LPH (61-78). Biochem Biophys Res Commun 1979; 86(4): 1002-13. [http://dx.doi.org/10.1016/0006-291X(79)90217-1] [PMID: 219857]

[27] Chrétien M, Lee CM, Sandberg BE, *et al.* Substrate specificity of the enzyme tonin: cleavage of substance P. FEBS Lett 1980; 113(2): 173-6. [http://dx.doi.org/10.1016/0014-5793(80)80585-0] [PMID: 6156083]

[28] Moreau T, Brillard-Bourdet M, Chagas J, Gauthier F. Pro-rat atrial natriuretic peptide-mimicking peptides as substrates for rat kallikreins rK2 (tonin) and rK9. Biochim Biophys Acta 1995; 1249(2): 168-72. [http://dx.doi.org/10.1016/0167-4838(95)00038-V] [PMID: 7599170]

[29] Thibault G, Genest J. Tonin, an esteroprotease from rat submaxillary glands. Biochim Biophys Acta 1981; 660(1): 23-9. [http://dx.doi.org/10.1016/0005-2744(81)90103-0] [PMID: 6268171]

[30] Lazure C, Leduc R, Seidah NG, Thibault G, Genest J, Chrétien M. The complete amino acid sequence of rat submaxillary gland tonin does contain the aspartic acid at the active site: confirmation by protein sequence analysis. Biochem Cell Biol 1987; 65(4): 321-37. [http://dx.doi.org/10.1139/o87-042] [PMID: 3038148]

[31] Lazure C, Seidah NG, Thibault G, Boucher R, Genest J, Chrétien M. Sequence homologies between tonin, nerve growth factor gamma-subunit, epidermal growth factor-binding protein and serine proteases. Nature 1981; 292(5821): 383-4. [http://dx.doi.org/10.1038/292383a0] [PMID: 6265796]

[32] Fujinaga M, James MN. Rat submaxillary gland serine protease, tonin. Structure solution and refinement at 1.8 A resolution. J Mol Biol 1987; 195(2): 373-96. [http://dx.doi.org/10.1016/0022-2836(87)90658-9] [PMID: 2821276]

[33] Gutkowska J, Corvol P, Figueiredo AF, Inagami T, Bouhnik J, Genest J. Kinetic studies of rat renin and tonin on purified rat angiotensinogen. Canadian journal of biochemistry and cell biology = Revue canadienne de biochimie et biologie cellulaire 1984; 62(2-3): 137-42. [http://dx.doi.org/10.1139/o84-020] [PMID: 6097352]

[34] Araujo GW, Silva AM, Pesquero JB, Lindsey CJ, Beraldo WT, Pesquero JL. Kininogenase activity of rSMT3, a rat submandibular gland tonin. Agents Actions Suppl 1992; 38(Pt 3): 23-30. [PMID: 1334352]

[35] Gualberto MP, Nunes RL, Beraldo WT, Pesquero JL. Tonin-like activity present in the human submandibular gland. Agents Actions Suppl 1992; 38(Pt 1): 392-400. [PMID: 1334624]

[36] Boucher R, Garcia R, Gutkowska J, Demassieux S, Genest J. Tonin--angiotensin II system in hypertension. Clin Sci Mol Med Suppl 1978; 4: 183s-6s. [PMID: 215373]

[37] Garcia R, Boucher R, Gutkowska J, Kondo K, Demassieux S, Genest J. Effect of antitonin on blood pressure in the one-kidney hypertensive rat. Clin Sci Mol Med 1978; 54(4): 457-61. [eng.]. [PMID: 205386]

[38] Garcia R, Schiffrin EL, Gutkowska J, Boucher R, Genest J. Reduction of hypertension in one-kidney one-clip rabbits by immunization with tonin. Proc Soc Exp Biol Med 1979; 162(2): 245-8. [http://dx.doi.org/10.3181/00379727-162-40658] [PMID: 229482]

[39] Kondo K, Garcia R, Boucher R, Genest J. Effects of intracerebroventricular administration of tonin on water intake and blood pressure in the rat. Brain Res 1980; 200(2): 437-41. [http://dx.doi.org/10.1016/0006-8993(80)90932-4] [PMID: 6158365]

[40] Schiffrin EL, Garcia R, Gutkowska J, Boucher R, Genest J. Pressor effect of tonin in anephric animals. Can J Physiol Pharmacol 1981; 59(8): 864-71. [http://dx.doi.org/10.1139/y81-129] [PMID: 6271377]

[41] Schiffrin EL, Garcia R, Gutkowska J, Lis M, Genest J. Effects of tonin on the adrenal secretion in the rat. Hypertension 1981; 3(6 Pt 2): II-9-II-13. [PMID: 6271674]

[42] Schiffrin EL, Garcia R, Gutkowska J, Genest J. Role of the pituitary in the effects of tonin on adrenal secretion of the rat. Can J Physiol Pharmacol 1983; 61(3): 201-6. [http://dx.doi.org/10.1139/y83-031] [PMID: 6301666]

[43] Garcia R, Schiffrin EL, Thibault G, Genest J. Effects of tonin, an angiotensin II-forming enzyme, on vascular smooth muscle in the normal rabbit. Hypertension 1981; 3(3 Pt 2): I101-6. [http://dx.doi.org/10.1161/01.HYP.3.3_Pt_2.I101] [PMID: 6266953]

[44] Cardoso CC, Alenina N, Ferreira AJ, *et al.* Increased blood pressure and water intake in transgenic mice expressing rat tonin in the brain. Biol Chem 2010; 391(4): 435-41. [http://dx.doi.org/10.1515/bc.2010.040] [PMID: 20180641]

[45] Pacheco DF, Pacheco CM, Lima MP, *et al.* Antinociceptive response in transgenic mice expressing rat tonin. Eur J Pharmacol 2013; 713(1-3): 1-5. [http://dx.doi.org/10.1016/j.ejphar.2013.04.032] [PMID: 23665491]

[46] Borges JC, Silva JA Jr, Gomes MA, *et al.* Tonin in rat heart with experimental hypertrophy. Am J Physiol Heart Circ Physiol 2003; 284(6): H2263-8. [http://dx.doi.org/10.1152/ajpheart.00416.2002] [PMID: 12543632]

[47] Damasceno DD, Lima MP, Motta DF, *et al.* Cardiovascular and electrocardiographic parameters after tonin administration in Wistar rats. Regul Pept 2013; 181: 30-6. [http://dx.doi.org/10.1016/j.regpep.2012.12.009] [PMID: 23318501]

[48] Yin FC, Spurgeon HA, Rakusan K, Weisfeldt ML, Lakatta EG. Use of tibial length to quantify cardiac hypertrophy: application in the aging rat. Am J Physiol 1982; 243(6): H941-7. [PMID: 6216817]

[49] Deschepper CF, Bouhnik J, Ganong WF. Colocalization of angiotensinogen and glial fibrillary acidic protein in astrocytes in rat brain. Brain Res 1986; 374(1): 195-8. [http://dx.doi.org/10.1016/0006-8993(86)90411-7] [PMID: 3521789]

[50] O'Callaghan EL, Bassi JK, Porrello ER, Delbridge LM, Thomas WG, Allen AM. Regulation of angiotensinogen by angiotensin II in mouse primary astrocyte cultures. J Neurochem 2011; 119(1): 18-26.
[http://dx.doi.org/10.1111/j.1471-4159.2011.07406.x] [PMID: 21797869]

[51] Dzau VJ, Ellison KE, Brody T, Ingelfinger J, Pratt RE. A comparative study of the distributions of renin and angiotensinogen messenger ribonucleic acids in rat and mouse tissues. Endocrinology 1987; 120(6): 2334-8.
[http://dx.doi.org/10.1210/endo-120-6-2334] [PMID: 3552634]

[52] Wolny A, Clozel JP, Rein J, *et al.* Functional and biochemical analysis of angiotensin II-forming pathways in the human heart. Circ Res 1997; 80(2): 219-27.
[http://dx.doi.org/10.1161/01.RES.80.2.219] [PMID: 9012744]

[53] Park S, Bivona BJ, Kobori H, *et al.* Major role for ACE-independent intrarenal ANG II formation in type II diabetes. Am J Physiol Renal Physiol 2010; 298(1): F37-48.
[http://dx.doi.org/10.1152/ajprenal.00519.2009] [PMID: 19846569]

CHAPTER 9

ACE Gene "Dosage" and Cardiovascular and Renal Disease

José Geraldo Mill[1,*], Alexandre Costa Pereira[2], Rebeca Caldeira Machado[1], Ludimila Forechi[1], Marcelo Perim Baldo[1] and **José Eduardo Krieger[2]**

[1] *Department of Physiological Sciences, Federal University of Espirito Santo, Vitória, Espirito Santo, Brazil*

[2] *Laboratory of Genetic and Molecular Cardiology, Heart Institute, University of Sao Paulo, Sao Paulo, Brazil*

Abstract: Complex phenotypes are those depending on a complex interaction between the genotype and environmental factors. Genetic studies on different human populations have shown a great variability in the genetic background due to the presence of genetic polymorphisms. The renin-angiotensin system (RAS) is closely involved in regulation of several physiological processes, such as body fluids homeostasis and blood pressure. Angiotensin-converting enzyme (ACE) plays a central role in the RAS functioning because this enzyme activates angiotensin II (Ang II) generation (vasoconstrictor) and inactivates bradykinin (vasodilator) simultaneously. ACE activity in plasma is variable in different families, and this variability is related with the genomic structure of the ACE gene dependent of a 287 base-pairs Insertion (presence) or Deletion (absence) in the DNA sequence. Variation in the number of copies of a single gene has been interpreted as representing different "dosage" of a specific gene product. Presence of D allele in ACE gene, mainly when in the DD polymorphism, has been associated with a higher generation of Ang II either in the systemic and in the local RAS leading to higher blood pressure levels and incidence of hypertension. These associations, however, have not been found in Caucasians, but are stronger in populations with Asiatic genetic background (where presence of the D allele is less frequent), such as the Amerindian populations. Individuals with DD polymorphism also have higher predisposition to development of accelerated atheroscl-

* **Corresponding author José Geraldo Mill:** Department of Physiological Sciences, Federal University of Espirito Santo, Av. Marechal Campos 1468 Vitória, ES, Brazil - 29042-755; E-mail: jgmill@npd.ufes.br.

Dulce Elena Casarini, Danielle Yuri Arita, Tatiana Sousa Cunha & Juliana Almada Colucci (Eds.)

erosis as compared with those presenting the DI and II ACE genes. However, these findings are not found in all studies because associations are generally weak and complex phenotypes, such as blood pressure levels and atherosclerosis development, depend on many genetic and environmental factors. Therefore, genetic polymorphisms may contribute to different phenotypes. Since the relationships between genes and the gene-environmental interactions are nonlinear, their practical use in medicine should be done with caution. However, they can give important insights in relation to different prevalence of diseases in populations with different genetic background.

Keywords: ACE polymorphism, Aldosterone, Angiotensinogen, Angiotensin converting enzyme, Angiotensin gene polymorphism, Angiotensin II, Atherosclerosis, Blood pressure, Bradykinin, Gene polymorphism, Hypertension, Potassium, Renin, Renin-angiotensin system, Sodium.

INTRODUCTION

The renin-angiotensin system (RAS) exerts a key role for the homeostatic regulation of the circulation since the main effector peptide of this system, angiotensin II (Ang II), are closely involved in the homeostasis of the body fluids and blood pressure. Classical components of RAS are the renin, angiotensinogen, angiotensin I (Ang I) and Ang II peptides. All effects of Ang II are mediated by its interaction with two membrane-bound receptors, named AT1 and AT2 receptors [1]. Renin is an intracellular protein produced in cells of the juxtaglomerular apparatus as a proenzyme (pro-renin). Once secreted into the plasma, the active enzyme (renin) cleaves the decapeptide Ang I from its precursor peptide angiotensinogen. Angiotensinogen is produced in many tissues and cells, but the liver accounts for the most circulating Ang I level [2]. Beyond the systemic or endocrine RAS, experimental research led to the description of several local or tissues RAS in different organs, including the brain, heart, kidneys and blood vessels [3]. Since these local systems are complete, that is, they have all the components of the systemic RAS, the entire downstream cascade of the RAS peptides can also be generated as paracrine or local secretions. Therefore, Ang I produced in plasma as well as locally in organs and tissues can be transformed locally in the highly active peptide Ang II by the angiotensin-converting enzyme (ACE). Ang II in turn shows ubiquitous actions in almost all tissues and organs of the body, particularly in the heart, blood vessels and kidneys.

The systemic RAS was originally described as a key component related to the control of body volume because Ang II shows an important participation on Na_+ and K_+ metabolism thus affecting the concentration of these minerals in the body fluids. The volume of the extracellular space and the Na_+ concentration outside and inside cells affect the systemic vascular resistance and the cardiac output, thus interfering in the long-term blood pressure regulation [1, 3 - 5]. Moreover, the local production of the biologically active peptides of the RAS has shown that, beyond their systemic effects, they exert also local regulatory actions related to the structure and function of several organs, such as the heart and blood vessels. These findings were relevant to understand the participation of some components of the RAS, mainly Ang II, in several physiological processes, such as cardiac and vascular remodeling after myocardial infarction [6, 7], the long term glomerular damages determined by diabetes and hypertension [8] and other tissue injuries occurring in several other systemic diseases, such as in sarcoidosis [9]. Ang II is the most powerful endogenous vasoconstrictor. It also retains Na_+ in the kidneys, stimulates twist and salt appetite and induces endothelial dysfunction by reducing nitric oxide availability in resistance arterioles. Furthermore, Ang II, mainly when produced locally in the heart and in the kidneys also stimulates cell proliferation and growth and the deposition of new molecules in the extracellular matrix, contributing to alter tissue structure and function. The development of orally active ACE inhibitors and lately the AT1 receptor blockers opened new perspectives for the treatment of several highly prevalent diseases, such as hypertension, heart failure, diabetic nephropathy, and others. More recently, another pathophysiologic and therapeutic perspectives are being opened with the description of physiological actions of new components of the RAS, such as angiotensin-1-7 (Ang 1-7), angiotensin converting enzyme 2 (ACE 2), angiotensin 2-5 (Ang 2-5) and MAS-receptors [10, 11]. Since all these substances are produced in many different sites of the organism, these new players may represent other important therapeutic targets with potential importance for the treatment of several diseases. However, even considering these new components of the classical RAS, ACE still represents the key step to our actual understanding of the multiple physiological and pathological processes influenced by a deregulation of the systemic RAS. Therefore, our aim in this chapter is to give an overview of the ACE gene expression and how the different forms of organization of this enzyme may interfere in the physiological effects of Ang II. Since Ang 1-7 can also be generated from Ang II by ACE 2 [11], it is conceivable to speculate that some actions today inferred to Ang II could be dependent on other components of the RAS. Indeed, the actual conception of the RAS suggests that the overall effect of this system depends on the balance between Ang II and Ang 1-7 production and on interaction with their specific receptors.

Angiotensin Converting Enzyme Gene

ACE is an enzyme that can be found in many tissues of different animal species. The human ACE gene is located in the long arm of chromosome 17 (17q23) comprising a sequence of 21 kilobases. A high number of specific variants have been found in this gene. To date, more than 160 single nucleotide polymorphisms (SNP) have been described [12]. Thirty four of these SNP are located in encoding regions while the others are found in regulatory regions of the gene.

ACE is a zinc metalloproteinase exhibiting two catalytic domains named as N- and C- domains. ACE gene is derived from an ancient duplication of single catalytic enzyme. The enzymatic form named somatic ACE is synthesized in the vascular endothelium as well as in other endothelial tissues (renal tubules, for example) and in other tissues.

The somatic ACE contains four domains, one intracellular, another trans-membrane and two extracellular containing the amino and carboxyl domains [13, 14]. Circulating ACE in plasma is derived from the endothelial isoenzyme by a selective protein cleavage [15]. Testis ACE is an isoenzyme similar to the C-domain portion of somatic ACE, only expressed in male germ cells. This ACE isoform is able to produce Ang II from its precursor angiotensinogen [14]. The effects of RAS peptides in maturation of the germinative epithelium are poorly understood until now. However, mice without the testis ACE produce fewer offspring than mice containing this ACE isoform [16]. Therefore, these data suggest that local production of RAS peptides is necessary for normal maturation of male reproductive system and for spermatozoid development.

ACE activity detected in the plasma is dependent on the continuous liberation of the enzyme from the vascular endothelium into the bloodstream thus reaching all parts of the body [13, 17]. The extracellular localization of ACE on the vascular endothelium facilitates the interaction between the enzyme with Ang I. ACE is highly expressed in the endothelium of pulmonary vessels, so that a single passage of blood through the pulmonary circulation is sufficient to fully convert Ang I into Ang II. In the heart, ACE is not only expressed in endothelial cells of the coronary vessels but also in cardiomyocytes and myofibroblasts [18]. The enzyme expression, however, is not uniformly distributed in the different regions of the organ [19]. In normal hearts, the enzyme expression is higher in atria than in ventricles and, as a rule, ACE is more expressed in the right heart chambers than in the left ones. A different expression pattern is observed diseased hearts. Thus, in chronically infarcted hearts, for example, the highest expression level, not only of ACE, but also of AT1 receptors, is observed in the infarct scar [20]. Therefore, the organized fibrous scar of chronically infarcted hearts seems to be an important source of Ang II to the surviving myocardium and it is likely that this production is important for the remodeling process occurring at remote regions of the heart in such conditions. Thus, the high expression of RAS in the infarct scar may influence the myocardial structure and function all over the heart because peptides leaving the scar may reach distant heart regions through the rich venous system of the scar tissue.

ACE Polymorphisms and ACE Activity

Single genetic polymorphism affects one of a few sequences of DNA nucleotides whereas variations in the copy number of a specific gene represent changes in large DNA sequences (generally more than 1 kb). A small nucleotide sequence can be either deleted or amplified, making possible the occurrence of different number of copies of a specific gene in an individual genome. These DNA rearrangements account for an important component of the inter-individual genetic variation [21]. Variation in the number of copies of a single gene has been interpreted as representing different "doses" of a specific gene product since the expression of the gene product (a protein, a peptide, *etc.*) varies as a function of the number of copies of the gene.

Serum ACE activity is relatively stable in one single individual when repeated measures are obtained at different times. However, large inter-individual variability can be observed in the general population suggesting the existence of modulating factors interfering on the gene expression or in posttranslational enzyme processing [22]. In 1990, Rigat *et al.* [23] reported that ACE activity variability in plasma was dependent of a specific familiar factor since variability of activity in serum was greater inter families than within families. Therefore, ACE activity variability was linked to different genetic background among families. The association of genomic structure and ACE activity showed that ACE activity variability could be correlated with insertion (I) or deletion (D) of a 287 base pair sequence of DNA [23]. Considering the action of Ang II in in various physiological and pathophysiological processes, the investigation of this polymorphism brought up great interest in the scientific community. Since then, this ACE deletion/insertion polymorphism is one of the most extensively studied because of its potential effects to the cardiovascular and renal physiology and the relationship with the pathophysiological aspects of several cardiovascular and renal diseases.

Experimental and clinical studies have been performed since the initial description of the ACE I/D polymorphism. Individuals homozygous to the D allele present higher serum ACE activity resulting in increased circulating levels of Ang II [24]. Thus, DD genotype would consist in the highest "dose" of genetic activation of the RAS whereas the II genotype would indicate the lowest "dosage". Further studies showed that the D/I polymorphism also affects ACE activity in the local RAS [25]. Therefore, paracrine or intracrine generation of Ang II in the heart, kidneys and blood vessels would also depend on the genetic background. Since ACE also is responsible for bradykinin inactivation, individuals with DD, DI, or II genotypes could also present different levels of this vasodilating peptide in body fluids and tissues [25, 26]. Individuals with the DD genotype show higher Ang II and lower bradykinin levels not only in plasma but also in the heart, kidneys and blood vessels. In view of Ang II and bradykinin participation in several physiological process (sodium and fluid retention, vasoconstriction, blood pressure increase, cell proliferation) an intense research was developed in an attempt to describe the involvement of this polymorphism in several diseases, including hypertension, atherosclerosis, heart failure, chronic kidney diseases and others [27].

Considering the different genetic background of populations, it is conceivable that the ACE polymorphisms may show variable prevalence across populations. It has been suggested that the different distribution of ACE polymorphisms across populations, may contribute, at least partially, to the different basal blood pressure values observed in large epidemiological studies [28]. Thus, 36% of the North American whites exhibit DD polymorphism [29] whereas in a Flemish sample of adults, only 22% showed this genotype [30]. In a sample of the Mexican population, prevalence of DD polymorphism was 29.7%, ID 53.7% and II only 16.6% [31]. Da Cruz *et al.*, [32] performed an interesting study in two southern Brazilian populations with different ancestry. In a sample of 525 "gaúchos" (a population with predominant European ancestry) the ID genotype was the most prevalent (44%), a value close to the DD polymorphism (42.5%), whereas the II was present in only 14% of this group. This distribution was compared in this same study in subsample of 364 Brazilian Japanese (individuals living in Brazil, however, born in Japan or with their parents born in Japan). In this latter group the II ACE polymorphism was the most prevalent, comprising 47% of the individuals, followed by the ID (41%). Therefore, insertion (presence of I allele) affected almost all individuals of this group. The DD polymorphism is found in only 12% and it is associated to higher levels ACE activity in plasma. These data confirm that important differences in D and I alleles distribution in populations are related to different ancestry. Another investigation was conducted by our research group in Espírito Santo State (southeast Brazilian coast) to determine proportion of several genetic polymorphisms in populations groups with different ancestry and trying to correlate these data with blood pressure phenotypes. One survey was performed in the general population of Vitória (State capital) where ancestry in quite diverse, with most individuals having a mixed genetic background (Caucasian, African and Indigenous). According to the Brazilian classification these individuals are termed "brown" or "pardos". In a sample of 1,425 individuals of the general population (49.6% of "pardos", 36.7% of whites, and 7.4% of blacks) we found that the D allele was present in almost 75% of the individuals (DD = 29.1% and DI = 54.9%) while the II genotype was found in only 15.9% of the studied sample [33]. A similar study was conducted in small group of a native Brazilians still living in the North of the Espírito Santo coast. This indigenous community is composed of two different Indigenous groups. A larger one, named "Tupinikin" (N= 496) and another smaller composed of "Guarani" (N = 60). A different genotype distribution was found in this indigenous population when compared to the general population of Vitoria. The II genotype was the most frequent and found in 50.5% of the studied individuals, followed by DI (43.9%) and DD (9.6%). Interestingly, the genotype frequency in the indigenous population was similar to the one found in the Japanese group studied in the southern Brazilian region, reinforcing the view that a common ancestry exists for Ameridians and the populations originated from the central Asia [34]. In this Indigenous community there was also 114 non-indigenous individuals (most of them "pardos" married to indigenous). The D/I distribution was similar to the values found in the general population of Vitória. Unlike other studies, we did not found any association between D/I ACE polymorphisms with basal blood pressure values or with presence of hypertension. These different findings in literature may depend on the complexity of the phenotype under evaluation. Blood pressure is quite complex phenotype because it depends on a complex interaction between many genotype variants and environmental factors. Therefore, the presence of an environmental pattern may prevent phenotype expressions. However, another RAS related polymorphism (MT polymorphism of the angiotensinogen gene) showed an important influence on blood pressure in both studied populations [33, 34]. In this case, presence of T polymorphism (higher angiotensinogen production) was associated with increased blood pressure values and prevalence of hypertension. These data reinforce the view that single genes cannot sometimes influence complex phenotypes, such as blood pressure, because gene effects can be masked by ambient factors.

Pathophysiological Significance of ACE Polymorphisms

Ang II and bradykinin are peptides involved in regulation of several physiological processes. Therefore, changes in the control of production and/or degradation may contribute to unbalance the presence of vasoconstrictor and vasodilator peptides in specific regions thus contributing to the development or worsening of several diseases. Since ACE polymorphisms are associated with the capacity of this enzyme to generate Ang II and to inactivate bradykinin either in plasma as in local tissues, a great research effort was developed in the last twenty years aiming to describe associations between specific ACE polymorphisms and the incidence or progression of cardiovascular and kidneys diseases. Some of this knowledge will be summarized in the next paragraphs.

Hypertension

Several studies tested the hypothesis that blood pressure levels and hypertension incidence was related to the presence of the D allele. No evidence of such association predicted from a pathophysiological point of view, however, was found in some large studies. In the Dutch Hypertension and Offspring Study for example, Schmidt *et al.*, [35] failed to find a significant relation between the D/I ACE polymorphism in parents and in their offspring. This negative association was also found in a population-based study developed in Brazil in which our research group was also unable to detect significant difference in the blood pressure of groups exhibiting different ACE polymorphisms [33]. However, a significant interference of the angiotensinogen MT polymorphism in blood pressure phenotypes was observed in this same study. The detected TT allele was correlated with significant higher levels of systolic and diastolic blood pressure when compared to the occurrence of MM allele in homozygous. Therefore, the association of T allele "dosage" and higher blood pressure levels suggested its contribution to hypertension incidence in the general population.

Other investigations, however, have found positive associations, although weak, between presence of D allele and blood pressure. A meta-analysis of 23 studies including 6,923 subjects showed a pooled odds ratio of 1.10 indicating 10% higher risk of hypertension in individuals presenting DD genotype as compared with those with the II one [36]. In this meta-analysis, however, there was strong evidence of heterogeneity among studies and sub-group analysis revealed that the main effect was almost exclusively due to the influence of D polymorphism in the blood pressure of individuals with an Asian ancestry. Another meta-analysis including only Caucasian populations [37] also showed only a marginal influence of the allele D on the systolic and diastolic blood pressure (+0.7 mmHg and +0.5 mmHg, respectively) in subjects with the DD genotype compared to those with II genotype. Interestingly, according to some studies included in the same meta-analysis, the Ang II levels in plasma were significantly higher in presence of DD genotype as compared to individuals presenting the I allele. Therefore, gene "dosage", albeit producing an effect in one proxy variable (plasma Ang II levels in this case) did not produce the expected effect when a more distant phenotype, such as blood pressure. Again, these data suggest that the same genetic variation may produce different phenotypes in view of diverse gene-to-gene interaction or environmental influences on gene expression or protein action.

In conclusion, the D/I polymorphism of the ACE gene shows different prevalence when different population are compared. It seems that in Asians, but not in Caucasians, presence of D allele leads to higher plasma levels of Ang II and blood pressure. Therefore, the influence of this polymorphism to the hypertension development seems to be more important in populations with an Asian genetic background. Considering the high number of genetic, behavioral and environmental factors which potentially contributes to the age dependent blood pressure increase [38], is conceivable to deduce that D/I ACE polymorphism has only a marginal importance for the epidemiological aspects of essential hypertension, except for people of Asian ancestry, such as the Brazilian Japanese and the Brazilian indigenous population where presence of D allele indicates increased risk of hypertension development. Presence of D allele in such individuals would suggest necessity of more rigorous efforts to control other factors predisposing to hypertension development.

Salt Sensitivity and Blood Pressure

Salt sensitivity is defined as the blood pressure response to diets with a high sodium content that vary among individuals. Blood pressure usually increases with a high sodium intake. However, the intensity of this response is not uniform, showing important variation from one individual to another. Individuals showing a high blood pressure increase in response to a high-sodium diet are named salt sensitive. Genetic factors have been described to be involved in this phenomenon. In this sense, the blood pressure response to increased salt consumption represents an important characteristic in the study of genetics of hypertension.

Many factors may influence the blood pressure response to salt intake, and the RAS was described to exert an important influence in this process. Studies analyzed ACE gene polymorphism and salt sensitivity in two Japanese groups with hypertension generating controversial results. In 1994 Kojima *et al.* [39] did not found any association between the I/D ACE gene polymorphism and salt sensitivity. However, in another study, patients with the I allele were more sensitive to a high salt intake. Association between ACE gene I/D and blood pressure response to increased sodium intake was also found in another study [40] what reinforces the view that salt sensitivity may be partially dependent on the genetic background [41]. A study with 114 hypertensive subjects, demonstrated that although a statistically significant association for the angiotensin T genotype was detected, it was not found the same profile for the ACE I/D polymorphism [42]. Studying Japanese male work-people, Zhang *et al.* [43] concluded that ACE I/D and hypertension are not associated. However, the interaction of ACE polymorphism and salt intake results in high blood pressure levels, thus predisposing a subject to hypertension. These observations suggest that subjects with the ID and II genotype are more sensitive to develop hypertension when receive a high sodium diet when compared to DD genotype [43].

Atheroscleroros is

Atherosclerosis is the most prevalent disease in the entire adult population. Despite to be a systemic disease, the distribution of the atherosclerotic plaques varies in different arterial territories. The atherosclerotic plaque results from a slow evolution of an inflammatory and proliferative disease affecting both large and small artery wall [44]. Endothelial dysfunction seems to be a key element for the initial vascular damage leading to a local inflammatory reaction followed by smooth muscle proliferation. Ang II seems to contribute to all steps of the atherosclerosis pathway and therefore polymorphisms of the RAS system may also play a role for atherosclerosis appearance and progression [45]. The carotid artery is a specific vascular territory in which atherosclerosis has been mostly investigated, once its wall is easily investigated by ultrasonography. Therefore, non-invasive images may reveal the disease at different points and at different stages. The intima-media thickness (IMT) of the common or of the inner carotid artery has been considered the gold standard measure to assess subclinical atherosclerosis. Media thickening results from an accelerated smooth muscle proliferation in the vascular wall [46]. In the literature studies described a positive association between D allele and IMT, mainly in high-risk individuals [12, 47].

Therefore, studies have demonstrated that the increased Ang II levels in individuals containing the D allele, may facilitate the stimulation of smooth muscle cells and fibroblast in the sub-intimal space of arteries. Interestingly, such association was observed mainly in individuals presenting other risk factors for cardiovascular diseases, such as smoking, diabetes and hypercholesterolemia. This finding in the carotid arteries seems to be extensive to other vascular beds. Thus, Angerholm-Larsen *et al.*, [37] performed a meta-analysis in Caucasians and individuals presenting the DD genotype showed an odds ratio of 1.21 ($P<0.001$) for myocardial infarction, 1.19 ($P<0.01$) for ischemic heart disease and 1.18 ($P<0.05$) for cerebrovascular disease when compared with the group presenting DI or II genotypes.

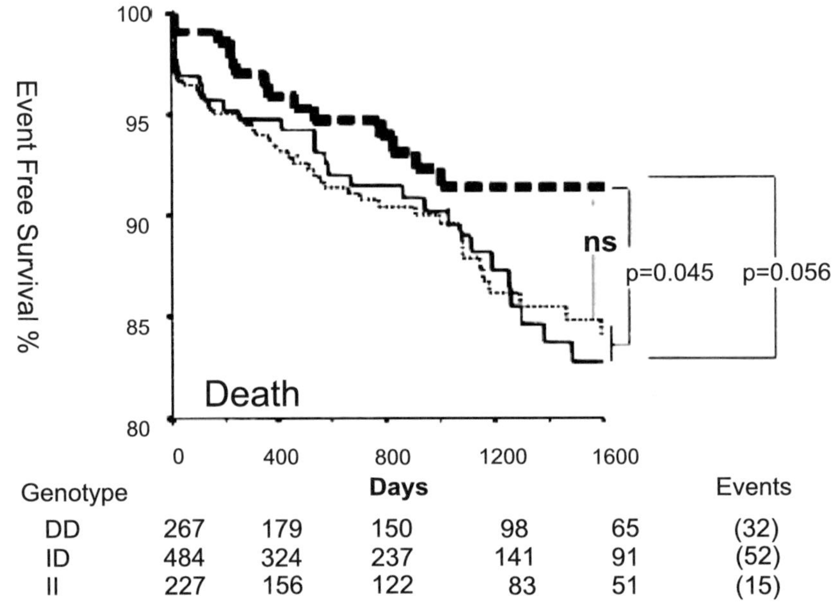

Fig. (1). Kaplan-Meyer survival curves for patients with myocardial infarction with different ACE polymorphisms. Mortality was lower (6.6%) in II group (dashed line) and higher in the DI and DD groups (10.7% and 12.0%, respectively). *Adapted from Palmer et al., 2003* [51].

The deleterious effects of Ang II to the post-infarction remodeling and heart failure development is well established in literature either in experimental animal models of myocardial infarction [48] as in clinical settings [49]. Association between detection of D allele and a bad prognostic after myocardial infarction has been obtained in several follow up studies. D allele identification in patients with idiopathic cardiomyopathy [50] and after myocardial infarction [51] was positively associated with hospitalization and mortality. In this last study, 976 patients with confirmed myocardial infarction were followed for up to five years. There was a significant association between presence of D allele and mortality, even after adjusting for several co-morbidities and treatments. Multivariate analysis showed that ACE genotype was a significant predictor of mortality after infarction in all subgroups (Fig. **1**). Considering the proliferative action of Ang II in the smooth muscle of vascular wall, it is conceivable that ACE polymorphism could also interfere in re-stenosis after invasive treatment of obstructive plaque.

Pharmacogenetics and ACE Polymorphism

An interesting conclusion emerged from the analysis of data obtained in the GRACE Study (Genetic Risk Assessment of Cardiac Events). A cohort of 479 individuals with systolic dysfunction (mean left ventricular ejection fraction = 25±8%) secondary to ischemic or non-ischemic heart diseases was followed for a median time of 3 years. The end points investigated in the cohort were cardiac death or cardiac transplantation [52]. Survival analysis showed similarity with data found previously in the Palmer *et al.*, [51] study, that is, gene "dosage" was strongly associated with outcomes. Therefore, a more detailed knowledge of genetic data makes possible to reach more precise prognosis. Presence of homozygous D allele determined the poorest prognosis while the II genotype was associated with less mortality or necessity of transplant, the DI genotype determining an intermediate phenotype. However, when subgroup analysis was performed, differences between genotypes were more important when patients were divided according the use of ß-blockers. Complex phenotypes are generally determined by fine interactions between the genetic background and environment. When a diseased organ is analyzed, the "environment" can be represented by presence of drugs or mediating peptides in the internal milieu. Influence of D allele was stronger in patients without β-blockade. The impact of the polymorphism was almost completely eliminated in the subgroup of patients treated with β-blockers (Fig. **2**). The interactions between the RAS and the sympathetic nervous system have been known for a long time. The systemic generation of Ang II depends on the renin liberation from the juxtaglomerular apparatus in the kidneys [2, 4]. Blockade of β-adrenergic receptors decreases the renin release, thus attenuating the positive effect of D allele for the systemic generation of Ang II. Low cardiac output determines a reflex activation of the sympathetic system and thus of the endocrine RAS. It is likely that this activation may also be influenced by presence of different ACE alleles.

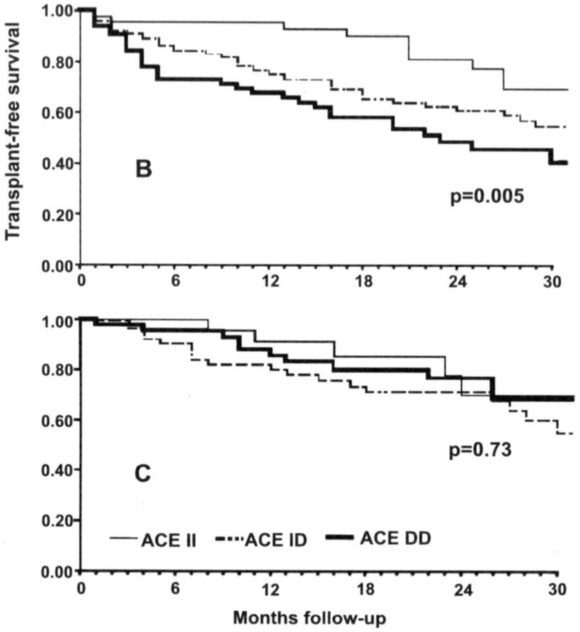

Fig. (2). Survival without cardiac transplant in patients with heart failure with different I/D ACE polymorphism. Upper panel: patients on chronic use of β- blockers. Lower panel: patients without β-blockade. *Adapted from McNamara, 2010 (Grace Study)* [27].

CONCLUSION

This chapter shows that single gene polymorphism may contribute to different phenotypes. However, given the complex relationship among different genes and gene-environmental interactions, the relation gene-phenotype is not linear. Thus, according to Ang II levels in plasma, it was expected that carriers of the polymorphism DD of the ACE gene should present higher blood pressure levels and higher risk of hypertension development. Robust population-based studies and meta-analysis, however, were unable to show such association. These apparent unexpected findings occur because the appearance of a particular phenotype depends on a complex interaction of different genes and the environment. However, our knowledge of specific genotypes may provide important information for the treatment of several diseases, such as the interaction between the RAS and the adrenergic system for the treatment of several diseases where the sympathetic system or the RAS are activated, such as after infarction and heart failure.

CONFLICT OF INTEREST

The authors confirm that they have no conflict of interest to declare for this publication.

ACKNOWLEDGEMENTS

The authors acknowledge the continuous support of CNPq [Grants No. 302296/2008 - 08-5 and 561959/2010-2] and FAPESP. Rebeca C Machado and Ludmila Forechi were recipients of fellowships from CAPES.

REFERENCES

[1] Herichova I, Szantoova K. Renin-angiotensin system: upgrade of recent knowledge and perspectives. Endocr Regul 2013; 47(1): 39-52. [http://dx.doi.org/10.4149/endo_2013_01_39] [PMID: 23363256]

[2] Deschepper CF. Angiotensinogen: hormonal regulation and relative importance in the generation of angiotensin II. Kidney Int 1994; 46(6): 1561-3. [http://dx.doi.org/10.1038/ki.1994.446] [PMID: 7700006]

[3] Baltatu OC, Campos LA, Bader M. Local renin-angiotensin system and the brain--a continuous quest for knowledge. Peptides 2011; 32(5): 1083-6. [http://dx.doi.org/10.1016/j.peptides.2011.02.008] [PMID: 21333703]

[4] Antunes-Rodrigues J, de Castro M, Elias LL, Valença MM, McCann SM. Neuroendocrine control of body fluid metabolism. Physiol Rev 2004; 84(1): 169-208. [http://dx.doi.org/10.1152/physrev.00017.2003] [PMID: 14715914]

[5] Bie P, Damkjaer M. Renin secretion and total body sodium: pathways of integrative control. Clin Exp Pharmacol Physiol 2010; 37(2): e34-42. [http://dx.doi.org/10.1111/j.1440-1681.2009.05316.x] [PMID: 19843096]

[6] Lindpaintner K, Jin M, Wilhelm M, Toth M, Ganten D. Aspects of molecular biology and biochemistry of the cardiac renin-angiotensin system. Br J Clin Pharmacol 1989; 27 (Suppl. 2): 159S-65S. [http://dx.doi.org/10.1111/j.1365-2125.1989.tb03477.x] [PMID: 2669912]

[7] de Resende MM, Mill JG. Effect of high salt intake on local renin-angiotensin system and ventricular dysfunction following myocardial infarction in rats. Clin Exp Pharmacol Physiol 2007; 34(4): 274-9. [http://dx.doi.org/10.1111/j.1440-1681.2007.04556.x] [PMID: 17324137]

[8] Sasaki M, Uehara S, Ohta H, *et al.* Losartan ameliorates progression of glomerular structural changes in diabetic KKAy mice. Life Sci 2004; 75(7): 869-80. [http://dx.doi.org/10.1016/j.lfs.2004.01.022] [PMID: 15183078]

[9] Baudin B. New aspects on angiotensin-converting enzyme: from gene to disease. Clinical chemistry and laboratory medicine : CCLM / FESCC 2002; 40(3): 256-65. [http://dx.doi.org/10.1515/CCLM.2002.042]

[10] Santos RA, Campagnole-Santos MJ. Central and peripheral actions of angiotensin-(1-7). Brazilian journal of medical and biological research = Revista brasileira de pesquisas medicas e biologicas / Sociedade Brasileira de Biofisica (et al) 1994; 27(4): 1033-47.

[11] Santos RA, Ferreira AJ, Verano-Braga T, Bader M. Angiotensin-converting enzyme 2, angiotensin-(--7) and Mas: new players of the renin-angiotensin system. J Endocrinol 2013; 216(2): R1-R17. [http://dx.doi.org/10.1530/JOE-12-0341] [PMID: 23092879]

[12] Sayed-Tabatabaei FA, Houwing-Duistermaat JJ, van Duijn CM, Witteman JC. Angiotensin-converting enzyme gene polymorphism and carotid artery wall thickness: a meta-analysis. Stroke 2003; 34(7): 1634-9. [http://dx.doi.org/10.1161/01.STR.0000077926.49330.64] [PMID: 12805498]

[13] Erdos EG, Skidgel RA. The angiotensin I-converting enzyme. Laboratory investigation; a journal of technical methods and pathology 1987; 56(4): 345-8.

[14] Riordan JF. Angiotensin-I-converting enzyme and its relatives. Genome Biol 2003; 4(8): 225. [http://dx.doi.org/10.1186/gb-2003-4-8-225] [PMID: 12914653]

[15] Ramchandran R, Kasturi S, Douglas JG, Sen I. Metalloprotease-mediated cleavage secretion of pulmonary ACE by vascular endothelial and kidney epithelial cells. Am J Physiol 1996; 271(2 Pt 2): H744-51. [PMID: 8770118]

[16] Bernstein KE, Shen XZ, Gonzalez-Villalobos RA, *et al.* Different in vivo functions of the two catalytic domains of angiotensin-converting enzyme (ACE). Curr Opin Pharmacol 2011; 11(2): 105-11. [ACE]. [http://dx.doi.org/10.1016/j.coph.2010.11.001] [PMID: 21130035]

[17] Arnal JF, Battle T, Rasetti C, *et al.* ACE in three tunicae of rat aorta: expression in smooth muscle and effect of renovascular hypertension. Am J Physiol 1994; 267(5 Pt 2): H1777-84. [PMID: 7977808]

[18] Sun Y, Weber KT. Angiotensin converting enzyme and myofibroblasts during tissue repair in the rat heart. J Mol Cell Cardiol 1996; 28(5): 851-8. [http://dx.doi.org/10.1006/jmcc.1996.0080] [PMID: 8762025]

[19] Mill JG, Milanez MdaC, Busatto VC, de Moraes AC, Gomes MdaG. [Activation of the cardiac angiotensin-converting enzyme after myocardial infarction and its role in ventricular remodeling]. Arq Bras Cardiol 1997; 69(2): 101-10. [PMID: 9567332]

[20] Busatto VC, Cunha V, Cicilini MA, Mill JG. Differential effects of isoproterenol on the activity of angiotensin-converting enzyme in the rat heart and aorta. Brazilian journal of medical and biological research = Revista brasileira de pesquisas medicas e biologicas / Sociedade Brasileira de Biofisica (et al) 1999; 32(3): 355-65. [http://dx.doi.org/10.1590/S0100-879X1999000300017]

[21] Stranger BE, Forrest MS, Dunning M, *et al.* Relative impact of nucleotide and copy number variation on gene expression phenotypes. Science 2007; 315(5813): 848-53. [http://dx.doi.org/10.1126/science.1136678] [PMID: 17289997]

[22] Alhenc-Gelas F, Richard J, Courbon D, Warnet JM, Corvol P. Distribution of plasma angiotensin I-converting enzyme levels in healthy men: relationship to environmental and hormonal parameters. J Lab Clin Med 1991; 117(1): 33-9. [PMID: 1846167]

[23] Rigat B, Hubert C, Alhenc-Gelas F, Cambien F, Corvol P, Soubrier F. An insertion/deletion polymorphism in the angiotensin I-converting enzyme gene accounting for half the variance of serum enzyme levels. J Clin Invest 1990; 86(4): 1343-6. [http://dx.doi.org/10.1172/JCI114844] [PMID: 1976655]

[24] Tiret L, Rigat B, Visvikis S, *et al.* Evidence, from combined segregation and linkage analysis, that a variant of the angiotensin I-converting enzyme (ACE) gene controls plasma ACE levels. Am J Hum Genet 1992; 51(1): 197-205. [PMID: 1319114]

[25] Danser AH, Schalekamp MA, Bax WA, *et al.* Angiotensin-converting enzyme in the human heart. Effect of the deletion/insertion polymorphism. Circulation 1995; 92(6): 1387-8. [http://dx.doi.org/10.1161/01.CIR.92.6.1387] [PMID: 7664416]

[26] Rigat B, Hubert C, Corvol P, Soubrier F. PCR detection of the insertion/deletion polymorphism of the human angiotensin converting enzyme gene (DCP1) (dipeptidyl carboxypeptidase 1). Nucleic Acids Res 1992; 20(6): 1433. [http://dx.doi.org/10.1093/nar/20.6.1433-a] [PMID: 1313972]

[27] McNamara DM. Genomic variation and neurohormonal intervention in heart failure. Heart Fail Clin 2010; 6(1): 35-43. [http://dx.doi.org/10.1016/j.hfc.2009.08.004] [PMID: 19945059]

[28] Corvol P, Soubrier F, Jeunemaitre X. Molecular genetics of the renin-angiotensin-aldosterone system in human hypertension. Pathol Biol (Paris) 1997; 45(3): 229-39. [PMID: 9296068]

[29] Beohar N, Damaraju S, Prather A, Yu QT, Raizner A, Kleiman NS, *et al.* Angiotensin-I converting enzyme genotype DD is a risk factor for coronary artery disease. Journal of investigative medicine : the official publication of the American Federation for Clinical Research 1995; 43(3): 275-80.

[30] Balkestein EJ, Wang JG, Struijker-Boudier HA, *et al.* Carotid and femoral intima-media thickness in relation to three candidate genes in a Caucasian population. J Hypertens 2002; 20(8): 1551-61. [http://dx.doi.org/10.1097/00004872-200208000-00018] [PMID: 12172317]

[31] Alvarez-Aguilar C, Enríquez-Ramírez ML, Figueroa-Nuñez B, *et al.* Association between angiotensin-

1 converting enzyme gene polymorphism and the metabolic syndrome in a Mexican population. Exp Mol Med 2007; 39(3): 327-34.
[http://dx.doi.org/10.1038/emm.2007.36] [PMID: 17603286]

[32] Da Cruz IB, Oliveira G, Taufer M, *et al.* Angiotensin I-converting enzyme gene polymorphism in two ethnic groups living in Brazil's southern region: association with age. J Gerontol A Biol Sci Med Sci 2003; 58(9): M851-6.
[http://dx.doi.org/10.1093/gerona/58.9.M851] [PMID: 14528043]

[33] Pereira AC, Mota GF, Cunha RS, Herbenhoff FL, Mill JG, Krieger JE. Angiotensinogen 235T allele "dosage" is associated with blood pressure phenotypes. Hypertension 2003; 41(1): 25-30.
[http://dx.doi.org/10.1161/01.HYP.0000047465.97065.15] [PMID: 12511525]

[34] Meyerfreund D. Estudo da Hipertensão Arterial e de outros fatores de risco cardiovascular nas comunidades indígenas do Espírito Santo: Universidade Federal do Espírito Santo. 2006.

[35] Schmidt S, van Hooft IM, Grobbee DE, Ganten D, Ritz E. Polymorphism of the angiotensin I converting enzyme gene is apparently not related to high blood pressure: Dutch Hypertension and Offspring Study. J Hypertens 1993; 11(4): 345-8.
[http://dx.doi.org/10.1097/00004872-199304000-00003] [PMID: 8390500]

[36] Staessen JA, Wang JG, Ginocchio G, *et al.* The deletion/insertion polymorphism of the angiotensin converting enzyme gene and cardiovascular-renal risk. J Hypertens 1997; 15(12 Pt 2): 1579-92.
[http://dx.doi.org/10.1097/00004872-199715120-00059] [PMID: 9488209]

[37] Agerholm-Larsen B, Nordestgaard BG, Tybjaerg-Hansen A. ACE gene polymorphism in cardiovascular disease: meta-analyses of small and large studies in whites. Arterioscler Thromb Vasc Biol 2000; 20(2): 484-92.
[http://dx.doi.org/10.1161/01.ATV.20.2.484] [PMID: 10669647]

[38] Knight BS, Sunn N, Pennell CE, Adamson SL, Lye SJ. Developmental regulation of cardiovascular function is dependent on both genotype and environment. Am J Physiol Heart Circ Physiol 2009; 297(6): H2234-41.
[http://dx.doi.org/10.1152/ajpheart.01338.2008] [PMID: 19783772]

[39] Kojima S, Inenaga T, Matsuoka H, *et al.* The association between salt sensitivity of blood pressure and some polymorphic factors. J Hypertens 1994; 12(7): 797-801.
[http://dx.doi.org/10.1097/00004872-199407000-00011] [PMID: 7963508]

[40] Giner V, Poch E, Bragulat E, *et al.* Renin-angiotensin system genetic polymorphisms and salt sensitivity in essential hypertension. Hypertension 2000; 35(1 Pt 2): 512-7.
[http://dx.doi.org/10.1161/01.HYP.35.1.512] [PMID: 10642351]

[41] Poch E, González D, Giner V, Bragulat E, Coca A, de La Sierra A. Molecular basis of salt sensitivity in human hypertension. Evaluation of renin-angiotensin-aldosterone system gene polymorphisms. Hypertension 2001; 38(5): 1204-9.
[http://dx.doi.org/10.1161/hy1101.099479] [PMID: 11711524]

[42] Caprioli J, Mele C, Mossali C, *et al.* Polymorphisms of EDNRB, ATG, and ACE genes in salt-sensitive hypertension. Can J Physiol Pharmacol 2008; 86(8): 505-10.
[http://dx.doi.org/10.1139/Y08-045] [PMID: 18758497]

[43] Zhang L, Miyaki K, Araki J, Song Y, Kimura T, Omae K, *et al.* Interaction of angiotensin I-converting enzyme insertion-deletion polymorphism and daily salt intake influences hypertension in Japanese men. Hypertension research: official journal of the Japanese Society of Hypertension 2006; 29(10): 751-8.

[44] Libby P, Ridker PM, Hansson GK. Leducq Transatlantic Network on Atherothrombosis. Inflammation in atherosclerosis: from pathophysiology to practice. J Am Coll Cardiol 2009; 54(23): 2129-38. [http://dx.doi.org/10.1016/j.jacc.2009.09.009] [PMID: 19942084]

[45] Sata M, Fukuda D. Crucial role of renin-angiotensin system in the pathogenesis of atherosclerosis. J Med Invest 2010; 57(1-2): 12-25. [http://dx.doi.org/10.2152/jmi.57.12] [PMID: 20299739]

[46] Simon A, Gariepy J, Chironi G, Megnien JL, Levenson J. Intima-media thickness: a new tool for diagnosis and treatment of cardiovascular risk. J Hypertens 2002; 20(2): 159-69. [http://dx.doi.org/10.1097/00004872-200202000-00001] [PMID: 11821696]

[47] Sayed-Tabatabaei FA, Oostra BA, Isaacs A, van Duijn CM, Witteman JC. ACE polymorphisms. Circ Res 2006; 98(9): 1123-33. [http://dx.doi.org/10.1161/01.RES.0000223145.74217.e7] [PMID: 16690893]

[48] Mill JG, Stefanon I, dos Santos L, Baldo MP. Remodeling in the ischemic heart: the stepwise progression for heart failure. Brazilian journal of medical and biological research = Revista brasileira de pesquisas medicas e biologicas / Sociedade Brasileira de Biofisica (et al) 2011; 44(9): 890-. [http://dx.doi.org/10.1590/S0100-879X2011007500096]

[49] Anavekar NS, Solomon SD. Angiotensin II receptor blockade and ventricular remodelling. J Renin Angiotensin Aldosterone Syst 2005; 6(1): 43-8. [http://dx.doi.org/10.3317/jraas.2005.006] [PMID: 16088851]

[50] Andersson B, Sylvén C. The DD genotype of the angiotensin-converting enzyme gene is associated with increased mortality in idiopathic heart failure. J Am Coll Cardiol 1996; 28(1): 162-7. [http://dx.doi.org/10.1016/0735-1097(96)00098-8] [PMID: 8752809]

[51] Palmer BR, Pilbrow AP, Yandle TG, *et al.* Angiotensin-converting enzyme gene polymorphism interacts with left ventricular ejection fraction and brain natriuretic peptide levels to predict mortality after myocardial infarction. J Am Coll Cardiol 2003; 41(5): 729-36. [http://dx.doi.org/10.1016/S0735-1097(02)02927-3] [PMID: 12628714]

[52] McNamara DM, Holubkov R, Postava L, *et al.* Effect of the Asp298 variant of endothelial nitric oxide synthase on survival for patients with congestive heart failure. Circulation 2003; 107(12): 1598-602. [http://dx.doi.org/10.1161/01.CIR.0000060540.93836.AA] [PMID: 12668492]

CHAPTER 10

The ACE2 – Angiotensin (1-7)-Mas Receptor Axis in the Kidney

Mark C. Chappell[1,*], Bryan A. Wilson[1], Allyson C. Marshall[1], Ebaa M. Al Zayadneh[1], James C. Rose[2], Debra I. Diz[1] and **Hossam A. Shaltout[1,2]**

[1] *Hypertension and Vascular Research Center, Department of Physiology & Pharmacology, Wake Forest University School of Medicine, Winston-Salem, NC, USA 27157-1032*

[2] *Department of Obstetrics and Gynecology, Wake Forest University School of Medicine, Winston-Salem North Carolina, USA*

Abstract: The renin-angiotensin-system (RAS) constitutes a key hormonal system in both the acute and long-term maintenance of blood pressure. Indeed, inappropriate regulation of this system is a major contributor to various pathologies that impact kidney function and blockade of the RAS either through attenuation of angiotensin converting enzyme (ACE) activity or angiotensin type 1 receptor (AT_1R)-dependent signaling has important therapeutic benefit. The RAS is no longer considered a monolithic peptidergic system whereby Ang II is the sole effector acting through the AT_1R, but a diverse system that reflects multiple peptides with distinct actions that are mediated by multiple receptors. The ACE-Ang II-AT_1R axis is considered the classic pathway of the RAS that upon activation contributes to a number of peripheral and central mechanisms to effectively regulate blood pressure. However, the dysregulation of the AT_1R axis may lead to sustained hypertension, inflammation, and an imbalance in redox mechanisms, cellular fibrosis, and other pathological responses. The ACE2-Ang-(1-7)-AT_7R axis is now defined as the non-classical pathway of the RAS that in many situations exhibits actions that are opposite those of the Ang II-AT_1R axis. The cellular actions of the Ang-(1-7)-AT_7R axis primarily reflect the stimulation of both nitric oxide and prostaglandin pathways that would contribute to lower blood pressure and attenuation of inflammation, fibrosis and cellular injury. Moreover, the progression of various pathologies attributed to a stimulated Ang II-AT_1R axis may, in part, reflect

* **Corresponding author Mark C. Chappell:** The Hypertension & Vascular Research Center, Department of Physiology & Pharmacology, Wake Forest University School of Medicine, Winston-Salem, NC, USA 27157-1032; Telephone: [336]-716-9236; FAX: [336]-716-2456; E-mail: mchappel@wakehealth.edu.

Dulce Elena Casarini, Danielle Yuri Arita, Tatiana Sousa Cunha & Juliana Almada Colucci (Eds.)

a reduced Ang-(1-7) tone. The current review assesses the non-classical axis of the RAS regarding the cellular and intracellular pathways for the expression and metabolism of Ang-(1-7), as well as the influence of the peptide in fetal-programmed hypertension.

Keywords: Angiotensin converting enzyme 2, Epithelial to mesenchymal transition, Fetal programming, Glucocorticoids, Natriuresis, Neprilysin, Peptide metabolism, Renin-angiotensin system, Thimet oligopeptidase.

INTRODUCTION

The concept of peptide pathways that are distinct from the Ang II-AT_1 receptor axis has emerged over the last two decades that ostensibly originated from our demonstration of the endogenous expression [1] and biological actions of Ang-(1-7) (Fig. **1**) [2 - 4]. Over the course of this period, key evidence has established a novel Ang-(1-7) receptor (Mas protein) that is widely distributed in cardiovascular tissues, identification of AT_7/Mas receptor antagonists and agonists, a selective peptidase (ACE2) that directly hydrolyzes Ang II to Ang-(--7), the ACE-dependent metabolism of Ang-(1-7), and the elucidation of various signaling pathways that are activated by Ang-(1-7) [5, 6]. Apart from the identification of the biochemical components of the Ang-(1-7)-AT_7 receptor (AT_7R) axis expressed throughout the body, accumulating data on the novel functions of the peptide add to the physiological significance of this system [7, 8]. Ang-(1-7) was originally investigated on the peptide's ability to elicit vasorelaxation and to reduce blood pressure, particularly in lieu of the higher circulating Ang-(1-7) levels following treatment with ACE inhibitors; however, the functional effects of the Ang-(1-7) axis that are not directly related to blood pressure regulation should be considered as well [2, 9, 10]. The functional arc of Ang-(1-7) appears to beneficially influence numerous pathological conditions including diabetes, cancer, vascular and skeletal muscle dysfunction, wound healing and cognitive decline [3, 6, 11]. The span of Ang-(1-7)'s actions is not altogether unexpected given that the RAS, and in particular, the Ang-(1-7) axis is widely expressed in the body and this system may be important in the buffering of the Ang II-AT_1R pathway [12]. In the current review, we critically assess recent studies on the ACE2-Ang-(1-7)-MasR axis as they pertain to the expression and metabolism of the peptide, the renal actions of the peptide and the emerging role of Ang-(1-7) in fetal-programmed hypertension.

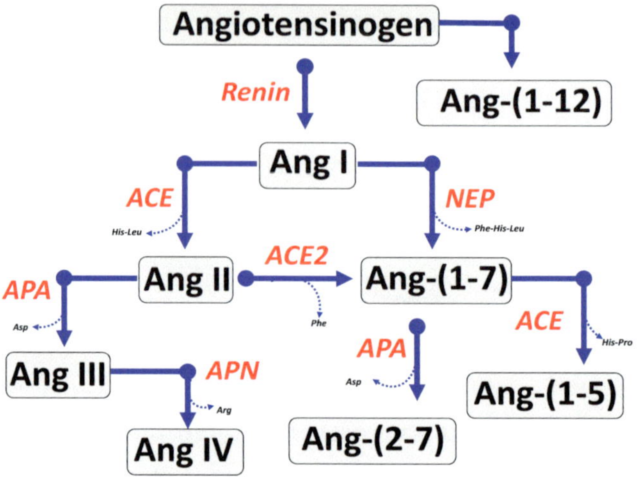

Fig. (1). Cascade of the renin-angiotensin system elucidating the peptide pathways. Angiotensinogen is initially hydrolyzed to angiotensin I (Ang I) by the aspartyl protease Renin. Angiotensin converting enzyme (ACE) hydrolyzes Ang I to Ang II. The carboxypeptidase ACE2 cleaves the Pro^7-Phe^8 bond of Ang II to Ang-(1-7). Alternatively, Ang I is hydrolyzed by endopeptidases (NEP - neprilysin, thimet oligopeptidases, prolyl oligopeptidase) to Ang-(1-7). Aminopeptidases including aminopeptidase A (APA) and aminopeptidase N (APN) process Ang II to Ang-(2-8) (Ang III) and Ang-(3-8) (Ang IV), respectively. ACE degrades Ang-(1-7) to the pentapeptide Ang-(1-5) and APA may contribute to the generation of Ang-(2-7). Angiotensinogen may undergo alternative processing by a non-renin dependent pathway to form Ang-(1-12) in rat.

Renal Angiotensin-(1-7)

Angiotensinogen, a 453 amino acid protein, is the sole precursor for all angiotensins [13]. Angiotensinogen is the only known substrate for the aspartyl protease renin that forms Ang I and des-[Ang I]-angiotensinogen; circulating Ang I is rapidly hydrolyzed by the metallopeptidase ACE to the active peptide Ang II (Fig. **1**). Following ACE inhibitor treatment, circulating Ang I and Ang-(1-7) are markedly higher [14]. The higher the expression of Ang-(1-7) in the circulation provided the first initial the evidence that the peptide may impart a therapeutic benefit to ACE inhibitors and that the peptide's actions may be distinct from that of the Ang II-AT_1R axis. Importantly, these data suggested that Ang-(1-7) formation in the circulation is likely independent from the generation of Ang II by ACE [4]. Subsequent studies revealed that the endopeptidase neprilysin, originally termed “enkephalinase” for its ability to degrade endogenous opiate peptides, converted Ang I directly to Ang-(1-7) [15 - 18]. Ang-(1-7) processing pathways likely include both ACE2 and neprilysin, as well as enzymes upstream (ACE, chymase) that process Ang I to Ang II and essentially compete for the Ang I substrate. Following the formation of Ang-(1-7), there are additional enzymatic pathways that are likely involved in the metabolism of the peptide. In the circulation and isolated proximal tubules, the inhibition of ACE protected the metabolism of Ang-(1-7) to the pentapeptide Ang-(1-5) [4, 19, 20]. These studies suggest that similar to bradykinin, higher Ang-(1-7) expression reflects, in part, blockade of a major route for metabolism of the peptide through ACE. More recent studies from our laboratory identified a soluble peptidase in the brain medulla and cerebrospinal fluid (CSF) of the sheep that hydrolyzed Ang-(1-7) [21, 22]. The peptidase activity was 3-fold greater in the fetal-programmed adult sheep arising from *in utero* betamethasone exposure. The increased peptidase activity correlated with a higher level of blood pressure as well as reduced content of Ang-(1-7) in the CSF of betamethasone exposed sheep. Partial purification of the peptidase from medullary tissue revealed a very high sensitivity to the metalloendopeptidase inhibitor JMV-390 (IC_{50} < 1 nM) [22]. Subsequent studies localized the peptidase activity to the sheep renal cortex, isolated proximal tubules and human HK-2 proximal tubule cells [23]. Interestingly, the peptidase was the primary, if not exclusive activity in the HK-2 cells that degraded Ang-(1-7) (Fig. **2**) [22]. The peptidase exhibited similar characteristics to the activity in brain regarding substrate preference and sensitivity to various inhibitors; the peptidase activity was also evident in the HK-2 cell media suggesting the enzyme may undergo secretion (Fig. **2**) [22]. We also identified an intracellular endopeptidase activity corresponding to thimet oligopeptidase that processed Ang I directly to Ang-(1-7) in the HK-2 proximal cells (Fig. **3**) [23]. In contrast to the contribution of endopeptidases that form Ang-(1-7), Other carboxypeptidases including prolyl carboxypeptidase (PC) and ACE2 may process Ang II directly to Ang-(1-7). Although ACE2 exhibits optimal activity at neutral pH, the optimal activity for PC is more acidic that would be comparable to the lysosomal compartment [24]. ACE2 is predominantly distributed to the apical face of the tubules and likely contributes to the extracellular processing of Ang II to Ang-(1-7) [25, 26]. Moreover, the efficiency constant (k_{cat}/K_m) of ACE2 for Ang II is significantly higher than other angiotensin substrates and a recombinant soluble form of ACE2 is proposed as an anti-hypertensive agent to ameliorate tissue injury [27 - 30]. However, it is not clear whether the addition of exogenous ACE2 can overcome the synthetic capacity of the Ang I-ACE pathway in the circulation over an extended period to chronically reduce the Ang II-Ang-(1-7) ratio.

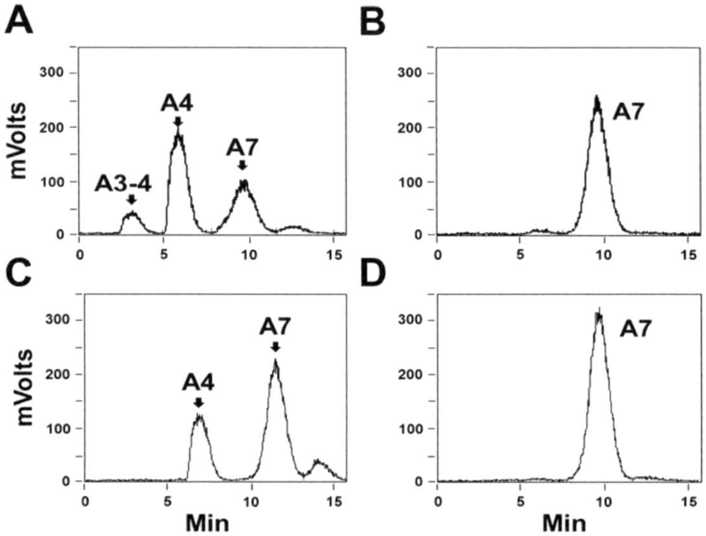

Fig. (2). Ang-(1-7) peptidase in HK-2 human proximal tubule cells. Conversion of Ang-(1-7) (A7) to the metabolite Ang-(3-4) (A4) in the cytosolic fraction (**Panel A**) and cell media (**Panel C**) of the HK-2 cells. The inhibitor JMV-390 (1 μM) blocked the metabolism of Ang-(1-7) in the cytosolic fraction (**Panel B**) and cell media (**Panel D**) of HK-2 cells. (Adapted from Wilson *et al.* [23]).

In general, the serum content of ACE2 is very low while that of ACE is higher [31]. Circulating ACE2, however, increases in pathological conditions such as diabetes and myocardial infarction in both experimental models and humans [32 - 35]. We recently assessed circulating ACE and ACE2 activities in female and male normotensive Lewis rats, as well as the hypertensive mRen2.Lewis strain. We utilized the peptides Ang II (ACE2) and Ang I (ACE) under comparable substrate conditions in serum to allow for the direct comparison of these enzymatic activities. As shown in (Fig. **4A**), ACE activity was markedly higher than ACE2 in the circulation across all groups [32]. Indeed, serum ACE2 activity was very low in the normotensive Lewis and the female mRen2.Lewis [32]. Circulating ACE activity was also higher in the hypertensive strain and increased in the diabetic groups by 50% and 75% for females and males, respectively (Fig. **4A**) [32]. In contrast, male mRen2.Lewis rats exhibited higher serum ACE2 activity as compared to male and female Lewis or the female hypertensive rats; however, circulating ACE2 increases 300% and 500% in male and female mRen2.Lewis, respectively, after streptozotocin-induced (STZ) diabetes in the hypertensive strain (Fig. **4A**) [32]. Increased expression of ACE2 in the male mRen2.Lewis or following induction of diabetes in the hypertensive groups may be an attempt to limit Ang II expression and preserve Ang-(1-7), particularly in lieu of higher ACE activity. Studies to date have not identified the cellular source of circulating ACE2 nor the extent that enzymatic shedding contributes to the soluble form of the enzyme. We consider it unlikely that the kidney is a major source of circulating ACE2 as the enzyme is localized to the tubular brush border and shedding of the enzyme would contribute exclusively to activity in the tubular fluid or urine. Apart from the kidney, other potential sources for circulating ACE2 in diabetes include the vasculature, heart and lung compartments, although pulmonary ACE2 activity in control and diabetic mRen2.Lewis males was quite low and was not different between the control and diabetic groups (*MC Chappell, unpublished observations*).

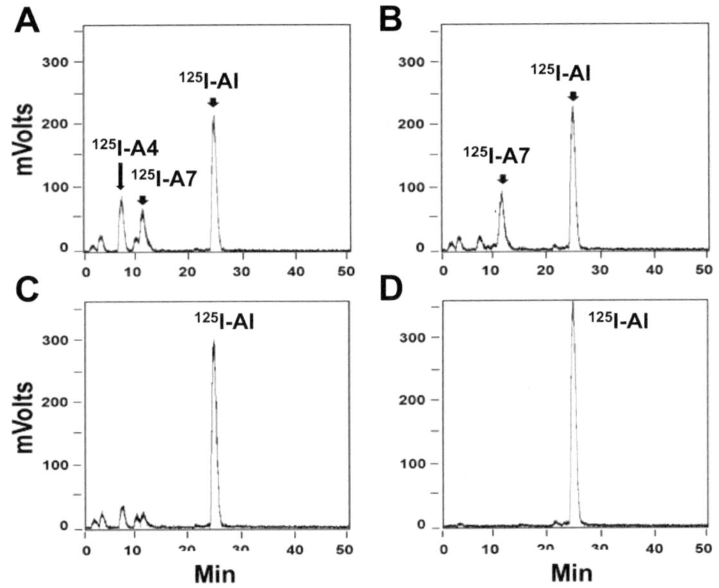

Fig. (3). Ang I to Ang-(1-7) conversion by thimet oligopeptidase in HK-2 cells. Panel A: Ang I (A1) is converted to Ang-(1-7) (A7) and Ang-(3-4) (A4) in the cytosolic fraction of HK-2 cells. **Panel B:** Addition of JMV-390 (1 nM) reduced A4 peak but did not inhibit A7. **Panel C:** The thimet oligopeptidase inhibitor c-phenylpropyl-Ala-Ala-aminobenzoate (cPAA, 10 μM) essentially abolished A7 and increased the A1 peak. **Panel D:** A1 metabolism is abolished by the thiol inhibitor *para*-chloromercuribenzoate (PCMB, 10 μM). (Adapted from Wilson *et al.* [23]).

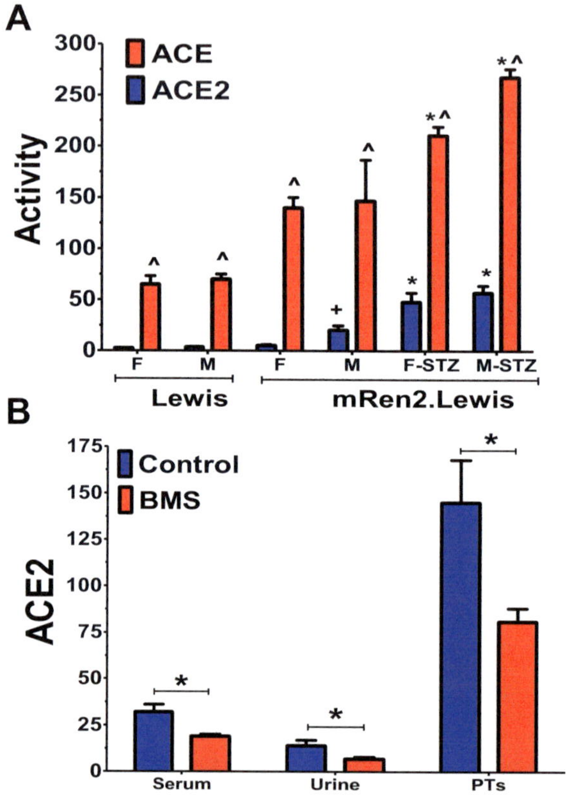

Fig. (4). Differential response of circulating ACE2 in diabetes and betamethasone-induced fetal programming events. Panel A: Comparison of circulating ACE2 and ACE activities in female (F) and male (M) normotensive Lewis, hypertensive mRen2.Lewis and diabetic (STZ) mRen2.Lewis rats. *$P<0.05$ *versus* non-diabetic mRen2.Lewis; ^$P<0.05$ *versus* ACE2; $^{+}P<0.05$ *versus* female mRen2.Lewis. Activity is expressed as fmol/minute/ml serum. Adapted from Yamaleyeva *et al.* [32] and Chappell and Westwood (unpublished results). **Panel B:** ACE2 activity is reduced in the circulation, urine and cortical proximal tubules from the kidney of betamethasone-exposed (BMS) sheep as compared to unexposed controls. *$P<0.05$ *versus* control. Activity is expressed as fmol/minute/ml serum, urine or mg tissue protein. (Adapted from Shaltout *et al.* [97]).

Intracellular Actions of Ang-(1-7)

The RAS has been long-viewed as a circulating system that comprises an enzymatic cascade to deliver bioactive peptides to receptors on various target organs; however, abundant evidence also favors a local RAS for Ang II and Ang-(1-7) expression [36]. Robertson and Khairallah initially demonstrated binding of Ang II to nuclear chromatin isolated from both cardiomyocytes and vascular smooth muscle cells [37]. Subsequent studies identified Ang II binding on nuclei isolated from rat liver [38 - 40]. Functional sites for Ang II on the isolated nuclei were supported by evidence that Ang II increased the rate of mRNA transcription for several proteins of the RAS including renin and angiotensinogen [41, 42]. Additional studies established AT_1R on the nuclear fraction isolated from rat cortex and medulla [43 - 45]. In this regard, the addition of Ang II to the renal nuclei stimulated the mRNA levels for angiotensinogen, the sodium-hydrogen transporter NHE3 and the monocyte chemoattractant protein (MCP-1) on renal nuclei [45]. Zhuo and colleagues further show that administration of Ang II to isolated nuclei or given intracellularly elicited a rapid calcium response [46]. In support of dynamic changes in nuclear calcium, we find that Ang II causes an immediate fluorescence signature for reactive oxygen species (ROS) using the molecular probe dichlorofluorescein (DCF) in renal nuclei; the Ang II response was abolished by diphenyleneiodonium (DPI) and the AT_1R antagonist losartan [47]. Moreover, pharmacological blockade of either phosphoinositol 3-kinase (PI3K) or protein kinase C (PKC) eliminated the increase in ROS to Ang II consistent with the localization of these kinase pathways and NAD(P)H oxidase NOX4 to the nucleus [47 - 51].

The aforementioned studies that demonstrate nuclear AT_1 receptors support the concept for the intracellular expression of G-protein coupled receptors (GPCRs) on intracellular organelle such as the nucleus and mitochondria [52 - 55]. Lee *et al.* identified a canonical nuclear localization sequence (NLS) on the human MasR gene in their study on the cellular distribution of the GPCRs [52]. Based on previous work that established the expression of functional AT_1R and AT_2R on isolated renal nuclei, we began a series of studies to assess the intracellular role for Ang-(1-7). Immunofluorescent (ICC) studies of the AT_7/MasR revealed striking expression of the protein to the tubular elements of the sheep kidney with complete blockade of receptor staining by an antigenic peptide to MasR (Fig. **5**). Western blotting revealed a protein band of 35 kDa in nuclei isolated from proximal tubules of the sheep kidney using the Mas antibody for ICC studies [56].

In addition, the antagonist [D-Ala[1]]-Ang-(1-7) [DALA or A779] significantly reduced ^{125}I-[Sarcorsine[1], Threonine[8]]-Ang II (Sarthran) binding on isolated nuclei [58]. Moreover, we find that Ang-(1-7) dose-dependently stimulated nitric oxide (NO) from the renal nuclei using the molecular probe 4-amino-5-methylam-no-2',7'-Difluorofluorescein (DAF); NO generation was abolished by L-NAME, a non-selective NOS inhibitor and DALA [56]. These data for Ang-(1-7) are consistent with previous studies that demonstrate a functional role for bradykinin to increase NO and cGMP from liver nuclei, as well the nuclear localization of type III or endothelial NOS (eNOS) and soluble guanylate cyclase (sGC) [57, 58]. Since one functional aspect of the Ang-(1-7) axis is to antagonize an activated Ang II-AT_1R pathway, additional studies addressed whether blockade of the nuclear ACE2-Ang-(1-7) axis influences Ang II signaling. Addition of an ACE2 inhibitor or DALA augmented oxidative stress to Ang II within isolated nuclei of the renal cortex [59]. It is presently unclear as to the exact mechanism that Ang-(1-7) antagonizes the pro-oxidative effects of Ang II on the nucleus. One potential mechanism is the activation by Ang-(1-7) of intracellular phosphatases including MKP-1 and SHP-1 that may attenuate Ang II-dependent stimulation of various kinase pathways that lead to an increase in ROS. Indeed, several types of phosphatases are known to reside or localize to the nucleus and these may contribute to the potential nuclear actions of Ang-(1-7) [60 - 62].

The previous studies focused on the demonstration of functional nuclear receptors for AT_1R, AT_2R and AT_7/MasR that mediate the release of ROS and NO, respectively on the nucleus. However, identification of pathways that may contribute to the expression of their peptide ligands within the cell and to target selective intracellular organelle such as the nucleus or mitochondria is unclear at this time. Casarini and colleagues demonstrated intracellular components of the RAS including Ang-(1-7) and Ang II within mesangial cells [63, 64]. Other investigators find that high glucose conditions markedly augment intracellular Ang II content in vascular smooth muscle cells (VSMC), cardiofibroblasts, myocytes, and mesangial cells, as well as enhance nuclear Ang II expression [65 - 69]. Moreover, exposure of VSMC to high glucose reduced the intracellular levels of Ang-(1-7) that may be linked to the downregulation of ACE2 [70]. In rat proximal tubule NRK-52 cells, Chou *et al.* demonstrated that the inhibitory effects on Ang-(1-7) expression by high glucose are likely mediated by TGFβ-dependent downregulation of ACE2 [71]. We also utilized the renal NRK-52E cell line to recently demonstrate the intracellular localization of both Ang-(1-7) and Ang II to the nucleus; peptide quantification of the nuclear fraction revealed comparable levels of Ang II and Ang-(1-7) in the 40-50 fmol/mg protein range [72].

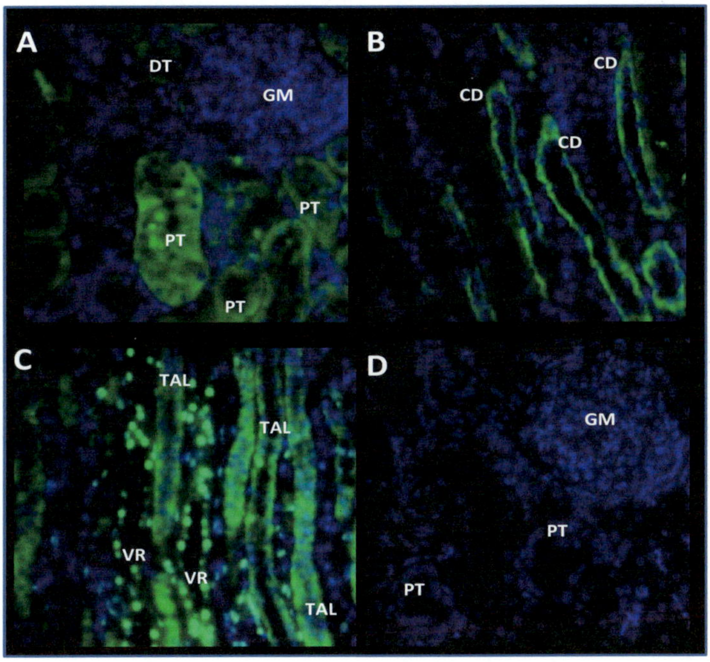

Fig. (5). Renal localization of the AT_7 /Mas receptor protein. Immunofluorescent (ICC) signature of the Mas protein by an affinity-purified antibody (Alomone, Israel) in the sheep kidney. **Panel A:** Positive staining is evident in the cortical proximal tubules (PT) and distal tubules (DT); however Mas staining was absent in the glomerulus (GM) in tissue sections of the renal cortex; **Panel B:** the collecting ducts (CD) exhibit positive staining for the Mas receptor; **Panel C:** medullary cells of the thick ascending limb of Henle (TAL) and vasa recta (VR) show the Mas receptor fluorescence; **Panel D:** the ICC Mas signal is blocked by the prior incubation with the peptide against the Mas receptor antibody. Adapted from Gwathmey *et al.* [58].

These studies further identified nuclear renin and prorenin expression, as well as aliskerin-sensitive processing of angiotensinogen to Ang I [72]. Moreover, the advanced glycation end product (AGE) methoxyl-glycated albumin (MGA) that is increased in diabetes and other pathologies, attenuated cellular levels of Ang-(1-7) but did not influence Ang I or Ang II expression in the NRK-52E cells [73]. Although we did not measure the impact of MGA exposure on ACE2 expression, the extent of Ang-(1-7) metabolism in the cytosolic fraction of the NRK-52E cells was significantly increased by MGA [73]. The peptidase activity that hydrolyzes Ang-(1-7) in the NRK-52E cells appears to be distinct from that characterized in the sheep tissues and the human HK-2 cells as the NRK-52 activity was not inhibited by JMV-390 (*Alzayadneh and Chappell, unpublished results*). The MGA-dependent reduction in intracellular Ang-(1-7) was associated with epithelial to mesenchymal transition (EMT) in the NRK-52E cells that may contribute to epithelial loss and enhanced fibrosis in diabetes [73]. In this case, treatment of the NRK-52 cells with extracellular Ang-(1-7) abolished the AGE-induced EMT [73] (Fig. **6**). The cytokine TGF-β plays a key role in EMT, tubular hypertrophy and fibrosis, and we find that MGA exposure significantly increased the release of TGF-β in the NRK-52E cells. Moreover, an inhibitor of the TGF-β receptor kinase blocked the EMT response to MGA, as well as to TGF-β [73]. Although Ang-(1-7) failed to attenuate TGF-β release in the MGA-exposed cells, the peptide blocked the MAP kinase activation to MGA [73]. In addition, Ang-(1-7) abolished the direct activation of the non-canonical MAP kinase pathway by TGF-β. Surprisingly, we failed to demonstrate that the AT_1R antagonist losartan exhibited any inhibitory actions towards the AGE-induced EMT, cell hypertrophy or MAP kinase activation [73]. In this regard, Zhang *et al.* demonstrated that Ang-(1-7) treatment of diabetic mice was superior to the AT_1 receptor antagonist regarding the progression of renal injury [74].

Finally, we recently reported evidence for the expression of an Ang-(1-7) system within the mitochondria of the sheep kidney [75]. Abadir *et al.* originally demonstrated that liver mitochondria express both AT_2 and AT_1 receptors [76]. In aged mice, the ratio of AT_1R to AT_2R increased as compared to younger mice and chronic treatment with an AT_1R antagonist prevented the decline in AT_2R expression suggesting that Ang II may influence mitochondrial health and cellular aging [76]. These investigators further showed that activation of AT_2R in isolated mitochondrial was coupled to an increase in NO [76]. Although our studies did not access AT_1R or AT_2R expression in cortical renal mitochondria, we find evidence for the AT_7/MasR, active renin and angiotensinogen in the sheep mitochondria [75]. We demonstrated peptide levels that range from 5 to 60 fmol/mg protein for Ang I, Ang II and Ang-(1-7) in the isolated mitochondria [75]. The mitochondrial preparation also processed ^{125}I-Ang I to ^{125}I-Ang-(1-7).

The formation of Ang-(1-7) was essentially abolished by inhibitors against the endopeptidases thimet oligopeptidase and neprilysin. Protein expression for both neprilysin and thimet oligopeptidase were also evident in the mitochondria [75]. However, we could not demonstrate processing of Ang I to Ang II in the isolated mitochondria, particularly under conditions in which the generation of Ang-(1-7) was effectively blocked [75]. In preliminary studies, Zhuo and colleagues demonstrate that the Ang II-AT_1R complex traffics to the mitochondria in proximal tubule cells; therefore, receptor-mediated internalization of Ang II may potentially be the mitochondrial source of the peptide [77].

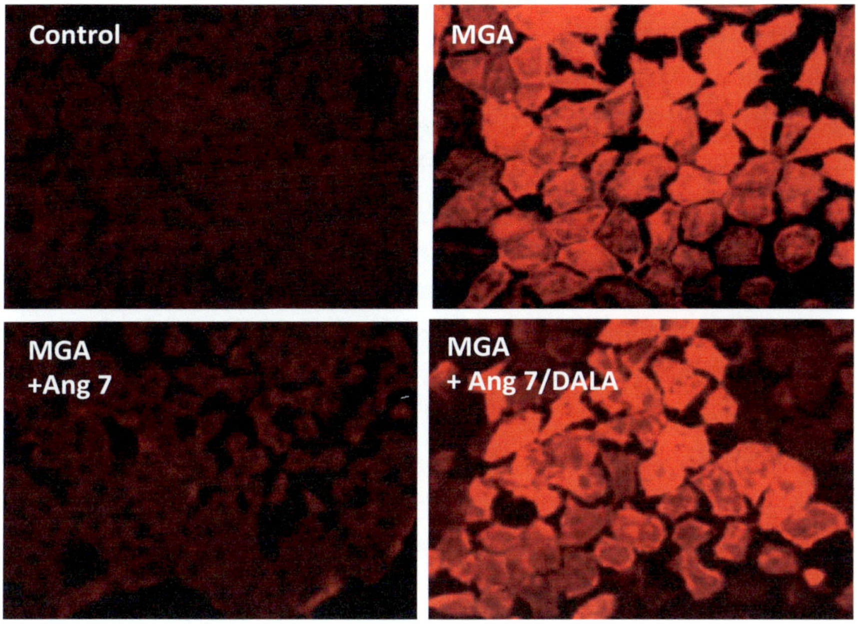

Fig. (6). Ang-(1-7) attenuates epithelial to mesenchymal transition in NRK-52E cells. Treatment with 100 nM Ang-(1-7) (Ang 7) abolished α-smooth muscle actin (α-SMA) expression, a canonical marker of epithelial to mesenchymal transition (EMT), in response to the advanced glycation end product (AGE) methoxylglycated albumin (MGA). Addition of the AT_7 receptor antagonist D-Ala^7-Ang-(1-7) (DALA, 10 μM) reversed the inhibitory effects of Ang 7 on MGA-dependent EMT. Adapted from Alzayadneh and Chappell [73].

Fetal Programming Events

Barker and colleagues advanced the hypothesis over 20 years ago that early intrauterine events may produce long-lasting cellular alterations that predispose adults to cardiovascular and/or metabolic pathologies [78]. One primary stimulus of these alterations in the fetus or fetal programming events is an inappropriate exposure *in utero* to glucocorticoids. Indeed, a number of experimental studies reveal that *in utero* exposure to exogenous glucocorticoids or conditions that increase endogenous glucocorticoid exposure to the fetus results in elevated blood pressure in the exposed adult [79 - 82]. The clinical relevance of fetal programing events is obvious regarding the current treatment of pregnant women with exogenous glucocorticoids who are in danger of premature delivery. In this case, glucocorticoid exposure *in utero* reduces mortality of the premature infant that likely reflects the accelerated maturation of pulmonary function. However, it is not clear as to the long-term consequences of the exposed infant to glucocorticoid-induced programming events. The clinical evidence is controversial as Doyle *et al.* reported that glucocorticoid-exposed young adults exhibited higher blood pressure than an unexposed cohort [81]; however, the Dessens study found no effect of glucocorticoid exposure on blood pressure [83]. These differences may reflect that the exposed group in the Doyle study was treated at an earlier mean gestational age than those in the Dessens study [28 *vs.* 32 weeks of gestation]. Although the mechanisms pertaining to fetal programing events and long-term alterations in the cardiovascular system are currently unresolved, various experimental studies have suggested a role of the ACE-Ang II-AT_1R axis [84 - 89]. In regards to programming events and the RAS, we developed a fetal programing model in which pregnant ewes are administered the glucocorticoid agonist betamethasone at the same dose as given to women in jeopardy of premature delivery and at approximately the same gestational age [90]. Both male and female exposed adults exhibit a lower nephron number and a ~15 mmHg increase in mean arterial blood pressure by 1 year of age [91]. The exposed sheep also exhibit an impaired baroreflex sensitivity that significantly precedes the increase in blood pressure and is evident as early as 6 weeks of age [91]. Blockade of the AT_1R in the betamethasone-exposed sheep normalized arterial blood pressure and improved the baroreflex. Blockade of the AT_7/MasR reduced the baroreflex sensitivity and increased arterial blood pressure in the saline-exposed or control sheep, but did not influence these indices in the betamethasone exposed sheep that may reflect an attenuated Ang-(1-7) axis as a programming event [92]. Indeed, we find evidence of lower protein expression of the AT_7/MasR in the brain medulla of the betamethasone exposed sheep; however, the protein expression of the AT_1R was not significantly different [93].

In regards to renal mechanisms that may contribute to a sustained increase in blood pressure, male exposed sheep exhibit an exacerbated response to Ang II that reflects both an increase in renal vascular resistance and enhanced sodium absorption [91, 94]. Moreover, the expected natriuretic response to Ang-(1-7) was abolished in the betamethasone-exposed males, but was essentially intact in the betamethasone-exposed females [91, 94]. Our recent studies have utilized isolated proximal tubule cells from both betamethasone and control adult sheep to elucidate the cellular mechanisms for the sodium response to Ang II [95]. Similar to the intact sheep, Ang II stimulated sodium uptake to a greater extent in proximal tubule cells from adult male betamethasone sheep than control males or the exposed and non-exposed females. The Ang II response in the male betamethasone tubule cells was associated with a marked decrease in NO levels. In contrast, the NO response was intact in the female betamethasone tubule cells [95]. The tubule cells from the betamethasone-exposed male sheep also exhibited a higher content of both the AT_1R and the sodium hydrogen exchanger (NHE3) than the non-exposed males [95]. The expression of the AT_2R tended to be higher in the females as compared to the males, but there was no significant effect of betamethasone exposure on the AT_2R isoform. Finally, our preliminary studies reveal reduced Ang-(1-7) responsiveness to attenuate sodium uptake in the proximal tubule cells from the betamethasone-exposed male sheep that was associated with a blunted NO response [96]. We find a significant reduction in protein expression of the AT_7/MasR in the tubule cells of the betamethasone-exposed males, but not in epithelial cells of the betamethasone females suggesting that the Ang-(1-7)-AT_7/MasR axis is preserved in the females [96]. Although these data clearly show that programming events target the Ang-(1-7) receptor axis in the proximal tubule cells, it is also likely that other signaling components downstream from AT_7/MasR may be attenuated by betamethasone exposure to promote greater sodium retention. In this regard, the proximal tubule expression of ACE2 was markedly reduced in the betamethasone exposed sheep (Fig. **4B**). Moreover, the soluble forms of circulating and urinary ACE2 were also attenuated in the betamethasone sheep suggesting that the shedding of the membrane form of the peptidase does not account for the lower expression of renal ACE2 (Fig. **4B**). In contrast, the tubular expression of ACE and neprilysin were not altered by betamethasone exposure clearly implying a differential effect of programming on the components of the RAS [97].

CONCLUSION

In the present review, we have discussed several aspects of the Ang-(1-7)-AT_7/MasR axis pertaining to the intracellular actions of the system and the role of the peptide in fetal programming events. The biochemical and functional evidence certainly establishes that the Ang-(1-7) axis is distinct from the ACE-Ang II-AT_1R pathway; however, evidence also suggests an interaction between these systems and an altered ratio of greater Ang II to Ang-(1-7) tone may contribute to greater cardiovascular pathologies than changes in one system alone. Furthermore, the evidence of an intracellular Ang-(1-7) axis is also consistent with overwhelming biochemical and functional data on a complete RAS within the cell and emphasizes that approaches to target the RAS should consider the overall effect to enhance Ang-(1-7) tone and attenuate the Ang II-AT_1R pathway. Finally, the recognition that fetal programing events target both the Ang II-AT_1R and the ACE2-Ang-(1-7)-AT_7/MasR pathways in brain and kidney clearly implies the functional importance of both systems in cardiovascular disease.

CONFLICT OF INTEREST

The authors confirm that they have no conflict of interest to declare for this publication.

ACKNOWLEDGEMENTS

These studies were supported in part by grants from the National Institute of Health grants (HL-56973, HL-51952, HD084227, HD-047584 and HD-017644 and the American Heart Association (AHA-151521 and AHA-355741). An unrestricted grant from the Farley-Hudson Foundation (Jacksonville, NC), Groskert Heart Fund and the Wake Forest Venture Fund is also acknowledged.

REFERENCES

[1] Chappell MC, Brosnihan KB, Diz DI, Ferrario CM. Identification of Angiotensin-(1-7) in rat brain. Evidence for differential processing of angiotensin peptides. J Biol Chem 1989; 264(28): 16518-23. [PMID: 277795]

[2] Chappell MC. Emerging evidence for a functional angiotensin-converting enzyme 2-angiotensin-(1-7)-MAS receptor axis: more than regulation of blood pressure? Hypertension 2007; 50(4): 596-9. [http://dx.doi.org/10.1161/HYPERTENSIONAHA.106.076216] [PMID: 17785634]

[3] Santos RA. Angiotensin-(1-7). Hypertension 2004; 63: 1138-44. [http://dx.doi.org/10.1161/HYPERTENSIONAHA.113.01274] [PMID: 24664288]

[4] Chappell MC. Biochemical evaluation of the renin-angiotensin system: the good, bad, and absolute? Am J Physiol Heart Circ Physiol 2016; 310(2): H137-52. [http://dx.doi.org/10.1152/ajpheart.00618.2015] [PMID: 26475588]

[5] Bader M, Ganten D. Update on tissue renin-angiotensin systems. J Mol Med 2008; 86(6): 615-21. [http://dx.doi.org/10.1007/s00109-008-0336-0] [PMID: 18414822]

[6] Ferrario CM, Ahmad S, Joyner J, Varagic J. Advances in the renin angiotensin system focus on angiotensin-converting enzyme 2 and angiotensin-(1-7). Adv Pharmacol 2010; 59: 197-233. [http://dx.doi.org/10.1016/S1054-3589(10)59007-0] [PMID: 20933203]

[7] Gomes ER, Santos RA, Guatimosim S. Angiotensin-(1-7)-mediated signaling in cardiomyocytes Int J Hypertens 2012; 2012: 493129.

[8] Ferreira AJ, Santos RA, Raizada MK. Angiotensin-(1-7)/angiotensin-converting enzyme 2/mas receptor axis and related mechanisms. Int J Hypertens 2012; 2012: 690785.

[9] Ferreira AJ, Murca TM, Fraga-Silva RA, Castro CH, Raizada MK, Santos RA. New cardiovascular and pulmonary therapeutic strategies based on the angiotensin-converting enzyme 2/angiotensin-(1-7)/ mas receptor axis. Int J Hypertens 2012; 2012: 147825.

[10] Ferreira AJ, Santos RA, Bradford CN, *et al.* Therapeutic implications of the vasoprotective axis of the renin-angiotensin system in cardiovascular diseases. Hypertension 2010; 55(2): 207-13. [http://dx.doi.org/10.1161/HYPERTENSIONAHA.109.140145] [PMID: 20038757]

[11] Santos RA, Ferreira AJ, Simões E Silva AC. Recent advances in the angiotensin-converting enzyme 2-angiotensin(1-7)-Mas axis. Exp Physiol 2008; 93(5): 519-27. [http://dx.doi.org/10.1113/expphysiol.2008.042002] [PMID: 18310257]

[12] Paul M, Poyan Mehr A, Kreutz R. Physiology of local renin-angiotensin systems. Physiol Rev 2006; 86(3): 747-803. [http://dx.doi.org/10.1152/physrev.00036.2005] [PMID: 16816138]

[13] Wu XC, Johns EJ. Nitric oxide modulation of neurally induced proximal tubular fluid reabsorption in the rat. Hypertension 2002; 39(3): 790-3. [http://dx.doi.org/10.1161/hy0302.105681] [PMID: 11897765]

[14] Campbell DJ, Kladis A, Duncan AM. Effects of converting enzyme inhibitors on angiotensin and bradykinin peptides. Hypertension 1994; 23(4): 439-49. [http://dx.doi.org/10.1161/01.HYP.23.4.439] [PMID: 8144213]

[15] Iyer SN, Ferrario CM, Chappell MC. Angiotensin-(1-7) contributes to the antihypertensive effects of blockade of the renin-angiotensin system. Hypertension 1998; 31(1 Pt 2): 356-61. [http://dx.doi.org/10.1161/01.HYP.31.1.356] [PMID: 9453328]

[16] Campbell DJ, Anastasopoulos F, Duncan AM, James GM, Kladis A, Briscoe TA. Effects of neutral endopeptidase inhibition and combined angiotensin converting enzyme and neutral endopeptidase inhibition on angiotensin and bradykinin peptides in rats. J Pharmacol Exp Ther 1998; 287(2): 567-77. [PMID: 9808682]

[17] Anastasopoulos F, Leung R, Kladis A, *et al.* Marked difference between angiotensin-converting enzyme and neutral endopeptidase inhibition in vivo by a dual inhibitor of both enzymes. J Pharmacol Exp Ther 1998; 284(3): 799-805. [PMID: 9495836]

[18] Allred AJ, Diz DI, Ferrario CM, Chappell MC. Pathways for angiotensin-(1-7) metabolism in pulmonary and renal tissues. Am J Physiol Renal Physiol 2000; 279(5): F841-50. [PMID: 11053044]

[19] Chappell MC, Pirro NT, Sykes A, Ferrario CM. Metabolism of angiotensin-(1-7) by angiotensin-converting enzyme. Hypertension 1998; 31(1 Pt 2): 362-7. [http://dx.doi.org/10.1161/01.HYP.31.1.362] [PMID: 9453329]

[20] Shaltout HA, Westwood BM, Averill DB, *et al.* Angiotensin metabolism in renal proximal tubules, urine, and serum of sheep: evidence for ACE2-dependent processing of angiotensin II. Am J Physiol Renal Physiol 2007; 292(1): F82-91. [http://dx.doi.org/10.1152/ajprenal.00139.2006] [PMID: 16896185]

[21] Marshall AC, Shaltout HA, Pirro NT, Rose JC, Diz DI, Chappell MC. Enhanced activity of an angiotensin-(1-7) neuropeptidase in glucocorticoid-induced fetal programming. Peptides 2014; 52: 74-81. [http://dx.doi.org/10.1016/j.peptides.2013.12.006] [PMID: 24355101]

[22] Marshall AC, Pirro NT, Rose JC, Diz DI, Chappell MC. Evidence for an angiotensin-(1-7) neuropeptidase expressed in the brain medulla and CSF of sheep. J Neurochem 2014; 130(2): 313-23. [http://dx.doi.org/10.1111/jnc.12720] [PMID: 24661079]

[23] Wilson BA, Cruz-Diaz N, Marshall AC, *et al.* An angiotensin-(1-7) peptidase in the kidney cortex, proximal tubules, and human HK-2 epithelial cells that is distinct from insulin-degrading enzyme. Am J Physiol Renal Physiol 2015; 308(6): F594-601. [http://dx.doi.org/10.1152/ajprenal.00609.2014] [PMID: 25568136]

[24] Grobe N, Weir NM, Leiva O, *et al.* Identification of prolyl carboxypeptidase as an alternative enzyme for processing of renal angiotensin II using mass spectrometry. Am J Physiol Cell Physiol 2013; 304(10): C945-53. [http://dx.doi.org/10.1152/ajpcell.00346.2012] [PMID: 23392115]

[25] Vickers C, Hales P, Kaushik V, *et al.* Hydrolysis of biological peptides by human angiotensin-converting enzyme-related carboxypeptidase. J Biol Chem 2002; 277(17): 14838-43. [http://dx.doi.org/10.1074/jbc.M200581200] [PMID: 11815627]

[26] Rice GI, Thomas DA, Grant PJ, Turner AJ, Hooper NM. Evaluation of angiotensin-converting enzyme

(ACE), its homologue ACE2 and neprilysin in angiotensin peptide metabolism. Biochem J 2004; 383(Pt 1): 45-51.
[http://dx.doi.org/10.1042/BJ20040634] [PMID: 15283675]

[27] Oudit GY, Liu GC, Zhong J, *et al.* Human recombinant ACE2 reduces the progression of diabetic nephropathy. Diabetes 2010; 59(2): 529-38.
[http://dx.doi.org/10.2337/db09-1218] [PMID: 19934006]

[28] Zhong J, Guo D, Chen CB, *et al.* Prevention of angiotensin II-mediated renal oxidative stress, inflammation, and fibrosis by angiotensin-converting enzyme 2. Hypertension 2011; 57(2): 314-22.
[http://dx.doi.org/10.1161/HYPERTENSIONAHA.110.164244] [PMID: 21189404]

[29] Wysocki J, Ye M, Rodriguez E, *et al.* Targeting the degradation of angiotensin II with recombinant angiotensin-converting enzyme 2: prevention of angiotensin II-dependent hypertension. Hypertension 2010; 55(1): 90-8.
[http://dx.doi.org/10.1161/HYPERTENSIONAHA.109.138420] [PMID: 19948988]

[30] Oudit GY, Penninger JM. Recombinant human angiotensin-converting enzyme 2 as a new renin-angiotensin system peptidase for heart failure therapy. Curr Heart Fail Rep 2011; 8(3): 176-83.
[http://dx.doi.org/10.1007/s11897-011-0063-7] [PMID: 21611889]

[31] Rice GI, Jones AL, Grant PJ, Carter AM, Turner AJ, Hooper NM. Circulating activities of angiotensin-converting enzyme, its homolog, angiotensin-converting enzyme 2, and neprilysin in a family study. Hypertension 2006; 48(5): 914-20.
[http://dx.doi.org/10.1161/01.HYP.0000244543.91937.79] [PMID: 17000927]

[32] Yamaleyeva LM, Gilliam-Davis S, Almeida I, Brosnihan KB, Lindsey SH, Chappell MC. Differential regulation of circulating and renal ACE2 and ACE in hypertensive mRen2.Lewis rats with early-onset diabetes. Am J Physiol Renal Physiol 2012; 302(11): F1374-84.
[http://dx.doi.org/10.1152/ajprenal.00656.2011] [PMID: 22378820]

[33] Epelman S, Shrestha K, Troughton RW, *et al.* Soluble angiotensin-converting enzyme 2 in human heart failure: relation with myocardial function and clinical outcomes. J Card Fail 2009; 15(7): 565-71.
[http://dx.doi.org/10.1016/j.cardfail.2009.01.014] [PMID: 19700132]

[34] Soler MJ, Riera M, Crespo M, *et al.* Circulating angiotensin-converting enzyme 2 activity in kidney transplantation: a longitudinal pilot study. Nephron Clin Pract 2012; 121(3-4): c144-50.
[http://dx.doi.org/10.1159/000345508] [PMID: 23257682]

[35] Tikellis C, Johnston CI, Forbes JM, *et al.* Characterization of renal angiotensin-converting enzyme 2 in diabetic nephropathy. Hypertension 2003; 41(3): 392-7.
[http://dx.doi.org/10.1161/01.HYP.0000060689.38912.CB] [PMID: 12623933]

[36] Kobori H, Nangaku M, Navar LG, Nishiyama A. The intrarenal renin-angiotensin system: from physiology to the pathobiology of hypertension and kidney disease. Pharmacol Rev 2007; 59(3): 251-87.
[http://dx.doi.org/10.1124/pr.59.3.3] [PMID: 17878513]

[37] Robertson AL Jr, Khairallah PA. Angiotensin II: rapid localization in nuclei of smooth and cardiac muscle. Science 1971; 172(3988): 1138-9.
[http://dx.doi.org/10.1126/science.172.3988.1138] [PMID: 4324923]

[38] Booz GW, Conrad KM, Hess AL, Singer HA, Baker KM. Angiotensin-II-binding sites on hepatocyte nuclei. Endocrinology 1992; 130(6): 3641-9.
[PMID: 1597161]

[39] Tang SS, Rogg H, Schumacher R, Dzau VJ. Characterization of nuclear angiotensin-II-binding sites in rat liver and comparison with plasma membrane receptors. Endocrinology 1992; 131(1): 374-80.
[PMID: 1612017]

[40] Re RN, Vizard DL, Brown J, LeGros L, Bryan SE. Angiotensin II receptors in chromatin. J Hypertens Suppl 1984; 2(3): S271-3.
[PMID: 6100740]

[41] Eggena P, Zhu JH, Clegg K, Barrett JD. Nuclear angiotensin receptors induce transcription of renin and angiotensinogen mRNA. Hypertension 1993; 22(4): 496-501.
[http://dx.doi.org/10.1161/01.HYP.22.4.496] [PMID: 8406654]

[42] Eggena P, Zhu JH, Sereevinyayut S, *et al.* Hepatic angiotensin II nuclear receptors and transcription of growth-related factors. J Hypertens 1996; 14(8): 961-8.
[http://dx.doi.org/10.1097/00004872-199608000-00005] [PMID: 8884550]

[43] Licea H, Walters MR, Navar LG. Renal nuclear angiotensin II receptors in normal and hypertensive rats. Acta Physiol Hung 2002; 89(4): 427-38.
[http://dx.doi.org/10.1556/APhysiol.89.2002.4.3] [PMID: 12489752]

[44] Pendergrass KD, Averill DB, Ferrario CM, Diz DI, Chappell MC. Differential expression of nuclear AT1 receptors and angiotensin II within the kidney of the male congenic mRen2. Lewis rat. Am J Physiol Renal Physiol 2006; 290(6): F1497-506.
[http://dx.doi.org/10.1152/ajprenal.00317.2005] [PMID: 16403834]

[45] Li XC, Zhuo JL. Intracellular ANG II directly induces in vitro transcription of TGF-beta1, MCP-1, and NHE-3 mRNAs in isolated rat renal cortical nuclei *via* activation of nuclear AT1a receptors. Am J Physiol Cell Physiol 2008; 294(4): C1034-45.
[http://dx.doi.org/10.1152/ajpcell.00432.2007] [PMID: 18256274]

[46] Zhuo JL, Li XC, Garvin JL, Navar LG, Carretero OA. Intracellular ANG II induces cytosolic Ca2+ mobilization by stimulating intracellular AT1 receptors in proximal tubule cells. Am J Physiol Renal Physiol 2006; 290(6): F1382-90.
[http://dx.doi.org/10.1152/ajprenal.00269.2005] [PMID: 16380461]

[47] Pendergrass KD, Gwathmey TM, Michalek RD, Grayson JM, Chappell MC. The angiotensin II-AT1 receptor stimulates reactive oxygen species within the cell nucleus. Biochem Biophys Res Commun 2009; 384(2): 149-54.
[http://dx.doi.org/10.1016/j.bbrc.2009.04.126] [PMID: 19409874]

[48] Kuroda J, Nakagawa K, Yamasaki T, *et al.* The superoxide-producing NAD(P)H oxidase Nox4 in the nucleus of human vascular endothelial cells. Genes Cells 2005; 10(12): 1139-51.
[http://dx.doi.org/10.1111/j.1365-2443.2005.00907.x] [PMID: 16324151]

[49] Hilenski LL, Clempus RE, Quinn MT, Lambeth JD, Griendling KK. Distinct subcellular localizations of Nox1 and Nox4 in vascular smooth muscle cells. Arterioscler Thromb Vasc Biol 2004; 24(4): 677-83.

[http://dx.doi.org/10.1161/01.ATV.0000112024.13727.2c] [PMID: 14670934]

[50] Spencer NY, Yan Z, Boudreau RL, *et al.* Control of hepatic nuclear superoxide production by glucose 6-phosphate dehydrogenase and NADPH oxidase-4. J Biol Chem 2011; 286(11): 8977-87. [http://dx.doi.org/10.1074/jbc.M110.193821] [PMID: 21212270]

[51] Ahmarani L, Avedanian L, Al-Khoury J, Perreault C, Jacques D, Bkaily G. Whole-cell and nuclear NADPH oxidases levels and distribution in human endocardial endothelial, vascular smooth muscle, and vascular endothelial cells. Can J Physiol Pharmacol 2013; 91(1): 71-9. [http://dx.doi.org/10.1139/cjpp-2012-0265] [PMID: 23368419]

[52] Gobeil F, Fortier A, Zhu T, *et al.* G-protein-coupled receptors signalling at the cell nucleus: an emerging paradigm. Can J Physiol Pharmacol 2006; 84(3-4): 287-97. [http://dx.doi.org/10.1139/y05-127] [PMID: 16902576]

[53] Vaniotis G, Allen BG, Hébert TE. Nuclear GPCRs in cardiomyocytes: an insider's view of β-adrenergic receptor signaling. Am J Physiol Heart Circ Physiol 2011; 301(5): H1754-64. [http://dx.doi.org/10.1152/ajpheart.00657.2011] [PMID: 21890692]

[54] Kumar R, Thomas CM, Yong QC, Chen W, Baker KM. The intracrine renin-angiotensin system. Clin Sci 2012; 123(5): 273-84. [http://dx.doi.org/10.1042/CS20120089] [PMID: 22590974]

[55] Ellis B, Li XC, Miguel-Qin E, Gu V, Zhuo JL. Evidence for a functional intracellular angiotensin system in the proximal tubule of the kidney. Am J Physiol Regul Integr Comp Physiol 2012; 302(5): R494-509. [http://dx.doi.org/10.1152/ajpregu.00487.2011] [PMID: 22170616]

[56] Gwathmey TM, Westwood BM, Pirro NT, *et al.* Nuclear angiotensin-(1-7) receptor is functionally coupled to the formation of nitric oxide. Am J Physiol Renal Physiol 2010; 299(5): F983-90. [http://dx.doi.org/10.1152/ajprenal.00371.2010] [PMID: 20810609]

[57] Savard M, Barbaz D, Bélanger S, *et al.* Expression of endogenous nuclear bradykinin B2 receptors mediating signaling in immediate early gene activation. J Cell Physiol 2008; 216(1): 234-44. [http://dx.doi.org/10.1002/jcp.21398] [PMID: 18264983]

[58] Gobeil F Jr, Zhu T, Brault S, *et al.* Nitric oxide signaling *via* nuclearized endothelial nitric-oxide synthase modulates expression of the immediate early genes iNOS and mPGES-1. J Biol Chem 2006; 281(23): 16058-67. [http://dx.doi.org/10.1074/jbc.M602219200] [PMID: 16574649]

[59] Gwathmey TM, Pendergrass KD, Reid SD, Rose JC, Diz DI, Chappell MC. Angiotensin-(1-7)-angiotensin converting enzyme 2 attenuates reactive oxygen species formation to angiotensin II within the cell nucleus. Hypertension 2010; 55(1): 166-71. [http://dx.doi.org/10.1161/HYPERTENSIONAHA.109.141622] [PMID: 19948986]

[60] Gava E, Samad-Zadeh A, Zimpelmann J, *et al.* Angiotensin-(1-7) activates a tyrosine phosphatase and inhibits glucose-induced signalling in proximal tubular cells. Nephrol Dial Transplant 2009; 24(6): 1766-73. [http://dx.doi.org/10.1093/ndt/gfn736] [PMID: 19144997]

[61] Gallagher PE, Ferrario CM, Tallant EA. MAP kinase/phosphatase pathway mediates the regulation of

ACE2 by angiotensin peptides. Am J Physiol Cell Physiol 2008; 295(5): C1169-74.
[http://dx.doi.org/10.1152/ajpcell.00145.2008] [PMID: 18768926]

[62] Sampaio WO, Henrique de Castro C, Santos RA, Schiffrin EL, Touyz RM. Angiotensin-(1-7) counterregulates angiotensin II signaling in human endothelial cells. Hypertension 2007; 50(6): 1093-8.
[http://dx.doi.org/10.1161/HYPERTENSIONAHA.106.084848] [PMID: 17984366]

[63] Camargo de Andrade MC, Di Marco GS, de Paulo Castro Teixeira V, *et al.* Expression and localization of N-domain ANG I-converting enzymes in mesangial cells in culture from spontaneously hypertensive rats. Am J Physiol Renal Physiol 2006; 290(2): F364-75.
[http://dx.doi.org/10.1152/ajprenal.00110.2005] [PMID: 16106038]

[64] Aragão DS, Cunha TS, Arita DY, *et al.* Purification and characterization of angiotensin converting enzyme 2 (ACE2) from murine model of mesangial cell in culture. Int J Biol Macromol 2011; 49(1): 79-84.
[http://dx.doi.org/10.1016/j.ijbiomac.2011.03.018] [PMID: 21470562]

[65] Cristovam PC, Arnoni CP, de Andrade MC, *et al.* ACE-dependent and chymase-dependent angiotensin II generation in normal and glucose-stimulated human mesangial cells. Exp Biol Med (Maywood) 2008; 233(8): 1035-43.
[http://dx.doi.org/10.3181/0708-RM-229] [PMID: 18480420]

[66] Vidotti DB, Casarini DE, Cristovam PC, Leite CA, Schor N, Boim MA. High glucose concentration stimulates intracellular renin activity and angiotensin II generation in rat mesangial cells. Am J Physiol Renal Physiol 2004; 286(6): F1039-45.
[http://dx.doi.org/10.1152/ajprenal.00371.2003] [PMID: 14722017]

[67] Singh VP, Le B, Bhat VB, Baker KM, Kumar R. High-glucose-induced regulation of intracellular ANG II synthesis and nuclear redistribution in cardiac myocytes. Am J Physiol Heart Circ Physiol 2007; 293(2): H939-48.
[http://dx.doi.org/10.1152/ajpheart.00391.2007] [PMID: 17483239]

[68] Singh VP, Baker KM, Kumar R. Activation of the intracellular renin-angiotensin system in cardiac fibroblasts by high glucose: role in extracellular matrix production. Am J Physiol Heart Circ Physiol 2008; 294(4): H1675-84.
[http://dx.doi.org/10.1152/ajpheart.91493.2007] [PMID: 18296558]

[69] Lavrentyev EN, Estes AM, Malik KU. Mechanism of high glucose induced angiotensin II production in rat vascular smooth muscle cells. Circ Res 2007; 101(5): 455-64.
[http://dx.doi.org/10.1161/CIRCRESAHA.107.151852] [PMID: 17626897]

[70] Lavrentyev EN, Malik KU. High glucose-induced Nox1-derived superoxides downregulate PKC-betaII, which subsequently decreases ACE2 expression and ANG(1-7) formation in rat VSMCs. Am J Physiol Heart Circ Physiol 2009; 296(1): H106-18.
[http://dx.doi.org/10.1152/ajpheart.00239.2008] [PMID: 18978194]

[71] Chou CH, Chuang LY, Lu CY, Guh JY. Interaction between TGF-β and ACE2-Ang-(1-7)-Mas pathway in high glucose-cultured NRK-52E cells. Mol Cell Endocrinol 2013; 366(1): 21-30.
[http://dx.doi.org/10.1016/j.mce.2012.11.004] [PMID: 23174757]

[72] Alzayadneh EM, Chappell MC. Nuclear expression of renin-angiotensin system components in NRK-

52E renal epithelial cells. J Renin Angiotensin Aldosterone Syst 2015; 16(4): 1135-48. [http://dx.doi.org/10.1177/1470320313515039] [PMID: 24961503]

[73] Alzayadneh EM, Chappell MC. Angiotensin-(1-7) abolishes AGE-induced cellular hypertrophy and myofibroblast transformation *via* inhibition of ERK1/2. Cell Signal 2014; 26(12): 3027-35. [http://dx.doi.org/10.1016/j.cellsig.2014.09.010] [PMID: 25246357]

[74] Zhang K, Meng X, Li D, *et al.* Angiotensin(1-7) attenuates the progression of streptozotocin-induced diabetic renal injury better than angiotensin receptor blockade. Kidney Int 2015; 87(2): 359-69. [http://dx.doi.org/10.1038/ki.2014.274] [PMID: 25075768]

[75] Wilson BA, Nautiyal M, Gwathmey TM, Rose JC, Chappell MC. Evidence for a mitochondrial Angiotensin-(1-7) system in the kidney. Am J Physiol Renal Physiol 2016; 310: F637-45.

[76] Abadir PM, Foster DB, Crow M, *et al.* Identification and characterization of a functional mitochondrial angiotensin system. Proc Natl Acad Sci USA 2011; 108(36): 14849-54. [http://dx.doi.org/10.1073/pnas.1101507108] [PMID: 21852574]

[77] Li XC, Sandoval RM, Molitoris BA, Zhuo JL. In vivo evidence of AT1a receptor mediated uptake of angiotensin II by the proximal tubule visualized by intravital multiphoton imaging. Hypertension 2015; 66: A077.

[78] Barker DJ. The fetal and infant origins of disease. Eur J Clin Invest 1995; 25(7): 457-63. [http://dx.doi.org/10.1111/j.1365-2362.1995.tb01730.x] [PMID: 7556362]

[79] Dodic M, Abouantoun T, O'Connor A, Wintour EM, Moritz KM. Programming effects of short prenatal exposure to dexamethasone in sheep. Hypertension 2002; 40(5): 729-34. [http://dx.doi.org/10.1161/01.HYP.0000036455.62159.7E] [PMID: 12411469]

[80] Zandi-Nejad K, Luyckx VA, Brenner BM. Adult hypertension and kidney disease: the role of fetal programming. Hypertension 2006; 47(3): 502-8. [http://dx.doi.org/10.1161/01.HYP.0000198544.09909.1a] [PMID: 16415374]

[81] Doyle LW, Ford GW, Davis NM, Callanan C. Antenatal corticosteroid therapy and blood pressure at 14 years of age in preterm children. Clin Sci 2000; 98(2): 137-42. [http://dx.doi.org/10.1042/cs0980137] [PMID: 10657267]

[82] Seckl JR, Holmes MC. Mechanisms of disease: glucocorticoids, their placental metabolism and fetal 'programming' of adult pathophysiology. Nat Clin Pract Endocrinol Metab 2007; 3(6): 479-88. [http://dx.doi.org/10.1038/ncpendmet0515] [PMID: 17515892]

[83] Dessens AB, Haas HS, Koppe JG. Twenty-year follow-up of antenatal corticosteroid treatment. Pediatrics 2000; 105(6): E77-84. [http://dx.doi.org/10.1542/peds.105.6.e77] [PMID: 10835090]

[84] Moritz KM, Johnson K, Douglas-Denton R, Wintour EM, Dodic M. Maternal glucocorticoid treatment programs alterations in the renin-angiotensin system of the ovine fetal kidney. Endocrinology 2002; 143(11): 4455-63. [http://dx.doi.org/10.1210/en.2002-220534] [PMID: 12399443]

[85] Wintour EM, Moritz KM, Johnson K, Ricardo S, Samuel CS, Dodic M. Reduced nephron number in adult sheep, hypertensive as a result of prenatal glucocorticoid treatment. J Physiol 2003; 549(Pt 3): 929-35.

[http://dx.doi.org/10.1113/jphysiol.2003.042408] [PMID: 12730337]

[86] Alexander BT. Fetal programming of hypertension. Am J Physiol Regul Integr Comp Physiol 2006; 290(1): R1-R10.
[http://dx.doi.org/10.1152/ajpregu.00417.2005] [PMID: 16352854]

[87] Goyal R, Lister R, Leitzke A, Goyal D, Gheorghe CP, Longo LD. Antenatal maternal hypoxic stress: adaptations of the placental renin-angiotensin system in the mouse. Placenta 2011; 32(2): 134-9.
[http://dx.doi.org/10.1016/j.placenta.2010.11.004] [PMID: 21130492]

[88] Rasch R, Skriver E, Woods LL. The role of the RAS in programming of adult hypertension. Acta Physiol Scand 2004; 181(4): 537-42.
[http://dx.doi.org/10.1111/j.1365-201X.2004.01328.x] [PMID: 15283768]

[89] Wyrwoll CS, Mark PJ, Waddell BJ. Developmental programming of renal glucocorticoid sensitivity and the renin-angiotensin system. Hypertension 2007; 50(3): 579-84.
[http://dx.doi.org/10.1161/HYPERTENSIONAHA.107.091603] [PMID: 17664394]

[90] Shaltout HA, Rose JC, Figueroa JP, Chappell MC, Diz DI, Averill DB. Acute AT(1)-receptor blockade reverses the hemodynamic and baroreflex impairment in adult sheep exposed to antenatal betamethasone. Am J Physiol Heart Circ Physiol 2010; 299(2): H541-7.
[http://dx.doi.org/10.1152/ajpheart.00100.2010] [PMID: 20543085]

[91] Tang L, Carey LC, Bi J, *et al.* Gender differences in the effects of antenatal betamethasone exposure on renal function in adult sheep. Am J Physiol Regul Integr Comp Physiol 2009; 296(2): R309-17.
[http://dx.doi.org/10.1152/ajpregu.90645.2008] [PMID: 19036827]

[92] Shaltout HA, Rose JC, Chappell MC, Diz DI. Angiotensin-(1-7) deficiency and baroreflex impairment precede the antenatal Betamethasone exposure-induced elevation in blood pressure. Hypertension 2012; 59(2): 453-8.
[http://dx.doi.org/10.1161/HYPERTENSIONAHA.111.185876] [PMID: 22215705]

[93] Marshall AC, Shaltout HA, Nautiyal M, Rose JC, Chappell MC, Diz DI. Fetal betamethasone exposure attenuates angiotensin-(1-7)-Mas receptor expression in the dorsal medulla of adult sheep. Peptides 2013; 44: 25-31.
[http://dx.doi.org/10.1016/j.peptides.2013.03.018] [PMID: 23538211]

[94] Tang L, Bi J, Valego N, *et al.* Prenatal betamethasone exposure alters renal function in immature sheep: sex differences in effects. Am J Physiol Regul Integr Comp Physiol 2010; 299(3): R793-803.
[http://dx.doi.org/10.1152/ajpregu.00590.2009] [PMID: 20554936]

[95] Su Y, Bi J, Pulgar VM, Figueroa J, Chappell M, Rose JC. Antenatal glucocorticoid treatment alters Na+ uptake in renal proximal tubule cells from adult offspring in a sex-specific manner. Am J Physiol Renal Physiol 2015; 308(11): F1268-75.
[http://dx.doi.org/10.1152/ajprenal.00047.2015] [PMID: 25834069]

[96] Su Y, Bi J, Pulgar VM, Chappell MC, Rose JC. Antenatal betamehtasone attenuates the Angiotensin-(1-7)/nitric oxide axis in adult male but not adult female renal proximal tubule cells. Hypertension 2015; 66: AP169.

[97] Shaltout HA, Westwood BM, Averill DB, *et al.* Angiotensin metabolism in renal proximal tubules, urine, and serum of sheep: evidence for ACE2-dependent processing of angiotensin II. Am J Physiol Renal Physiol 2007; 292(1): F82-91.
[http://dx.doi.org/10.1152/ajprenal.00139.2006] [PMID: 16896185]

CHAPTER 11

Renin Receptors in Cardiovascular and Renal Diseases

A.H. Jan Danser*

Division of Pharmacology and Vascular Medicine, Department of Internal Medicine, Erasmus MC, Rotterdam, The Netherlands

Abstract: Local angiotensin generation depends on the uptake of circulating renin and/or its precursor prorenin. Such uptake may involve binding to a receptor. In the past 3 decades, three potential receptor candidates have been evaluated: a renin-binding protein, the mannose 6-phosphate/insulin-like growth factor II receptor, and the (pro)renin receptor. The most promising candidate seemed to be the (pro)renin receptor; however its affinity for renin and prorenin is several orders of magnitude above their actual levels in blood, raising doubt on whether this interaction truly occurs *in vivo*. In addition, conflicting *in-vivo* data have been reported regarding the putative (pro)renin receptor blocker, handle region peptide, while (pro)renin receptor knockout studies revealed lethal consequences that are (pro)renin-independent. The latter is most likely due to the fact that the (pro)renin receptor colocalizes with vacuolar H^+-ATPase, and possibly determines the stability of this vital enzyme. This chapter briefly discusses the various receptors, and ends with the conclusion that (pro)renin-(pro)renin receptor interaction, if it occurs *in vivo*, is limited to (pro)renin-synthesizing organs like the kidney.

Keywords: Angiotensin, Cyclo-oxygenase-2, ATP6AP2, Extracellular signal-regulated kinase, Glomerulosclerosis, Handle region peptide, Kidney, Mannose 6-phosphate/insulin-like growth factor II, Plasminogen-activator inhibitor-1, Prorenin, (Pro)renin receptor, Renin, Renin-binding protein, Transforming growth factor ß1, Vacuolar H^+-ATPase, Wnt signaling.

* **Corresponding author A.H.J. Danser:** Division of Pharmacology and Vascular Medicine, Department of Internal Medicine Erasmus MC, Dr. Molewaterplein 50, room EE1418b 3015 GE Rotterdam, The Netherlands; Telephone: 31-10-7043540; Fax: 31-10-7044733; E-mail: a.danser@erasmusmc.nl.

Dulce Elena Casarini, Danielle Yuri Arita, Tatiana Sousa Cunha & Juliana Almada Colucci (Eds.)

INTRODUCTION

Renin is formed from its precursor, prorenin, by cleavage of a 43-amino acid aminoterminal prosegment in the juxtaglomerular cells of the kidney. It is then either secreted into the circulation or stored in granules. Prorenin is also secreted from the kidney, without storage, and, unlike renin, originates simultaneously from several other organs, like the adrenal, eye and ovaries [1]. In general, plasma prorenin concentrations are much higher than plasma renin concentrations [2].

It is widely accepted that angiotensin (Ang) II, the end-product of the renin-angiotensin system (RAS), is generated not only in the circulation, but also locally. Given the exclusive synthesis of renin in the kidney, 2 scenarios have emerged to explain such tissue angiotensin generation: either renal renin accumulates at tissue sites (*e.g.*, through binding to a receptor), or prorenin (of renal or extrarenal origin) is activated at tissue sites. In support of renin uptake, tissue renin levels (expressed per g wet weight), *e.g.* in the heart, are too high to be explained based upon the amount of renin- and prorenin-containing extracellular fluid in tissue [3, 4]. In addition, studies in rat and pigs have shown that part of tissue renin is membrane-associated [3, 5]. Moreover, isolated perfused hearts of rats transgenic for human angiotensinogen release Ang I during renin infusion and this release continues after stopping the renin infusion [6].

These data strongly support the idea that circulating renin binds to a renin-binding protein/receptor, and that bound renin is catalytically active. It would be of even greater interest if such receptors would also bind prorenin, particularly if this would result in prorenin activation. Three potential renin/prorenin (here together denoted as (pro)renin) receptors have been described in the past 3 decades, a renin-binding protein, the mannose 6-phosphate/insulin-like growth factor II receptor, and the (pro)renin receptor ((P)RR). This chapter, based on a recent review [7], describes each of these receptors.

Renin-Binding Protein

An intracellular renin-binding protein (RnBP) was discovered almost thirty years ago in humans, rats and pigs [8 - 10]. Binding of renin to this RnBP strongly inhibited its capacity to convert angiotensinogen to Ang I, suggesting a role as an *in-vivo* renin inhibitor. Later it was discovered that RnBP is the enzyme N-acy--D-glucosamine 2-epimerase [11, 12]. *In-vitro* studies subsequently showed that RnBP not only inhibited renin, but that the reverse is also true [13]. Yet, mice lacking RnBP were normotensive and did not display any major alteration in their circulating or renal RAS [14]. Moreover, RnBP was located in the collecting duct and tubules, as opposed to the juxtaglomerular location of renin, and this situation did not change following renin induction in two kidney, one clip (2K1C) rats [15]. Taken together therefore, a role for the RnBP in the regulation of renin/prorenin and/or RAS activity in plasma or kidney seems unlikely.

Mannose 6-Phosphate/Insulin-Like Growth Factor II Receptor

Lysosomal enzymes, following their synthesis in the endoplasmic reticulum, are targeted to their destination *via* a mechanism involving phosphomannosyl residues. These residues are recognized by so-called mannose 6-phosphate (M6P) receptors. The secretory granules of the juxtaglomerular cells resemble lysosomes, and renin transport in these cells involves the M6P receptor [16]. Extracellular lysosomal enzymes bind to cell surface M6P receptors and are subsequently internalized *via* clathrin-coated pits. They dissociate from the receptor in acidified endosomal compartments and are delivered to lysosomes.

M6P receptors are divided in two groups: the large M6P receptors are cation-independent and bind ligands independently of divalent cations; the small M6P receptors are cation-dependent and require divalent cations for optimal binding [17]. The large M6P receptor is identical to the insulin-like growth factor II (IGFII) receptor [18], and hence this receptor is now known as the M6P/IGFII receptor [19, 20].

The M6P/IGFII receptor binds phosphomannosylated (*i.e.*, M6P-containing) renin and prorenin. Such binding resulted in their internalization in a variety of cells, including cardiomyocytes, fibroblasts, vascular smooth muscle cells and endothelial cells [21 - 26]. Moreover, after internalization, prorenin was converted to renin by an as yet unidentified enzyme [23]. Thus, at least theoretically, M6P/IGFII receptors might contribute to the uptake of M6P-containing (pro)renin from the circulation at tissue sites, as well as the local activation of this prorenin.

Yet, evidence for the release of internalized renin and prorenin into the medium could not be obtained - instead, intracellular degradation of renin, presumably in lysosomes, occurred [22, 23, 25]. Moreover, no role for M6P/IGFII receptor-bound renin or prorenin in angiotensin generation could be demonstrated [27]. It therefore appears that M6P/IGFII receptor-mediated prorenin and renin internalization represents (pro)renin clearance rather than a mechanism allowing tissue angiotensin generation.

(Pro) Renin Receptor

The (P)RR is a 350-amino acid, ubiquitously expressed transmembrane protein, discovered in 2002, that can bind both renin and prorenin [28 - 30]. (P)RR binding is supposed to induce a conformational change in prorenin, by which the prosegment is moved out of the catalytic cleft and the active site is exposed, leading to non-proteolytic activation of prorenin. Remarkably, (pro)renin binding to the (P)RR also results in the activation of signaling pathways, independent from the formation of angiotensins. The affinity of prorenin for the human (P)RR is 3-4-fold higher than that of renin [31]. Therefore, it seems reasonable to assume that the prosegment facilitates binding. A peptidic antagonist has been designed based on the idea that the prosegment of prorenin contains a 'handle region' (10P-19P) which binds to the receptor, allowing prorenin activation [32]. This so-called 'handle region peptide' (HRP) mimicks the handle region and will thus bind competitively to the receptor, thereby preventing receptor-mediated prorenin activation.

Effects in the Kidney

Ubiquitous overexpression of the human (P)RR in rats resulted in proteinuria, glomerulosclerosis [33] and renal cyclooxygenase-2 (COX-2) upregulation [34]. It also led to increased levels of aldosterone in blood plasma. The latter was not due to (pro)renin-induced (P)RR stimulation, since neither renin nor prorenin affected aldosterone synthesis in human adrenocortical cells [35]. These elevated aldosterone levels may thus be a direct consequence of (P)RR overexpression, independently of the RAS. HRP prevented the development of glomerulosclerosis in human (P)RR transgenic rats [33].

In diabetic rats, HRP normalized the elevated renal angiotensin content [36], without affecting blood pressure. Concomitantly, the development of diabetic nephropathy was prevented. Since this effect also occurred in Ang II type 1A (AT_{1A}) receptor-deficient mice [37], the effect of HRP could not be explained on the basis of suppression of local angiotensin generation. Interestingly, extracellular signal-regulated kinase 1 and 2 (ERK1/2) as well as phospho-p38 mitogen-activated protein kinase (MAPK) and phospho-Jun N-terminal kinase (JNK) MAPK were upregulated in the diabetic kidney, both in wild-type mice and in AT_{1A} receptor-deficient mice, and HRP fully normalized this increased phosphorylation [37]. Thus, HRP exerted beneficial effects in an Ang II-independent manner.

In vitro, renin induced ERK1/2 activation in mesangial cells. This activation resulted in transforming growth factor ß1 (TGFß1) release and the subsequent upregulation of genes coding for profibrotic molecules such as plasminogen-activator inhibitor-1 (PAI-1), fibronectin and collagens [28, 38]. Effects started to occur at renin levels below 1 nmol/L, and could be fully prevented by (P)RR si-RNA. Similar results were observed in human embryonic kidney (HEK) cells with both renin and prorenin, although now concentrations of 100 nmol/L were required [39]. Remarkably, in podocytes, 2 nmol/L human prorenin increased ERK1/2 without affecting TGFß1 or PAI-1 [40]. (P)RR suppression with si-RNA, but not RAS blockade, prevented this effect. Apparently therefore, the (P)RR-ERK1/2-mediated activation of profibrotic pathways does not occur in all cells and does not require Ang II.

COX-2 overexpression in podocytes exacerbated diabetic nephropathy by increasing (P)RR expression [41]. Thus, not only does (P)RR overexpression result in COX-2 upregulation [34, 42], but the reverse is also true, possibly because COX-2 products promote (P)RR activation. Indeed, Huang *et al.* [43] confirmed this positive feedback loop. First, they demonstrated that high glucose in rat mesangial cells upregulates (P)RR (*via* protein kinase C, ERK1/2 and JNK [44]) and (pro)renin, thereby facilitating Ang II generation. This Ang II subsequently induced COX-2 and interleukin-1ß, although a direct (Ang II-independent) effect of (P)RR stimulation on COX-2 activation is also feasible [42]. Second, COX-2 inhibition reduced the glucose-induced (P)RR upregulation, suggesting that COX-2 products directly upregulate (P)RR. In summary, various studies support a link between the (P)RR and COX-2, and this link involves, at least in part, Ang II.

HRP did not affect hypertensive nephrosclerosis in Goldblatt (2 kidney, 1 clip; 2K1C) rats [45]. Ryuzaki [46] confirmed this finding, but simultaneously demonstrated that HRP after 12 weeks of infusion reduced the glomerulosclerosis index, tubulointerstitial damage, TGFß1 expression and Ang II levels in the non-clipped kidney (but not in the clipped kidney). Under no condition did HRP affect blood pressure or proteinuria. Krebs *et al.* [47] also did not observe effects of HRP in the clipped kidney of 2K1C rats. Since damage in the clipped kidney usually occurs acutely (in a renin-dependent manner), these data suggest that HRP is unable to interfere with renin-(P)RR interaction in the clipped kidney. The mechanism of its long-term effects in the non-clipped kidney remains to be determined.

Effects in the Heart and Vessel Wall

Overexpression of the human (P)RR in rat vascular smooth muscle cells resulted in hypertension [48], without altering the levels of RAS components. HRP diminished cardiac fibrosis in high-salt fed stroke-prone spontaneously hypertensive rats (SHR) [49], without affecting blood pressure or the circulating RAS. No such effects occurred in SHR fed a normal salt diet [50]. Unexpectedly, in SHR on a normal salt diet treated with the renin inhibitor aliskiren, HRP diminished both the blood pressure-lowering effect of aliskiren and its beneficial effects on coronary endothelial function and cardiomyocyte area [51]. These latter effects of HRP occurred in an angiotensin-independent manner. Similarly, HRP counteracted the beneficial effects of renin inhibition on vascular dysfunction in diabetic hypertensive rats, *i.e.*, it allowed the return of a contractile factor generated by COX-2 [52].

These findings raise doubt on whether HRP truly acts as an inhibitor of (pro)renin-(P)RR interaction outside the kidney. In fact, Leckie and Bottrill were unable to find a binding site for HRP in human endothelial cells [53], and HRP even bound to embryonic stem cells lacking the transmembrane region of the

(P)RR [54]. Moreover, although Feldt *et al.* observed increased ERK1/2 phosphorylation in U937 monocytes following exposure to human renin or prorenin [54], human HRP did not block this phenomenon. In contrast, mouse HRP did block the mouse prorenin-induced ERK1/2 phosphorylation in mouse endothelial cells at concentrations of 10 and 100 µmol/L [55], *i.e.*, at concentrations that are several orders of magnitude above the levels obtained *in vivo* during HRP infusion [56]. To explain these discrepancies, it has been proposed that, in certain cells, and possibly particularly *in vitro*, the (P)RR is not or only scarcely located on the cell surface, thus not allowing an easy access for HRP [55].

Indeed, Yoshikawa *et al.* [57], like Batenburg *et al.* [29], observed that the majority of (P)RR in vascular smooth muscle cells is located in the endoplasmic reticulum and the Golgi, and not on the cell membrane. Similar observations were made in neonatal rat cardiomyocytes [58]. Nevertheless, renin and/or prorenin, when applied at high concentrations (up to 100 nmol/L) did bind to VSMC in a (P)RR-dependent manner [59] and induced ERK1/2 phosphorylation, DNA and protein synthesis, and PAI-1 release [59 - 61]. (P)RR knockdown with si-RNA prevented these effects [59, 62]. The (pro)renin-induced effects on PAI-1 release were additive to those of Ang II [59, 61], and angiotensin generation following (pro)renin-(P)RR interaction tended to occur at lower (pro)renin levels than direct signaling. Prorenin-induced MAPK p38 activation followed by heat shock protein 27 phosphorylation and an alteration in actin filament dynamics were described in neonatal rat cardiomyocytes [58]. Taken together, these data do support (pro)renin-(P)RR interaction in vascular smooth muscle cells and cardiomyocytes at exceptionally high (pro)renin levels *in vitro*. The conflicting results obtained with HRP *in vivo* and *in vitro* argue against the idea that this drug truly blocks (pro)renin-(P)RR interaction in the intact animal.

Implications

Despite 3 decades of research, none of the currently proposed receptors fulfils the ideal concept of a (pro)renin receptor, *i.e.*, a receptor that sequesters circulating renin and/or prorenin with high affinity at tissue sites, and subsequently facilitates angiotensin generation. The RnBP most likely is unrelated to the RAS, and the

M6P/IGFII receptor may, at most, function as a clearance receptor for renin and prorenin. This leaves the (P)RR as the most promising candidate. However, as outlined above, >10 years of research have not resulted in a clear picture of (pro)renin-(P)RR interaction *in vivo*. Confusingly, renin and prorenin may even act as agonists of this receptor, exerting angiotensin-independent effects. Importantly, the affinity of the receptor for renin and prorenin is in the high nanomolar range (possibly even 20 nmol/L for renin [31]), which is difficult to reconcile with the low picomolar levels of renin and prorenin in extracellular fluid [2]. It is however in full agreement with the observations that (P)RR overexpression in rats did not result in changes in RAS component levels [34, 48], and that in most *in-vitro* studies investigating (pro)renin-(P)RR interaction high nanomolar (up to 100 nmol/L [39]) (pro)renin concentrations were required to observe effects.

Moreover, prorenin overexpression, elevating plasma prorenin levels up to 400-fold in rodents, did raise blood pressure in an angiotensin-dependent manner [63 - 65]. Yet, it did not result in the fibrosis and/or glomerulosclerosis that were expected based upon *in-vitro* studies showing direct profibrotic responses to renin and prorenin. Possibly, for such direct effects prorenin rises of >1000-fold are required, and renin rises of >100.000-fold. However, such rises do not occur *in vivo*, at least in non-(pro)renin synthesizing organs. Whether they occur in (pro)renin-synthesizing tissues (*e.g.*, in renal interstitial fluid) remains to be proven. The maximum plasma (pro)renin rises that have been described in humans (*e.g.*, in severe heart failure or during RAS blockade) are around 50-100 - fold for renin (but usually well below 10-fold), and 2-3-fold for prorenin [2, 66, 67]. Consequently, although the 400-fold rise in circulating prorenin in prorenin-overexpressing rodents may have resulted in (P)RR-dependent Ang II formation (thus explaining the Ang II-dependent phenotype in these animals) [63 - 65], this observation is unlikely to reflect normal physiology.

Therefore, the phenotype that develops in response to (P)RR overexpression per se must represent (P)RR effects that are RAS-independent [68, 69]. In fact, it has recently been reported that the (P)RR co-localizes with vacuolar H^+-ATPase (V-ATPase) in the kidney [70]. This may relate to the observation that the 8.9 kDa accessory protein ATP6AP2 of vacuolar H^+-ATPase is a post-translationally truncated version of the (P)RR, resembling its C-terminal domain [31]. V-ATPases play an important role in the acidification of subcellular compartments. The (P)RR is indispensable for V-ATPase integrity, as in cardiomyocyte-specific (P)RR knock-out mice, the abundance of several V-ATPase subunits is decreased in cardiomyocytes, resulting in the development of heart failure due to defective autophagy and ultimately cell death [68]. Furthermore, the (P)RR plays a role on V-ATPase and Wnt receptors functions, affecting several signaling molecules [69]. These findings clearly indicate the importance of the (P)RR beyond prorenin binding, and raise doubt on the (P)RR as a (pro)renin binder/activator *in vivo*. This does not rule out that the (P)RR is an important player in tissue damage, and/or that RAS blockade exerts beneficial effects by reducing its expression. The current data with HRP are inconclusive, mainly because no *in-vivo* study has convincingly shown that this drug blocks (P)RR-(pro)renin interaction. It is even possible that HRP is a partial (P)RR agonist, independently of renin/prorenin, thus explaining some of its conflicting results. (P)RR blockade per se, given its interference with V-ATPase, might well be detrimental.

Future studies should now rigorously address whether (pro)renin-(P)RR interaction truly occurs *in vivo*, and if so, where. Clearly, such interaction seems impossible in organs not synthesizing (pro)renin, like the heart and vessel wall, where the (pro)renin levels (per gram tissue), at most, are comparable to those in plasma (per mL plasma). This leaves the kidney and extrarenal prorenin-synthesizing organs like the ovary as the most likely sites of interaction.

CONFLICT OF INTEREST

The authors confirm that they have no conflict of interest to declare for this publication.

ACKNOWLEDGEMENTS

Declare none.

REFERENCES

[1] Krop M, Danser AH. Circulating *versus* tissue renin-angiotensin system: on the origin of (pro)renin. Curr Hypertens Rep 2008; 10(2): 112-8. [http://dx.doi.org/10.1007/s11906-008-0022-1] [PMID: 18474177]

[2] Danser AH, Derkx FH, Schalekamp MA, Hense HW, Riegger GA, Schunkert H. Determinants of interindividual variation of renin and prorenin concentrations: evidence for a sexual dimorphism of (pro)renin levels in humans. J Hypertens 1998; 16(6): 853-62.
[http://dx.doi.org/10.1097/00004872-199816060-00017] [PMID: 9663926]

[3] Danser AH, van Kats JP, Admiraal PJ, *et al.* Cardiac renin and angiotensins. Uptake from plasma *versus in situ* synthesis. Hypertension 1994; 24(1): 37-48.
[http://dx.doi.org/10.1161/01.HYP.24.1.37] [PMID: 8021006]

[4] Katz SA, Opsahl JA, Lunzer MM, Forbis LM, Hirsch AT. Effect of bilateral nephrectomy on active renin, angiotensinogen, and renin glycoforms in plasma and myocardium. Hypertension 1997; 30(2 Pt 1): 259-66.
[http://dx.doi.org/10.1161/01.HYP.30.2.259] [PMID: 9260990]

[5] Campbell DJ, Valentijn AJ. Identification of vascular renin-binding proteins by chemical cross-linking: inhibition of binding of renin by renin inhibitors. J Hypertens 1994; 12(8): 879-90.
[http://dx.doi.org/10.1097/00004872-199408000-00005] [PMID: 7814847]

[6] Müller DN, Fischli W, Clozel JP, *et al.* Local angiotensin II generation in the rat heart: role of renin uptake. Circ Res 1998; 82(1): 13-20.
[http://dx.doi.org/10.1161/01.RES.82.1.13] [PMID: 9440700]

[7] Batenburg WW, Danser AH. (Pro)renin and its receptors: pathophysiological implications. Clin Sci 2012; 123(3): 121-33.
[http://dx.doi.org/10.1042/CS20120042] [PMID: 22494159]

[8] Tada M, Takahashi S, Miyano M, Miyake Y. Tissue-specific regulation of renin-binding protein gene expression in rats. J Biochem 1992; 112(2): 175-82.
[PMID: 1400260]

[9] Takahashi S, Inoue H, Miyake Y. The human gene for renin-binding protein. J Biol Chem 1992; 267(18): 13007-13.
[PMID: 1618798]

[10] Takahashi S, Ohsawa T, Miura R, Miyake Y. Purification of high molecular weight (HMW) renin from porcine kidney and direct evidence that the HMW renin is a complex of renin with renin binding protein (RnBP). J Biochem 1983; 93(1): 265-74.
[PMID: 6341368]

[11] Takahashi S, Takahashi K, Kaneko T, Ogasawara H, Shindo S, Kobayashi M. Human renin-binding protein is the enzyme N-acetyl-D-glucosamine 2-epimerase. J Biochem 1999; 125(2): 348-53.
[http://dx.doi.org/10.1093/oxfordjournals.jbchem.a022293] [PMID: 9990133]

[12] Takahashi S, Takahashi K, Kaneko T, *et al.* Identification of cysteine-380 as the essential residue for the human N-acetyl-D-glucosamine 2-epimerase (renin binding protein). J Biochem 1999; 126(4): 639-42.
[http://dx.doi.org/10.1093/oxfordjournals.jbchem.a022496] [PMID: 10502668]

[13] Takahashi S, Kumagai M, Shindo S, Saito K, Kawamura Y. Renin inhibits N-acetyl-D-glucosamine 2-epimerase (renin-binding protein). J Biochem 2000; 128(6): 951-6.
[http://dx.doi.org/10.1093/oxfordjournals.jbchem.a022846] [PMID: 11098137]

[14] Schmitz C, Gotthardt M, Hinderlich S, *et al.* Normal blood pressure and plasma renin activity in mice lacking the renin-binding protein, a cellular renin inhibitor. J Biol Chem 2000; 275(20): 15357-62. [http://dx.doi.org/10.1074/jbc.275.20.15357] [PMID: 10809771]

[15] Leckie BJ, Lacy PS, Lidder S. The expression of renin-binding protein and renin in the kidneys of rats with two-kidney one-clip hypertension. J Hypertens 2000; 18(7): 935-43. [http://dx.doi.org/10.1097/00004872-200018070-00016] [PMID: 10930192]

[16] Faust PL, Chirgwin JM, Kornfeld S. Renin, a secretory glycoprotein, acquires phosphomannosyl residues. J Cell Biol 1987; 105(5): 1947-55. [http://dx.doi.org/10.1083/jcb.105.5.1947] [PMID: 2960682]

[17] Dahms NM, Lobel P, Breitmeyer J, Chirgwin JM, Kornfeld S. 46 kd mannose 6-phosphate receptor: cloning, expression, and homology to the 215 kd mannose 6-phosphate receptor. Cell 1987; 50(2): 181-92. [http://dx.doi.org/10.1016/0092-8674(87)90214-5] [PMID: 2954652]

[18] Morgan DO, Edman JC, Standring DN, *et al.* Insulin-like growth factor II receptor as a multifunctional binding protein. Nature 1987; 329(6137): 301-7. [http://dx.doi.org/10.1038/329301a0] [PMID: 2957598]

[19] Ludwig T, Tenscher K, Remmler J, Hoflack B, Lobel P. Cloning and sequencing of cDNAs encoding the full-length mouse mannose 6-phosphate/insulin-like growth factor II receptor. Gene 1994; 142(2): 311-2. [http://dx.doi.org/10.1016/0378-1119(94)90282-8] [PMID: 8194771]

[20] Szebenyi G, Rotwein P. The mouse insulin-like growth factor II/cation-independent mannose 6-phosphate (IGF-II/MPR) receptor gene: molecular cloning and genomic organization. Genomics 1994; 19(1): 120-9. [http://dx.doi.org/10.1006/geno.1994.1021] [PMID: 8188212]

[21] Admiraal PJ, van Kesteren CA, Danser AH, Derkx FH, Sluiter W, Schalekamp MA. Uptake and proteolytic activation of prorenin by cultured human endothelial cells. J Hypertens 1999; 17(5): 621-9. [http://dx.doi.org/10.1097/00004872-199917050-00005] [PMID: 10403605]

[22] van Kesteren CA, Danser AH, Derkx FH, *et al.* Mannose 6-phosphate receptor-mediated internalization and activation of prorenin by cardiac cells. Hypertension 1997; 30(6): 1389-96. [http://dx.doi.org/10.1161/01.HYP.30.6.1389] [PMID: 9403558]

[23] Saris JJ, Derkx FH, De Bruin RJ, *et al.* High-affinity prorenin binding to cardiac man-6-P/IGF-II receptors precedes proteolytic activation to renin. Am J Physiol Heart Circ Physiol 2001; 280(4): H1706-15. [PMID: 11247783]

[24] Saris JJ, Derkx FH, Lamers JM, Saxena PR, Schalekamp MA, Danser AH. Cardiomyocytes bind and activate native human prorenin : role of soluble mannose 6-phosphate receptors. Hypertension 2001; 37(2 Pt 2): 710-5. [http://dx.doi.org/10.1161/01.HYP.37.2.710] [PMID: 11230361]

[25] van den Eijnden MM, Saris JJ, de Bruin RJ, *et al.* Prorenin accumulation and activation in human endothelial cells: importance of mannose 6-phosphate receptors. Arterioscler Thromb Vasc Biol 2001;

21(6): 911-6.
[http://dx.doi.org/10.1161/01.ATV.21.6.911] [PMID: 11397696]

[26] Batenburg WW, de Bruin RJ, van Gool JM, *et al.* Aliskiren-binding increases the half life of renin and prorenin in rat aortic vascular smooth muscle cells. Arterioscler Thromb Vasc Biol 2008; 28(6): 1151-7.
[http://dx.doi.org/10.1161/ATVBAHA.108.164210] [PMID: 18388329]

[27] Saris JJ, van den Eijnden MM, Lamers JM, Saxena PR, Schalekamp MA, Danser AH. Prorenin-induced myocyte proliferation: no role for intracellular angiotensin II. Hypertension 2002; 39(2 Pt 2): 573-7.
[http://dx.doi.org/10.1161/hy0202.103002] [PMID: 11882610]

[28] Nguyen G, Delarue F, Burcklé C, Bouzhir L, Giller T, Sraer JD. Pivotal role of the renin/prorenin receptor in angiotensin II production and cellular responses to renin. J Clin Invest 2002; 109(11): 1417-27.
[http://dx.doi.org/10.1172/JCI0214276] [PMID: 12045255]

[29] Batenburg WW, Krop M, Garrelds IM, *et al.* Prorenin is the endogenous agonist of the (pro)renin receptor. Binding kinetics of renin and prorenin in rat vascular smooth muscle cells overexpressing the human (pro)renin receptor. J Hypertens 2007; 25(12): 2441-53.
[http://dx.doi.org/10.1097/HJH.0b013e3282f05bae] [PMID: 17984666]

[30] Nabi AH, Kageshima A, Uddin MN, Nakagawa T, Park EY, Suzuki F. Binding properties of rat prorenin and renin to the recombinant rat renin/prorenin receptor prepared by a baculovirus expression system. Int J Mol Med 2006; 18(3): 483-8.
[PMID: 16865234]

[31] Lu X, Danser AH, Meima ME. HRP and prorenin: focus on the (pro)renin receptor and vacuolar H+-ATPase. Front Biosci (Schol Ed) 2011; 3: 1205-15.
[http://dx.doi.org/10.2741/221] [PMID: 21622266]

[32] Suzuki F, Hayakawa M, Nakagawa T, *et al.* Human prorenin has "gate and handle" regions for its non-proteolytic activation. J Biol Chem 2003; 278(25): 22217-22.
[http://dx.doi.org/10.1074/jbc.M302579200] [PMID: 12684512]

[33] Kaneshiro Y, Ichihara A, Sakoda M, *et al.* Slowly progressive, angiotensin II-independent glomerulosclerosis in human (pro)renin receptor-transgenic rats. J Am Soc Nephrol 2007; 18(6): 1789-95.
[http://dx.doi.org/10.1681/ASN.2006091062] [PMID: 17494887]

[34] Kaneshiro Y, Ichihara A, Takemitsu T, *et al.* Increased expression of cyclooxygenase-2 in the renal cortex of human prorenin receptor gene-transgenic rats. Kidney Int 2006; 70(4): 641-6.
[http://dx.doi.org/10.1038/sj.ki.5001627] [PMID: 16807542]

[35] Jansen PM, Hofland J, van den Meiracker AH, de Jong FH, Danser AH. Renin and prorenin have no direct effect on aldosterone synthesis in the human adrenocortical cell lines H295R and HAC15. J Renin Angiotensin Aldosterone Syst 2012; 13(3): 360-6.
[http://dx.doi.org/10.1177/1470320312438792] [PMID: 22396488]

[36] Ichihara A, Hayashi M, Kaneshiro Y, *et al.* Inhibition of diabetic nephropathy by a decoy peptide corresponding to the "handle" region for nonproteolytic activation of prorenin. J Clin Invest 2004;

114(8): 1128-35.
[http://dx.doi.org/10.1172/JCI21398] [PMID: 15489960]

[37] Ichihara A, Suzuki F, Nakagawa T, *et al.* Prorenin receptor blockade inhibits development of glomerulosclerosis in diabetic angiotensin II type 1a receptor-deficient mice. J Am Soc Nephrol 2006; 17(7): 1950-61.
[http://dx.doi.org/10.1681/ASN.2006010029] [PMID: 16738017]

[38] Huang Y, Wongamorntham S, Kasting J, *et al.* Renin increases mesangial cell transforming growth factor-beta1 and matrix proteins through receptor-mediated, angiotensin II-independent mechanisms. Kidney Int 2006; 69(1): 105-13.
[http://dx.doi.org/10.1038/sj.ki.5000011] [PMID: 16374430]

[39] Clavreul N, Sansilvestri-Morel P, Magard D, Verbeuren TJ, Rupin A. (Pro)renin promotes fibrosis gene expression in HEK cells through a Nox4-dependent mechanism. Am J Physiol Renal Physiol 2011; 300(6): F1310-8.
[http://dx.doi.org/10.1152/ajprenal.00119.2010] [PMID: 21411480]

[40] Sakoda M, Ichihara A, Kurauchi-Mito A, *et al.* Aliskiren inhibits intracellular angiotensin II levels without affecting (pro)renin receptor signals in human podocytes. Am J Hypertens 2010; 23(5): 575-80.
[http://dx.doi.org/10.1038/ajh.2009.273] [PMID: 20075844]

[41] Cheng H, Fan X, Moeckel GW, Harris RC. Podocyte COX-2 exacerbates diabetic nephropathy by increasing podocyte (pro)renin receptor expression. J Am Soc Nephrol 2011; 22(7): 1240-51.
[http://dx.doi.org/10.1681/ASN.2010111149] [PMID: 21737546]

[42] Gonzalez AA, Luffman C, Bourgeois CR, Vio CP, Prieto MC. Angiotensin II-independent upregulation of cyclooxygenase-2 by activation of the (Pro)renin receptor in rat renal inner medullary cells. Hypertension 2013; 61(2): 443-9.
[http://dx.doi.org/10.1161/HYPERTENSIONAHA.112.196303] [PMID: 23184385]

[43] Huang J, Siragy HM. Glucose promotes the production of interleukine-1beta and cyclooxygenase-2 in mesangial cells *via* enhanced (Pro)renin receptor expression. Endocrinology 2009; 150(12): 5557-65.
[http://dx.doi.org/10.1210/en.2009-0442] [PMID: 19861503]

[44] Huang J, Siragy HM. Regulation of (pro)renin receptor expression by glucose-induced mitogen-activated protein kinase, nuclear factor-kappaB, and activator protein-1 signaling pathways. Endocrinology 2010; 151(7): 3317-25.
[http://dx.doi.org/10.1210/en.2009-1368] [PMID: 20444941]

[45] Müller DN, Klanke B, Feldt S, *et al.* (Pro)renin receptor peptide inhibitor "handle-region" peptide does not affect hypertensive nephrosclerosis in Goldblatt rats. Hypertension 2008; 51(3): 676-81.
[http://dx.doi.org/10.1161/HYPERTENSIONAHA.107.101493] [PMID: 18212268]

[46] Ryuzaki M, Ichihara A, Ohshima Y, *et al.* Involvement of activated prorenin in the pathogenesis of slowly progressive nephropathy in the non-clipped kidney of two kidney, one-clip hypertension. Hypertens Res 2011; 34(3): 301-7.
[http://dx.doi.org/10.1038/hr.2010.230] [PMID: 21107335]

[47] Krebs C, Weber M, Steinmetz O, *et al.* Effect of (pro)renin receptor inhibition by a decoy peptide on renal damage in the clipped kidney of Goldblatt rats. Kidney Int 2008; 74(6): 823-4.

[http://dx.doi.org/10.1038/ki.2008.315] [PMID: 18756297]

[48] Burcklé CA, Jan Danser AH, Müller DN, *et al.* Elevated blood pressure and heart rate in human renin receptor transgenic rats. Hypertension 2006; 47(3): 552-6.
[http://dx.doi.org/10.1161/01.HYP.0000199912.47657.04] [PMID: 16401765]

[49] Ichihara A, Kaneshiro Y, Takemitsu T, *et al.* Nonproteolytic activation of prorenin contributes to development of cardiac fibrosis in genetic hypertension. Hypertension 2006; 47(5): 894-900.
[http://dx.doi.org/10.1161/01.HYP.0000215838.48170.0b] [PMID: 16585419]

[50] Susic D, Zhou X, Frohlich ED, *et al.* Cardiovascular effects of prorenin blockade in genetically hypertensive rats (SHR) on normal and high salt diet. Am J Physiol Heart Circ Physiol in press

[51] van Esch JH, van Veghel R, Garrelds IM, Leijten F, Bouhuizen AM, Danser AH. Handle region peptide counteracts the beneficial effects of the Renin inhibitor aliskiren in spontaneously hypertensive rats. Hypertension 2011; 57(4): 852-8.
[http://dx.doi.org/10.1161/HYPERTENSIONAHA.110.169060] [PMID: 21321303]

[52] Batenburg WW, van den Heuvel M, van Esch JH, *et al.* The (pro)renin receptor blocker handle region peptide upregulates endothelium-derived contractile factors in aliskiren-treated diabetic transgenic (mREN2)27 rats. J Hypertens 2013; 31(2): 292-302.
[http://dx.doi.org/10.1097/HJH.0b013e32835c1789] [PMID: 23303354]

[53] Leckie BJ, Bottrill AR. A specific binding site for the prorenin propart peptide Arg10-Arg20 does not occur on human endothelial cells. J Renin Angiotensin Aldosterone Syst 2011; 12(1): 36-41.
[http://dx.doi.org/10.1177/1470320310370610] [PMID: 20826507]

[54] Feldt S, Batenburg WW, Mazak I, *et al.* Prorenin and renin-induced extracellular signal-regulated kinase 1/2 activation in monocytes is not blocked by aliskiren or the handle-region peptide. Hypertension 2008; 51(3): 682-8.
[http://dx.doi.org/10.1161/HYPERTENSIONAHA.107.101444] [PMID: 18212269]

[55] Satofuka S, Ichihara A, Nagai N, *et al.* (Pro)renin receptor-mediated signal transduction and tissue renin-angiotensin system contribute to diabetes-induced retinal inflammation. Diabetes 2009; 58(7): 1625-33.
[http://dx.doi.org/10.2337/db08-0254] [PMID: 19389828]

[56] Wilkinson-Berka JL, Heine R, Tan G, *et al.* RILLKKMPSV influences the vasculature, neurons and glia, and (pro)renin receptor expression in the retina. Hypertension 2010; 55(6): 1454-60.
[http://dx.doi.org/10.1161/HYPERTENSIONAHA.109.148221] [PMID: 20368504]

[57] Yoshikawa A, Aizaki Y, Kusano K, *et al.* The (pro)renin receptor is cleaved by ADAM19 in the Golgi leading to its secretion into extracellular space. Hypertens Res 2011; 34(5): 599-605.
[http://dx.doi.org/10.1038/hr.2010.284] [PMID: 21270819]

[58] Saris JJ, 't Hoen PA, Garrelds IM, *et al.* Prorenin induces intracellular signaling in cardiomyocytes independently of angiotensin II. Hypertension 2006; 48(4): 564-71.
[http://dx.doi.org/10.1161/01.HYP.0000240064.19301.1b] [PMID: 16940215]

[59] Batenburg WW, Lu X, Leijten F, Maschke U, Müller DN, Danser AH. Renin- and prorenin-induced effects in rat vascular smooth muscle cells overexpressing the human (pro)renin receptor: does (pro)renin-(pro)renin receptor interaction actually occur? Hypertension 2011; 58(6): 1111-9.

[http://dx.doi.org/10.1161/HYPERTENSIONAHA.111.180737] [PMID: 22025376]

[60] Liu G, Hitomi H, Hosomi N, *et al.* Prorenin induces vascular smooth muscle cell proliferation and hypertrophy *via* epidermal growth factor receptor-mediated extracellular signal-regulated kinase and Akt activation pathway. J Hypertens 2011; 29(4): 696-705.
[http://dx.doi.org/10.1097/HJH.0b013e328343c62b] [PMID: 21252698]

[61] Zhang J, Noble NA, Border WA, Owens RT, Huang Y. Receptor-dependent prorenin activation and induction of PAI-1 expression in vascular smooth muscle cells. Am J Physiol Endocrinol Metab 2008; 295(4): E810-9.
[http://dx.doi.org/10.1152/ajpendo.90264.2008] [PMID: 18664599]

[62] Sakoda M, Ichihara A, Kaneshiro Y, *et al.* (Pro)renin receptor-mediated activation of mitogen-activated protein kinases in human vascular smooth muscle cells. Hypertens Res 2007; 30(11): 1139-46.
[http://dx.doi.org/10.1291/hypres.30.1139] [PMID: 18250563]

[63] Peters B, Grisk O, Becher B, *et al.* Dose-dependent titration of prorenin and blood pressure in Cyp1a1ren-2 transgenic rats: absence of prorenin-induced glomerulosclerosis. J Hypertens 2008; 26(1): 102-9.
[http://dx.doi.org/10.1097/HJH.0b013e3282f0ab66] [PMID: 18090546]

[64] Campbell DJ, Karam H, Ménard J, Bruneval P, Mullins JJ. Prorenin contributes to angiotensin peptide formation in transgenic rats with rat prorenin expression targeted to the liver. Hypertension 2009; 54(6): 1248-53.
[http://dx.doi.org/10.1161/HYPERTENSIONAHA.109.138495] [PMID: 19841286]

[65] Mercure C, Prescott G, Lacombe MJ, Silversides DW, Reudelhuber TL. Chronic increases in circulating prorenin are not associated with renal or cardiac pathologies. Hypertension 2009; 53(6): 1062-9.
[http://dx.doi.org/10.1161/HYPERTENSIONAHA.108.115444] [PMID: 19364992]

[66] Campbell DJ, Nussberger J, Stowasser M, *et al.* Activity assays and immunoassays for plasma Renin and prorenin: information provided and precautions necessary for accurate measurement. Clin Chem 2009; 55(5): 867-77.
[http://dx.doi.org/10.1373/clinchem.2008.118000] [PMID: 19264850]

[67] Klotz S, Burkhoff D, Garrelds IM, Boomsma F, Danser AH. The impact of left ventricular assist device-induced left ventricular unloading on the myocardial renin-angiotensin-aldosterone system: therapeutic consequences? Eur Heart J 2009; 30(7): 805-12.
[http://dx.doi.org/10.1093/eurheartj/ehp012] [PMID: 19223317]

[68] Kinouchi K, Ichihara A, Sano M, *et al.* The (pro)renin receptor/ATP6AP2 is essential for vacuolar H+-ATPase assembly in murine cardiomyocytes. Circ Res 2010; 107(1): 30-4.
[http://dx.doi.org/10.1161/CIRCRESAHA.110.224667] [PMID: 20570919]

[69] Cruciat CM, Ohkawara B, Acebron SP, *et al.* Requirement of prorenin receptor and vacuolar H+-ATPase-mediated acidification for Wnt signaling. Science 2010; 327(5964): 459-63.
[http://dx.doi.org/10.1126/science.1179802] [PMID: 20093472]

[70] Advani A, Kelly DJ, Cox AJ, *et al.* The (Pro)renin receptor: site-specific and functional linkage to the vacuolar H^+-ATPase in the kidney. Hypertension 2009; 54(2): 261-9.

CHAPTER 12

Renal Physiology and Immune System: The Role of Renin-Angiotensin System, Nitric Oxide and Catecholamines

Tatiana Sousa Cunha[1], **Danielle Yuri Arita**[2], **Ingrid Kazue Mizuno Watanabe**[2], **Juliana Dinéia Perez Brandão**[2], **Lys Angela Favaroni Mendes Salgado Ribeiro**[2], **Danielle Sanches Aragão**[2] and **Dulce Elena Casarini**[2,*]

[1] *Science and Technology Institute, Federal University of Sao Paulo, Sao Jose dos Campos, Brazil*

[2] *Department of Medicine, Nephrology Division, Escola Paulista de Medicina, Universidade Federal de São Paulo, Sao Paulo, Brazil*

Abstract: The renin-angiotensin system (RAS) affects both the innate and adaptive immune responses. Since hyperactive RAS has been associated with several diseases, the contribution of tissue RAS to the progression of immune and non-immune conditions has been considered in the recent years. It has a well-established role in fibrinogenesis, leukocyte infiltration, activity of T cells and has been shown to be chemotactic to macrophages, T cells, and natural killer cells. Nitric oxide (NO) is synthesized by many cell types involved in immunity and inflammation and plays an important role in hypotension and regulates the functional activity, growth and death of many immune and inflammatory cell types. Current evidences suggest that catecholamines (CAs) play a key role in activating and limiting inflammatory and immune reactions. In this chapter, we will discuss some aspects related to the role of these molecules in inflammatory process and immunologically mediated conditions.

Keywords: Catecholamines, HPA axis, Immune system, Nitric oxide, Renal physiology, Renin-angiotensin system, Sympathetic nervous system.

* **Corresponding author Dulce Elena Casarini:** Rua Botucatu, 740 – 2° andar, Department of Medicine/Nephrology Division, Vila Clementino – Sao Paulo/SP, Brazil, CEP 04023-900; Phone: +55 11 5904-1687; E-mail: casarini.elena@unifesp.br.

Dulce Elena Casarini, Danielle Yuri Arita, Tatiana Sousa Cunha & Juliana Almada Colucci (Eds.)

RENIN-ANGIOTENSIN SYSTEM

Since its discovery, the renin-angiotensin system (RAS) is recognized as a hormone system by which the kidney influences systemic cardiovascular regulation. Several studies on into molecular biology of RAS revealed that angiotensin II (Ang II), a potent vasoconstrictor, is synthesized not only in the circulation but also locally in tissues [1]. Accumulating data indicates that RAS participates in the induction and progression of several diseases, including immune and inflammatory conditions. Several clinical and experimental observations suggest that activated local RAS is involved in the pathogenesis of renal damage.

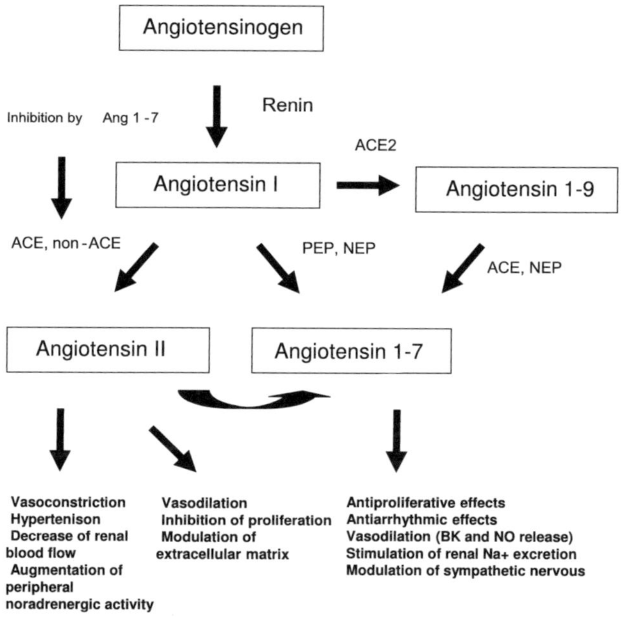

Fig. (1). Pathways for the formation of biologically active angiotensin peptides. Abbreviations: ACE, angiotensin-converting enzyme; ACE2, angiotensin-converting enzyme 2; NEP, neutral endopeptidase; PEP, prolylendopetidase. (Adapted from Schindler *et al.* 2007 [62]).

The classical RAS has important molecules that participate in several aspects of physiology and pathophysiology including renin, angiotensin converting enzyme (ACE), angiotensins I (Ang I) and II and Ang II type 1 and 2 (AT_1 and AT_2) receptors. The identification of new angiotensins, such as angiotensin-(1-7) (Ang

1-7) and angiotensin IV (Ang IV), renin/prorenin receptors, Mas receptor and angiotensin-converting enzyme 2 (ACE2) increased the complexity of the system, suggesting that further investigations are necessary to better understand the role of RAS (Fig. **1**) [2, 3].

Circulating angiotensinogen (AGT) concentration is an important factor for the RAS tone being the precursor of the angiotensin peptides [4]. Apart from important role of renin in the generation of circulating angiotensin peptides, several other enzymes convert AGT to either Ang I or Ang II directly, and non-ACE enzymes may convert Ang I to Ang II, which is able to increase AGT expression *via* nuclear factor-kappa B (NF- κB) activation in hepatocytes and other tissues [5] particularly at inflammation sites.

Both local and circulating Ang II exert their activities through AT_1 receptor, a protein with a typical structure of 7-transmembrane G protein-coupled receptors [6], or AT_2 receptor, which is highly expressed in fetal stage, and is up-regulated in response to injury in the adult [7]. AT_2 receptor is known to stimulate the production of bradykinin, nitric oxide (NO) and cGMP, thus, mediating vasodilatation, cell differentiation, and apoptosis [8]. Stimulation of AT_1 receptors activates downstream effectors including phospholipase A_2, C and D. Activation of phospholipase C produces inositol-1,4,5- triphosphate (IP_3) and diacylglycerol inducing calcium efflux into the cytoplasm and a cascade of events causing contraction of vascular smooth muscle cell (VSMC). Diacylglycerol is an effector of the RAS, mitogen activated protein kinase (MAPK) and MEK pathways. AT_1 receptor also activates kinases such as PKC and MAPK including ERK1/2, p38MAPK and c-Jun NH2-terminal kinase that are implicated in inflammation and hypertrophy [9].

Recently, new angiotensin receptors were described including Mas and angiotensin AT_4 receptors, which are able to bind Ang 1-7 and Ang IV peptides, respectively [10, 11]. The AT_4 receptor has been implicated in sodium transport in proximal tubules [12] and promotes thrombosis and fibrosis *via* induction of plasminogen activator inhibitor-I shown in both endothelial and vascular smooth muscle cells [13]. Mas receptor induces natriuresis and diuresis, [14] and mediates the effect of Ang 1–7 on prostaglandins and NO release [10].

In addition to the well-known hemodynamic effects, over a decade of research leads to the recognition of Ang II as a cytokine, capable of promoting the expression of many hormones, including other cytokines, chemokines, and growth factors involved in oxidative stress, inflammation and fibrosis. Ang II is a key factor in the inflammatory process and has been shown to increase vascular permeability, to recruit inflammatory cells (regulation of adhesion molecules and chemotaxis), and to induce differentiation and proliferation of immunocompetent cells.

It is well recognized that immunocompetent cell infiltrates are present in the kidney, especially in the interstitium, and RAS blockade has been shown to decrease interstitial cell infiltration in several cases of non-immune primary injury, attenuating chemokynes, adhesion molecules and other mediators. In fact, cytokine production (tumor necrosis factor- α, IL-1, IL-6 and IL-15) are suppressed by ACE inhibitors and AT_1 antagonists [15]. It has already been demonstrated that Ang II increases IL-6 expression in VSMC and renal cells, and the generation of IL-6 is also increased in kidney from Ang II infused rats [16]. Moreover, IL-6 stimulates the generation of AGT, leading to increased Ang II formation, and inflammation. Satou *et al.* (2009) reported that Ang II and IL-6 synergistically induce human AGT expression through the activation of NF- kB and STAT3 in immortalized human renal proximal tubular cells [17].

In the initial phase of inflammation characterized by an alteration of local vascular permeability, Ang II can influence it *via* endothelium mechanical injury caused by increased pressure, and *via* non hemodynamic actions, stimulating the synthesis and release of second mediators, such as prostaglandins and vascular endothelial growth factor (VEGF). Ang II induces VEGF expression in vascular and renal cells and AT_1 receptor blocker prevented Ang II-induced VEGF protein excretion in mesangial cells [18].

Ang II influences other inflammatory phases, including immune cell proliferation and differentiation. Ang II can induce proliferation of T cells *via* AT_1 receptor by a calcineurin- dependent pathway [19] and participates in the differentiation of bone marrow- derived cells, such as macrophage and dendritic cells (DC) [20, 21].

It is well recognized that immune cell infiltration plays an important role in the development and progression of several renal diseases. In addition to an over expression of chemotactic factors by resident renal cells [22], several groups have demonstrated the involvement of Ang II in recruitment of immune cells through its chemotactic properties supported by the observation of directional migration of monocytes, T cells, natural killer (NK) cells and DC [23, 24].

Beside the induction of RANTES expression [25], Ang II promotes the release of monocyte chemotactic protein-1 (MPC-1), the main chemokyne involved in monocyte infiltration into the kidney [26], which is expressed by various renal cell types, including mesangial and tubular epithelial cells. Also, Ang II causes overexpression of osteopontin and increases IL-8 and interferon gamma inducible protein-10 [27], related to neutrophil recruitment and activation.

In addition to its involvement in cell recruitment, apparently, Ang II participates in the adhesion of immune cells. Adhesion of monocytes and neutrophils to endothelial and mesangial cells is improved by Ang II [28], and this peptide also induces leukocyte-endothelial cell interaction *via* AT_1 and AT_2 receptors mediated P-selectin upregulation [29].

Several groups have demonstrated that immunocompetent cells express components of RAS and can generate Ang II [15]. Mononuclear lymphocytes have been found to produce Ang II, T cells and NK cells possess a complete enzymatic system to synthesize their own Ang II, and neutrophils and mast cells were shown to convert Ang I to Ang II [24]. The presence of AT_1 and AT_2 receptors has been observed in various immune cells, including T cells, NK cells and DC [24]. The capacity of producing and releasing Ang II locally, in addition to the existence of Ang II binding sites in immune cells, indicates that Ang II can activate inflammatory cells leading to an autocrine/paracrine-reinforcing loop and, consequently, an inflammatory vicious cycle.

Ang II induces cellular responses through several pathways, including free radical generation and nuclear transcriptional factors. Recent data suggest that NF-κB plays a pivotal role in AngII-induced inflammatory process. NF-κB activation leads to the production of cytokines and adhesion molecules, such as TNF-α, IL-6,

IL-8, MCP-1, VCAM-1, E-selectin, and transforming growth factor (TGF)-β. Both AT_1 and AT_2 receptors activate the NF-κB pathway [15]. Despite AT_2 receptor has been thought to counterbalance the actions of AT1R, recent studies demonstrated that AT_2 receptor may complement AT_1 receptor mediated effects. Depending on the cell type, different Ang II receptors and signaling pathways may predominate. In mesangial cells, NF-κB activation is mediated by both receptors, whereas in tubuloepithelial cells, this is mainly by AT_1 receptor. *In vivo*, renal NF-κB activation was only completely abolished by the combined therapy of both receptor antagonists [15].

Ang II also participates in reactive oxygen species (ROS) generation *via* NADPH oxidase activation or *via* uncoupled eNOS. In turn, ROS act as signal transduction messengers for transcription factors and have an important role in biologic process, such as phagocytosis.

Ang II is also involved in tissue repair process characterized partially by replacement of injured cells by connective tissue. Several clinical trials and experimental studies have shown a significant decrease of fibrosis progression through Ang II blockade. Indeed, Ang II regulates extracellular matrix accumulation mediated by AT1R- mediated production of profibrotic growth factors, such as TGF-β. TGF-β1 stimulates the production of several matrix components (chondroitin/dermatan sulfate proteoglycans, decorin, and biglycan) by mesangial cells and glomerular epithelial cells and may be useful for assessing the efficiency of RAS blockade in chronic kidney diseases. Ang II may be also involved in the expression of connective tissue growth factor (CTGF) [15], which is upregulated in many renal diseases. In addition, recent data suggest a new cellular participant in renal fibrosis named fibrocytes, which are downregulated by AT_1 receptor antagonist [30].

Besides Ang II, other RAS peptides play a critical role in the inflammatory process, especially when AT_1 receptor is blocked. Ang III increases MCP-1 expression *via* NF-κB activation in mesangial and mononuclear cells, and enhances AP-1 binding activity related to matrix accumulation factors, including TGF-β and fibronectin [15]. Additionally, Ang 1-7 increases immune cell infiltration, matrix deposition, cytokine production and NF-κB activity *via* Mas receptor in the kidney, under physiological and pathological conditions [15].

In summary, besides Ang II and AT_1 receptor, other angiotensins peptides and receptors elicit cellular responses through several molecular pathway contributing to the maintenance of inflammatory process. Accumulating data on RAS support the emerging idea of the synergism between immunological and resident cells in locally synthesized angiotensins in inflammation.

NITRIC OXIDE

Until the mid-80's, the free radical nitric oxide (NO) was considered as a common air pollutant, with the potential to cause acid rain and destroy the ozone layer. The notion that NO could be endogenously produced and could play a role as a major signaling molecule in mammals was indeed surprising at the time and resulted in the 1998 Nobel Prize for Medicine [31]. Since the identification of 'endothelium - derived relaxing factor' (EDRF) as NO, several studies have been conducted to explore the complex chemistry and biochemistry of this molecule, and today NO is considered as one of the most important mediators of biological processes in the heart and blood vessels.

NO is a simple diatomic gas and free radical that acts as a key biological messenger for general physiological solutions. This molecule is produced enzymatically by three nitric oxide synthase (NOS) isoforms: neuronal NOS (nNOS, NOS-1), inducible NOS (iNOS, NOS-2) and endothelial NOS (eNOS, NOS-3) [32]. It has already been described that the availability of L-arginine [33] and cofactors, the presence of the endogenous NOS inhibitor, and also the amount of NOS protein influence the enzymatic production rate.

NOS are expressed in a variety of tissues throughout the body, and are particularly prominent in the nervous and cardiovascular systems. Expression of these three NOS isoforms has also been reported in renal tissue. Studies have demonstrated the presence of eNOS in the renal vasculature, while expression of nNOS was identified in the macula densa, efferent arteriole and several other distal tubular cells, and it has been shown to modulate tubuloglomerular feedback activity. iNOS is constitutively expressed in several segments of the renal tubule and glomeruli, and NO produced by iNOS may have a pathophysiological role, since this isoform is upregulated in glomerular, mesangial, smooth muscle, and tubular epithelial cells, in response to inflammation. Indeed, systemic inhibition of iNOS reduces tubulo-interstitial injury in renal allograft rejection and prevents renal ischemia-reperfusion injury [34]. The topographical distribution of the NOS isoforms throughout the nephron segments and other renal structures confers a greater level of complexity to the regulation of NO synthesis in the kidney than is found in other organs, and this characteristic is only the first step in understanding how this molecule regulates renal function [35].

The biological effects of NO are variable, and this fact is becoming increasingly evident as our knowledge of this wonder molecule expands. Since it is a free radical, NO can react with a large number of molecules in the body and the fact that it is a gas allows for easy passage between cells and tissues [36]. Several studies were able to show the role of NO as a signaling molecule in endothelial and nerve cells. However, its biochemical properties not only enable NO to be an ideal signaling molecule, but also result in a wide range of biological effects. NO influences tubular electrolyte transport, regulates vascular tone and blood perfusion in most capillary beds, including the kidneys, and is also a potent competitive inhibitor of mitochondrial respiration [33]. Moreover, it contributes to blood pressure regulation, neuronal communication and immune defense [37, 38]. NO production is also important in protecting the kidney from inappropriate reductions of medullar blood flow and ischemia in response to physiological increases of circulating vasoconstrictor agents [39, 40].

While NO is vital to healthy function it is also a highly reactive molecule, known as a double-edged sword. Uncontrolled production of this molecule is associated with severe diseases including several forms of chronic inflammation and kidney dysfunction. In the rat model of autoimmune interstitial nephritis, inhibition of iNOS aggravated renal injury and may function as a negative feedback regulator of the autoimmune TH1 cell response, protecting host against immunopathological sequelae. In chronic kidney disease (CKD) NO reduced bioavailability has been shown to contribute to the progression of the disease [41] and NOS inhibition causes systemic and glomerular hypertension, glomerular ischemia, glomerulosclerosis, tubulo-interstitial injury, and protein-uria. On the other hand, endogenous as well as exogenous NO contributes to renal injury through apoptosis of tubular epithelial cells by the activation of caspase-8 [42]. Moreover, high levels of NO seems to be associated with acute rejection, since inhibition of iNOS in rats receiving renal allograft protected the graft from tubulo-interstitial injury and improved graft function and survival [43].

An emerging theme in the understanding of the biochemistry and physiology of NO, particularly within the kidney, is the profound interrelationship between NO and products of oxidative stress. Under physiological conditions, the kidney produces reactive oxygen species (ROS), which are neutralized by antioxidant defense systems, including superoxide dismutase (SOD), catalase, glutathione peroxidase (GPX) – and non-enzymatic (glutathione, vitamins C and E) systems. NO and ROS participate in normal kidney and vascular function, contributing to maintenance of vascular tone and tubular function. Increased renal ROS is associated with bio-inactivation of NO, affecting afferent arteriolar tone, tubuloglomerular feedback responses, and sodium reabsorption, and blood pressure regulation [44].

Multiple recent studies have provided evidence that oxidative stress is associated with several renal disease states and is amplified as the disease progresses. The interaction of NO and oxidative stress influences the extent of renal damage and may offer a target for therapies [45], since the increase on ROS formation is strongly associated with renal injury. ROS can stimulate the expression of proinflammatory and profibrotic molecules, which are crucial to the progression of renal disease and the subsequent development of fibrosis and kidney failure [46].

CATECHOLAMINES

Catecholamines (CAs), which include dopamine (DA), norepinephrine (noradrenaline, NE), and epinephrine (adrenaline, EPI), are important neurotransmitters and hormones that play an important role in water and salt metabolism and in blood pressure (BP) regulation, have complex interactions with other hormones and systems, such as renin-angiotensin-aldosterone system, vasopressin and atrial natriuretic factor, and stimulate the prostaglandin system. These monoamines are released by the body in response to acute and chronic stress situations.

CAs are formed mainly in brain, adrenal chromaffin cells and postganglionic fibers of sympathetic nervous system (SNS). The precursor is mainly the amino acid tyrosine, but phenylalanine can be converted to tyrosine in the liver. Tyrosine enters the cell *via* blood circulation and extracellular fluid. In the cytosol, tyrosine is converted to L– dopa by an oxygenase, tyrosine hydroxylase (TH). TH is the rate-limiting step in CA pathway, regulated by negative feedback, and requires the tetrahydrobiopterin (BH4) as a cofactor. L-dopa is converted to DA by an aromatic L-amino acid decarboxylase, DOPA decarboxylase (DCC). DA enters the secretory granule where it is converted into NE by dopamine-β-hydroxylase (DβH).

In contrast with the traditional concept of a unitary sympathoadrenal system, three distinct peripheral CA systems, have been established. The three systems are the SNS, adrenomedullary hormonal system, and DOPA-dopamine autocrine/paracrine system [47].

CAs carries a variety of physiological processes both in the central nervous system (CNS) and peripheral tissues. DA modulates various functions including behavior, movement, synthesis and hormone release, BP and salt and water homeostasis. DA plays a significant role in the pathogenesis of hypertension by interacting with the RAS and SNS and also by regulating the production of reactive oxygen species, contractility of vascular smooth muscle and epithelial sodium transport. In the SNS and in adrenal glands, EPI is the predominant hormone. NE is present in organs with sympathetic innervation and even in the sympathetic nerves, as well as in the adrenal medulla and urine. The kidney has been considered an extraneural source of CAs. DA is largely produced in tubular cells and there are also evidences that mesangial and epithelial cells along the nephron presented the complete biosynthetic machinery, such as the synthesis enzymes and the cofactor BH4, being able to store/release levels of NE, EPI and DA, with significant physiological effects [48 - 51].

DA increases blood flow by renal afferent arteriole dilatation, decreasing renal vascular resistance with increased filtration and ultrafiltration coefficient, and it also has natriuretic and diuretic actions. In acute renal failure, at low doses (0.5-3.0 μg/kg/min), DA predominantly stimulates DA receptors (DRs), increasing glomerular filtration, renal blood flow and sodium excretion. At high doses (5.0-20.0 μg/kg/min), it can lead to splanchnic and glomerular vasoconstriction and a significant increase in renal plasma flow, being stimulated by α- and β-adrenergic receptors [52].

DRs have been identified in different regions of the CNS, the endings of neurons pre-and post-ganglionic sympathetic nervous system, heart, gastrointestinal tract and kidney. These G-proteins receptors and classified into D_1- like (D_1 and D_5) and D_2-like (D_2, D_3 and D_4) subtypes. The two D_1-like activate adenyl cyclase stimulation, leading to an increase in the cyclase-adenosine monophosphate (cAMP); whereas the three D_2-like receptors are inhibit adenyl cyclase and Ca^{2+} channels and activate potassium channels, reducing cAMP. Abnormalities, regulation changes or deletion of any of the DRs subtypes can result in hypertension, being important in this pathogenesis. DA also acts on α- and β-adrenergic receptors [52 - 54].

DA acts as an autocrine/paracrine substance, promoting natriuresis by inhibition of Na^+/K^+ ATPase in the proximal tubule, thick ascending loop of Henle and cortical collecting duct [47]. Moreover, reports suggest that D_1-like receptors not only oppose the actions of Ang II *via* AT_1 receptors but also require AT_2 receptors to reduce renal sodium reabsorption. The activation of D_2 family receptors leads to NE inhibition in adrenergic neurons, aldosterone inhibition in adrenal cells, prolactin inhibition in neurohypophysis and renin in juxtaglomerular cells. DA receptors are widely expressed in the CNS, influencing the neuroendocrine secretion and also the control of locomotion, cognition and emotion. In the periphery, these receptors are present in kidney, blood vessels and pituitary, which mainly affect the homeostasis, vascular tone and hormone secretion [54 - 56].

NE has strong vasopressor properties although it also has some β-adrenergic effects enabling to maintain cardiac output. NE is an antinatriuretic and antidiuretic factor. EPI corresponds to 80% of adrenal medulla production. It is also considered a significant antinatriuretic factor. Reduced renal blood flow by 40%, increases renal vascular resistance, filtration fraction and renin secretion, maintains the glomerular filtration rate, decreases sodium excretion, potassium and chlorine, and little interference with the urine volume.

The adrenergic receptors (ARs) are important contributors to modulate SNS activity and cardiovascular homeostasis as well as a site of action for many therapeutic agents. Both NE and EPI mediate their biological actions *via* G-protein-coupled adrenergic receptor subtypes: α_1-receptors (α_{1A}, α_{1B}, α_{1D}), α_2-receptors (α_{2A}, α_{2B}, α_{2C}) and β-receptors (β_1, β_2 and β_3). The α_1-ARs are the prime mediators of smooth muscle contraction and hypertrophic growth, by increasing intracellular calcium. On the other hand, α_2-ARs coupled to inhibitory G protein causes a decrease of cAMP activity; the role of the α_2- ARs includes presynaptic inhibition of neurotransmitter release, diminished sympathetic efferent traffic, vasodilation and vasoconstriction resulting in smooth muscle relaxation. Central activation of α_{2A}-ARs lowers blood pressure and decreases plasma NE levels; activation of peripheral α_{2B}-ARs induces sodium retention and vasoconstriction, and α2C-ARs activation causes cold-induced vasoconstriction. β-Rs increase intracellular cAMP activity through adenyl ciclase, resulting in heart muscle contraction, smooth muscle relaxation and glycogenolysis [57]. During stress, EPI prepares the muscles, lungs and heart to more intense activity. CAs stimulates muscular and hepatic glycogenolysis, increasing plasma glucose level. They also stimulate lipolysis in adipose tissue, leading to increased plasma levels of fatty-acids. It promotes increased strength of muscle contraction and increased heart rate. It also results in an enhanced BP and a bronchodilator, promoting greater availability of O_2 [58].

The immune and neuroendocrine systems are linked through the SNS and this communication is essential for the maintenance of homeostatic function. During inflammation, the SNS is activated, releasing of CAs in the periphery. Both α- and β-adrenergic receptor subtypes are expressed in innate immune cells and NE regulates the level of CD4+ T and B lymphocyte activity *via* these adrenergic receptors. Several human autoimmune diseases have been associated with changes in lymphocyte AR expression and such alterations may reflect changes in sympathetic activity and CA availability [59, 60]. DA decreases serum concentration, such as prolactin, growth hormone, and thyrotropin releasing hormone, resulting in effects on the immune system, anabolism, and lipid and glucose metabolism [55].

Septic shock, systemic inflammation or pharmacological vasodilatation are associated with hypotension, despite normal or increased cardiac output. Considering that in these situations systemic hypotension may persist despite vigorous volume expansion, some potent systemic vasopressor agents, such as NE or high-dose DA can then be used to restore mean arterial blood pressure. Under these conditions, renal dysfunction is common and the use of NE is typically fraught with controversy [61].

Stress can occur in a variety of forms and depending on the type and intensity of the stressor, differential responses of the sympathetic nervous and adrenomedullary hormonal systems can be observed [60]. Chronic sympathetic nervous stimulation of the cardiovascular system could promote cardiovascular hypertrophy, "splinting" arterial baroreceptors in stiff blood vessel walls, in turn contributing to systolic hypertension and the risk of heart failure, kidney failure, and stroke [47]. Adrenergic stress may affect several organ systems and the heart seems to be most susceptible to sympathetic overstimulation. Adverse CA effects have been observed in the lungs, the coagulation, gastrointestinal, endocrinologic and immune systems, and metabolism, bone marrow, and skeletal muscles.

CONCLUSION

In conclusion, although the immune system may be directly influenced by RAS activation and NO and CAs production in some settings, the role of these substances in non-specific and specific immunity *in vivo* and in immunologically mediated diseases and inflammation is not fully understood. Future studies will focus on mechanisms of action of these substances, their target molecules and their role in infection and immunologically mediated diseases.

CONFLICT OF INTEREST

The authors confirm that they have no conflict of interest to declare for this publication.

ACKNOWLEDGEMENTS

The authors thank FAPESP, CNPq, CAPES for research grants.

REFERENCES

[1] Danser AH. Local renin-angiotensin systems: the unanswered questions. Int J Biochem Cell Biol 2003; 35(6): 759-68.
[http://dx.doi.org/10.1016/S1357-2725(02)00178-4] [PMID: 12676161]

[2] Santos RA, Ferreira AJ. Angiotensin-(1-7) and the renin-angiotensin system. Curr Opin Nephrol Hypertens 2007; 16(2): 122-8.
[http://dx.doi.org/10.1097/MNH.0b013e328031f362] [PMID: 17293687]

[3] Nguyen G, Delarue F, Burcklé C, Bouzhir L, Giller T, Sraer JD. Pivotal role of the renin/prorenin receptor in angiotensin II production and cellular responses to renin. J Clin Invest 2002; 109(11): 1417-27.
[http://dx.doi.org/10.1172/JCI0214276] [PMID: 12045255]

[4] Corvol P, Jeunemaitre X. Molecular genetics of human hypertension: role of angiotensinogen. Endocr Rev 1997; 18(5): 662-77.
[PMID: 9331547]

[5] Brasier AR, Jamaluddin M, Han Y, Patterson C, Runge MS. Angiotensin II induces gene transcription through cell-type-dependent effects on the nuclear factor-kappaB (NF-kappaB) transcription factor. Mol Cell Biochem 2000; 212(1-2): 155-69.
[http://dx.doi.org/10.1023/A:1007133710837] [PMID: 11108147]

[6] Tamura K, Tanaka Y, Tsurumi Y, *et al.* The role of angiotensin AT1 receptor-associated protein in renin-angiotensin system regulation and function. Curr Hypertens Rep 2007; 9(2): 121-7.
[http://dx.doi.org/10.1007/s11906-007-0022-6] [PMID: 17442223]

[7] Ardaillou R. [Does angiotensin II increase or decrease prostaglandin synthesis?]. Nephrologie 1999; 20(7): 391-2. [Does angiotensin II increase or decrease prostaglandin synthesis?].
[PMID: 10671149]

[8] Siragy HM. The angiotensin II type 2 receptor and the kidney. J Renin Angiotensin Aldosterone Syst 2009.
[PMID: 19861347]

[9] Lemarié CA, Paradis P, Schiffrin EL. New insights on signaling cascades induced by cross-talk between angiotensin II and aldosterone. J Mol Med 2008; 86(6): 673-8.
[http://dx.doi.org/10.1007/s00109-008-0323-5] [PMID: 18368382]

[10] Santos RA, Simoes e Silva AC, Maric C, *et al.* Angiotensin-(1-7) is an endogenous ligand for the G protein-coupled receptor Mas. Proc Natl Acad Sci USA 2003; 100(14): 8258-63.
[http://dx.doi.org/10.1073/pnas.1432869100] [PMID: 12829792]

[11] Vanderheyden PM. From angiotensin IV binding site to AT4 receptor. Mol Cell Endocrinol 2009; 302(2): 159-66.
[http://dx.doi.org/10.1016/j.mce.2008.11.015] [PMID: 19071192]

[12] Handa RK, Krebs LT, Harding JW, Handa SE. Angiotensin IV AT4-receptor system in the rat kidney. Am J Physiol 1998; 274(2 Pt 2): F290-9.
[PMID: 9486224]

[13] Kerins DM, Hao Q, Vaughan DE. Angiotensin induction of PAI-1 expression in endothelial cells is mediated by the hexapeptide angiotensin IV. J Clin Invest 1995; 96(5): 2515-20.
[http://dx.doi.org/10.1172/JCI118312] [PMID: 7593643]

[14] DelliPizzi AM, Hilchey SD, Bell-Quilley CP. Natriuretic action of angiotensin(1-7). Br J Pharmacol 1994; 111(1): 1-3.
[http://dx.doi.org/10.1111/j.1476-5381.1994.tb14014.x] [PMID: 8012686]

[15] Suzuki Y, Ruiz-Ortega M, Lorenzo O, Ruperez M, Esteban V, Egido J. Inflammation and angiotensin II. Int J Biochem Cell Biol 2003; 35(6): 881-900.
[http://dx.doi.org/10.1016/S1357-2725(02)00271-6] [PMID: 12676174]

[16] Ruiz-Ortega M, Ruperez M, Lorenzo O, *et al.* Angiotensin II regulates the synthesis of proinflammatory cytokines and chemokines in the kidney. Kidney Int Suppl 2002; (82): S12-22.
[http://dx.doi.org/10.1046/j.1523-1755.62.s82.4.x] [PMID: 12410849]

[17] Satou R, Gonzalez-Villalobos RA, Miyata K, *et al.* IL-6 augments angiotensinogen in primary cultured renal proximal tubular cells. Mol Cell Endocrinol 2009; 311(1-2): 24-31.
[http://dx.doi.org/10.1016/j.mce.2009.06.013] [PMID: 19583994]

[18] Gruden G, Thomas S, Burt D, *et al.* Interaction of angiotensin II and mechanical stretch on vascular endothelial growth factor production by human mesangial cells. J Am Soc Nephrol 1999; 10(4): 730-7.
[PMID: 10203356]

[19] Nataraj C, Oliverio MI, Mannon RB, *et al.* Angiotensin II regulates cellular immune responses through a calcineurin-dependent pathway. J Clin Invest 1999; 104(12): 1693-701.
[http://dx.doi.org/10.1172/JCI7451] [PMID: 10606623]

[20] Lapteva N, Nieda M, Ando Y, *et al.* Expression of renin-angiotensin system genes in immature and mature dendritic cells identified using human cDNA microarray. Biochem Biophys Res Commun 2001; 285(4): 1059-65.
[http://dx.doi.org/10.1006/bbrc.2001.5215] [PMID: 11467860]

[21] Strawn WB, Dean RH, Ferrario CM. Novel mechanisms linking angiotensin II and early atherogenesis. J Renin Angiotensin Aldosterone Syst 2000; 1(1): 11-7.
[http://dx.doi.org/10.3317/jraas.2000.001] [PMID: 11967786]

[22] Schlöndorff D. The role of chemokines in the initiation and progression of renal disease. Kidney Int Suppl 1995; 49: S44-7.
[PMID: 7674593]

[23] Kintscher U, Wakino S, Kim S, Fleck E, Hsueh WA, Law RE. Angiotensin II induces migration and Pyk2/paxillin phosphorylation of human monocytes. Hypertension 2001; 37(2 Pt 2): 587-93.
[http://dx.doi.org/10.1161/01.HYP.37.2.587] [PMID: 11230339]

[24] Jurewicz M, McDermott DH, Sechler JM, *et al.* Human T and natural killer cells possess a functional renin-angiotensin system: further mechanisms of angiotensin II-induced inflammation. J Am Soc Nephrol 2007; 18(4): 1093-102.

[http://dx.doi.org/10.1681/ASN.2006070707] [PMID: 17329576]

[25] Wolf G, Bohlender J, Bondeva T, Roger T, Thaiss F, Wenzel UO. Angiotensin II upregulates toll-like receptor 4 on mesangial cells. J Am Soc Nephrol 2006; 17(6): 1585-93. [http://dx.doi.org/10.1681/ASN.2005070699] [PMID: 16675600]

[26] Rovin BH, Rumancik M, Tan L, Dickerson J. Glomerular expression of monocyte chemoattractant protein-1 in experimental and human glomerulonephritis. Lab Invest 1994; 71(4): 536-42. [PMID: 7967509]

[27] Ortego M, Bustos C, Hernández-Presa MA, *et al.* Atorvastatin reduces NF-kappaB activation and chemokine expression in vascular smooth muscle cells and mononuclear cells. Atherosclerosis 1999; 147(2): 253-61. [http://dx.doi.org/10.1016/S0021-9150(99)00193-8] [PMID: 10559511]

[28] Krejcy K, Eichler HG, Jilma B, *et al.* Influence of angiotensin II on circulating adhesion molecules and blood leukocyte count *in vivo.* Can J Physiol Pharmacol 1996; 74(1): 9-14. [http://dx.doi.org/10.1139/y95-218] [PMID: 8963958]

[29] Piqueras L, Kubes P, Alvarez A, *et al.* Angiotensin II induces leukocyte-endothelial cell interactions *in vivo via* AT(1) and AT(2) receptor-mediated P-selectin upregulation. Circulation 2000; 102(17): 2118-23. [http://dx.doi.org/10.1161/01.CIR.102.17.2118] [PMID: 11044430]

[30] Sakai N, Wada T, Matsushima K, *et al.* The renin-angiotensin system contributes to renal fibrosis through regulation of fibrocytes. J Hypertens 2008; 26(4): 780-90. [http://dx.doi.org/10.1097/HJH.0b013e3282f3e9e6] [PMID: 18327089]

[31] Ignarro LJ, Buga GM, Wood KS, Byrns RE, Chaudhuri G. Endothelium-derived relaxing factor produced and released from artery and vein is nitric oxide. Proc Natl Acad Sci USA 1987; 84(24): 9265-9. [http://dx.doi.org/10.1073/pnas.84.24.9265] [PMID: 2827174]

[32] Singh S, Evans TW. Nitric oxide, the biological mediator of the decade: fact or fiction? Eur Respir J 1997; 10(3): 699-707. [PMID: 9073009]

[33] Palm F, Teerlink T, Hansell P. Nitric oxide and kidney oxygenation. Curr Opin Nephrol Hypertens 2009; 18(1): 68-73. [http://dx.doi.org/10.1097/MNH.0b013e32831c4cdf] [PMID: 19077692]

[34] Mattson DL, Wu F. Nitric oxide synthase activity and isoforms in rat renal vasculature. Hypertension 2000; 35(1 Pt 2): 337-41. [http://dx.doi.org/10.1161/01.HYP.35.1.337] [PMID: 10642321]

[35] Mount PF, Power DA. Nitric oxide in the kidney: functions and regulation of synthesis. Acta Physiol (Oxf) 2006; 187(4): 433-46. [http://dx.doi.org/10.1111/j.1748-1716.2006.01582.x] [PMID: 16866775]

[36] Bredt DS. Nitric oxide signaling specificity--the heart of the problem. J Cell Sci 2003; 116(Pt 1): 9-15. [http://dx.doi.org/10.1242/jcs.00183] [PMID: 12456711]

[37] Moncada S, Higgs A. The L-arginine-nitric oxide pathway. N Engl J Med 1993; 329(27): 2002-12.

[http://dx.doi.org/10.1056/NEJM199312303292706] [PMID: 7504210]

[38] Bryan NS, Bian K, Murad F. Discovery of the nitric oxide signaling pathway and targets for drug development. Front Biosci (Landmark Ed) 2009; 14: 1-18. [http://dx.doi.org/10.2741/3228] [PMID: 19273051]

[39] Cowley AW Jr, Mori T, Mattson D, Zou AP. Role of renal NO production in the regulation of medullary blood flow. Am J Physiol Regul Integr Comp Physiol 2003; 284(6): R1355-69. [http://dx.doi.org/10.1152/ajpregu.00701.2002] [PMID: 12736168]

[40] Cowley AW Jr. Renal medullary oxidative stress, pressure-natriuresis, and hypertension. Hypertension 2008; 52(5): 777-86. [http://dx.doi.org/10.1161/HYPERTENSIONAHA.107.092858] [PMID: 18852392]

[41] Baylis C. Nitric oxide deficiency in chronic kidney disease. Am J Physiol Renal Physiol 2008; 294(1): F1-9. [http://dx.doi.org/10.1152/ajprenal.00424.2007] [PMID: 17928410]

[42] Du C, Guan Q, Diao H, Yin Z, Jevnikar AM. Nitric oxide induces apoptosis in renal tubular epithelial cells through activation of caspase-8. Am J Physiol Renal Physiol 2006; 290(5): F1044-54. [http://dx.doi.org/10.1152/ajprenal.00341.2005] [PMID: 16352744]

[43] Goligorsky MS. Immune system in renal injury and repair: burning the candle from both ends? Pharmacol Res 2008; 58(2): 122-8. [http://dx.doi.org/10.1016/j.phrs.2008.05.011] [PMID: 18588980]

[44] Araujo M, Welch WJ. Oxidative stress and nitric oxide in kidney function. Curr Opin Nephrol Hypertens 2006; 15(1): 72-7. [http://dx.doi.org/10.1097/01.mnh.0000191912.65281.e9] [PMID: 16340670]

[45] Himmelfarb J. Linking oxidative stress and inflammation in kidney disease: which is the chicken and which is the egg? Semin Dial 2004; 17(6): 449-54. [http://dx.doi.org/10.1111/j.0894-0959.2004.17605.x] [PMID: 15660575]

[46] Rodríguez-Iturbe B, Vaziri ND, Herrera-Acosta J, Johnson RJ. Oxidative stress, renal infiltration of immune cells, and salt-sensitive hypertension: all for one and one for all. Am J Physiol Renal Physiol 2004; 286(4): F606-16. [http://dx.doi.org/10.1152/ajprenal.00269.2003] [PMID: 15001451]

[47] Goldstein DS. Catecholamines and stress. Endocr Regul 2003; 37(2): 69-80. [PMID: 12932192]

[48] Di Marco GS, Vio CP, Dos Santos OF, Schor N, Casarini DE. Catecholamine production along the nephron. Cell Physiol Biochem 2007; 20(6): 919-24. [http://dx.doi.org/10.1159/000110452] [PMID: 17982274]

[49] Arita DY, Di Marco GS, Schor N, Casarini DE. Purification and characterization of the active form of tyrosine hydroxylase from mesangial cells in culture. J Cell Biochem 2002; 87(1): 58-64. [http://dx.doi.org/10.1002/jcb.10277] [PMID: 12210722]

[50] Di Marco GS, Naffah-Mazzacoratti Md MdaG, Vio CP, Dos Santos OF, Schor N, Casarini DE. Mesangial cells are able to produce catecholamines *in vitro*. J Cell Biochem 2003; 89(1): 144-51. [http://dx.doi.org/10.1002/jcb.10485] [PMID: 12682915]

[51] Aperia A, Bertorello A, Hokfert T. Dopamine: an intrarenal renal hormone. Hormones, Autacoids, and the Kidney. 1. 1991; pp. 315-38.

[52] Vincent JL, Biston P, Devriendt J, Brasseur A, De Backer D. Dopamine *versus* norepinephrine: is one better? Minerva Anestesiol 2009; 75(5): 333-7.
[PMID: 19412154]

[53] Vallone D, Picetti R, Borrelli E. Structure and function of dopamine receptors. Neurosci Biobehav Rev 2000; 24(1): 125-32.
[http://dx.doi.org/10.1016/S0149-7634(99)00063-9] [PMID: 10654668]

[54] Zeng C, Zhang M, Asico LD, Eisner GM, Jose PA. The dopaminergic system in hypertension. Clin Sci 2007; 112(12): 583-97. [Lond].
[http://dx.doi.org/10.1042/CS20070018] [PMID: 17492945]

[55] Banday AA, Lokhandwala MF. Dopamine receptors and hypertension. Curr Hypertens Rep 2008; 10(4): 268-75.
[http://dx.doi.org/10.1007/s11906-008-0051-9] [PMID: 18625155]

[56] Wang X, Villar VA, Armando I, Eisner GM, Felder RA, Jose PA. Dopamine, kidney, and hypertension: studies in dopamine receptor knockout mice. Pediatr Nephrol 2008; 23(12): 2131-46.
[http://dx.doi.org/10.1007/s00467-008-0901-3] [PMID: 18615257]

[57] Kanagy NL. Alpha(2)-adrenergic receptor signalling in hypertension. Clin Sci 2005; 109(5): 431-7. [Lond].
[http://dx.doi.org/10.1042/CS20050101] [PMID: 16232127]

[58] Barth E, Albuszies G, Baumgart K, *et al.* Glucose metabolism and catecholamines. Crit Care Med 2007; 35(9) (Suppl.): S508-18.
[http://dx.doi.org/10.1097/01.CCM.0000278047.06965.20] [PMID: 17713401]

[59] Madden KS. Catecholamines, sympathetic innervation, and immunity. Brain Behav Immun 2003; 17 (Suppl. 1): S5-S10.
[http://dx.doi.org/10.1016/S0889-1591(02)00059-4] [PMID: 12615180]

[60] Webster Marketon JI, Glaser R. Stress hormones and immune function. Cell Immunol 2008; 252(1-2): 16-26.
[http://dx.doi.org/10.1016/j.cellimm.2007.09.006] [PMID: 18279846]

[61] Bellomo R, Giantomasso DD. Noradrenaline and the kidney: friends or foes? Crit Care 2001; 5(6): 294-8.
[http://dx.doi.org/10.1186/cc1052] [PMID: 11737909]

CHAPTER 13

Cardiovascular and Behavioral Effects of Emotional Stress: The Participation of Renin-Angiotensin System

Fernanda Klein Marcondes[1,*], **Vander José das Neves**[2], **Rafaela Costa**[1], **Andrea Sanches**[1], **Tatiana Sousa Cunha**[3], **Maria José Costa Sampaio Moura**[4] and **Dulce Elena Casarini**[5]

[1] *Department of Physiological Sciences, Piracicaba Dental School, University of Campinas, Brazil*

[2] *School of Physical Education and Sports, University of Sao Paulo, Brazil*

[3] *Science and Technology Institute, Universidade Federal de Sao Paulo, Brazil*

[4] *Life Sciences Center, Pontifical Catholic University of Campinas, Brazil*

[5] *Department of Medicine, Nephrology Division, Escola Paulista de Medicina, Federal University of Sao Paulo, Sao Paulo, Brazil*

Abstract: Stress reaction aims to preserve body homeostasis. During stress, the renin-angiotensin system (RAS) increases the effects of the sympathetic nervous system and the hypothalamic-pituitary- adrenal (HPA) axis so that the organism will adapt to stressors. However, during chronic stress, these responses are sustained, adaptation does not occur and pathologies might be developed. In this chapter, we address evidences towards the correlation between RAS and the negative effects that stress has on behavior and cardiovascular system. Both circulating and local RAS are involved in stress – related hypertension. Among the mechanisms involved, it has been demonstrated that RAS activates HPA axis, catecholamines upregulate the renin synthesis and RAS activity in the peripheral organs, and vascular effects of angiotensin II (Ang II) impair the balance between vascular relaxing and contracting agents. Considering cardiac hypertrophy, hyperactivity of RAS and SNS promotes growth factors increase, fibroblast proliferation and collagen synthesis in the myocardium. Ang

* **Corresponding author Fernanda Klein Marcondes:** Departamento de Ciencias Fisiologicas, Faculdade de Odontologia de Piracicaba Av. Limeira, 901 – Piracicaba, SP – Brazil CEP 13414-903; Phone/Fax: 55 – 19 – 2106 5380 / 2106 5212; E-mail: ferklein@unicamp.br.

Dulce Elena Casarini, Danielle Yuri Arita, Tatiana Sousa Cunha & Juliana Almada Colucci (Eds.)

II triggers the production of superoxide and acts as a pro-inflammatory molecule in the blood vessels, and, consequently, might initiate and aggravate the process of atherosclerosis. Considering emotional and cognitive effects of stress, there is a link between depression and dysfunction of stress response systems involving the activation of RAS. In treating hypertension, patients having depression might also benefit from RAS blockers as these agents are known to have antidepressant effects. Inhibitors of ACE have been reported to improve cognition and memory, *via* Ang II conversion to Ang IV in the central nervous system. Stress-induced brain RAS has also been suggested as having a role in Alzheimer's disease.

Keywords: Anxiety, Atherosclerosis, Cognition, Depression, Emotion, Stress, Hypertension, Hypothalamic-pituitary-adrenal axis, Memory, Renin-angiotensin system, Sympathoadrenal axis.

INTRODUCTION

According to the modern concept of stress, our regulatory physiological systems fluctuate within operating ranges to match environmental challenges. Such condition is known as allostasis. The stress is initiated by sensory pathways, which trigger adaptive responses in the central nervous system and, subsequently, hormonal secretion by the hypothalamic-pituitary-adrenal and sympathoadrenal axes [1].

During stress, the circulating and local renin-angiotensin systems (RAS) are also stimulated, increasing plasma renin activity [2], concentration of angiotensin II (Ang II) in blood [3], and expression of Ang II type 1 receptors (AT1R) [3]. Most organs are capable of producing Ang II, and many tissues express Ang II receptors. Therefore, Ang II can be considered a multitask peptide that regulates many systemic functions, including those involved in stress reactions [1].

Activates the peripheral and central responses to preserve body homeostasis [4]. These responses depend on genetic factors, underlying diseases, and stressors' intensity and frequency. Such conditions might cause hyperactivity in the hypothalamic-pituitary-adrenal and sympathoadrenal axes and RAS, resulting in a variety of stress-related diseases, such as hypertension, coronary heart disease, pathological cardiac hypertrophy, atherosclerosis, depression, anxiety [3, 5, 6].

Clinical and experimental data show that RAS is involved in stress-related diseases [2]. In animals and humans, the inhibition or blockade of the AT_1R has been reported to have positive effects on the treatment of atherosclerosis and hypertension-induced organ injury [7, 8], improves hypertensive patients quality of life [9], and decreases anxiety and depression in diabetic patients [10]. In addition, AT_1R receptors antagonists and angiotensin-converting enzyme (ACE) inhibitors improve mood and well-being [11, 12], increase the efficacy of antidepressants [13] and decrease anxiety and depression in normotensive subjects [14].

Moreover, the actions of aldosterone in the brain and other organs *via* mineralocorticoid receptors seem to induce deleterious effects like myocardial necrosis and fibrosis, endothelial dysfunction, catecholamine release and cardiac arrhythmias on depressive patients at risk of cardiovascular dysfunction [15 - 17]. Besides increasing the renin-angiotensin activity, chronic mild and unpredictable stress can also induce anhedonia, hypothalamic-pituitary-adrenal (HPA) axis dysfunction and activation of proinflammatory cytokines in laboratory animals [18].

Circulating and Local Renin-Angiotensin System

Circulating and local RAS are stimulated during acute and chronic stress. During stress, the renin-angiotensin system (RAS) increases the effects of the sympathetic nervous system (SNS) and the hypothalamic-pituitary- adrenal to maintain the homeostasis. In this way, the brain RAS stimulates the SNS, and consequently there is an increase in the secretion of renin and epinephrine in the kidney and blood [19], peripheral and central Ang II concentrations, AT1R expression in the HPA axis [2]. The renin released from kidney circulates in plasma and cleaves angiotensinogen to form angiotensin I. In the pulmonary vasculature, angiotensin I is converted to angiotensin II, which is transported by blood and activates specific angiotensin II receptors in the peripheral tissues. Also, the function of the circulating RAS is carry renin and angiotensinogen to the tissues, which produces locally the most angiotensin II by action of ACE. In the brain, stressful events can upregulates the AT_1R expression in the hypothalamic paraventricular nucleus (PVN) and anterior pituitary [20], and these effects induces synthesis and releasing of corticotrophin hormone (CRH), which stimulates releasing of adrenocorticotropic hormone (ACTH) and secretion of adrenal corticosteroid hormones in the circulation. Thus the AT1R present in the HPA axis and brain modulate the responses to stressors, and prolonged hyperactivity of RAS by stress may lead to a disease state [20].

Considering the local RAS, many tissues produce Ang II, such as juxtaglomerular cells, brain, heart, walls of blood vessels, pituitary, adrenal and sex glands. All these tissues possess angiotensin II receptors and exhibit angiotensin-mediated responses. The Ang II in the hypothalamus, myocardium and blood vessels of chronically stressed animals are higher than those acutely stressed [3]. This indicates that changes in local and circulating Ang II are essential to initiate illness in chronically stressed animals.

The local RAS, in agreement with Dzau [21], may play a more important role in the vasculature than other tissues in the regulation of blood pressure. The tissue RAS has tonic influence on the arteries, veins, heart, and kidney during persistent stress [3, 22].

The Ang II is a potent vasoconstrictor peptide capable of promotes endothelial dysfunction, growth and proliferation of vascular smooth muscle cells [23], and hypertension [24] in situations of chronic stress. In blood vessels, angiotensin receptors are found both in the endothelial and smooth muscle cells, while ACE is found only in the endothelial cells.

The production of renin has been reported to occur in the aorta and larger arteries. This renin in the blood vessel may be taking up from the circulation and generated by local synthesis [22]. Similarly, angiotensinogen may be circulating derived or locally expressed, since high angiotensinogen mRNA levels were demonstrated in the blood vessels [22]. In the heart, the local RAS was evidenced by renin enzymatic activity in homogenates of whole hearts, and both renin and angiotensinogen mRNAs were expressed in the atrial and ventricular myocytes [21]. In isolated heart of rat perfused with angiotensin I, it is promptly conversed to angiotensin II, and addition of ACE inhibitors prevents this conversion [25].

Tissue Ang II modulates the vascular functions by paracrine or autocrine mechanisms. Ang II modulates the contraction of vascular smooth muscle cells

(VSMC) and the secretion of prostacyclin by endothelial cells. Prostacyclin, an important vasodilator, inhibits platelet aggregation, growth of fibrous tissue, and intimal accumulation of lipids [26]. In a cluster of VSMC, Ang II activates the angiotensin receptors, which induces constriction of one or more VSMC. Also, Ang II may impair the NO production by the endothelium, inducing pronounced and sustained hypertension [8]. Beside this, the local Ang II increases the norepinephrine production by noradrenergic nerve endings in blood vessels. These local effects show the importance of the RAS in the regulation of vascular tone, pathogenesis of chronic hypertension, development of vascular hypertrophy, and pathogenesis of atherosclerosis [21]. Therefore, the presence of a circulating and local RAS may contribute to an overall stress reaction, and development of cardiovascular diseases.

Participation of Stress and Renin-Angiotensin System in the Pathogenesis of Hypertension

In our body, the homeostatic systems present environmental and internal variations. In this way, the body uses efficient adaptive process to maintain stability. Then, in front of an acute aggressive agent, the body quickly responds mobilizing energy to fight with the stressor, and returns to previous state, after the end of stressor. However, in front of repeated stress the body may not adapt and then fail to shut-off and returns to baseline [27]. When the system does not shut-off in time, the adaption not occurs, which may cause pathologies. Thus, since the hyperactivity of RAS may be maintained by chronic stress, illness as hypertension may initiates or is aggravated by stress.

The Ang II acts with other neurotransmitters and neuromodulators, controlling the activity of the HPA axis and the secretion of vasopressin and CRH [19]. During stress, the circulating Ang II activates AT1R in the anterior pituitary, adrenal gland and sympathetic nerves, increasing the secretion of ACTH, glucocorticoid, aldosterone and catecholamines. Also, the circulating Ang II activates stress pathways in the brain by interaction with Ang II receptors in areas outside the blood brain barrier, the circunventricular organs, such as the subfornical organ (SFO), intimately connected to the hypothalamic paraventricular nucleus (PVN), a crucial site in the HPA axis [1]. The AT_1R-expressing tract with direct connection among SFO, the PVN and the median eminence of the hypothalamus is a central pathway of interaction between circulating Ang II and HPA axis response to stress [28]. In addition, the direct connection between PVN, nucleus of the solitary tract and ventrolateral medulla, with high presence of the AT_1R, supports the evidence that Ang II exerts important role in the cardiovascular baroreceptors and sympathetic output baroreflex [19]. During stress, AT1R in the PVN and median eminence increase mediates the synthesis and release of CRH from median eminence and ACTH from the anterior pituitary, leading to the releasing of glucocorticoid from adrenal gland. Beside this, the central actions of the Ang II also increase the activity of peripheral sympathetic endings, leading to higher levels of circulating renin and Ang II, which increase fluid retention, vasoconstriction, arterial blood pressure and cardiac chronotropism [28]. Moreover, the actions of Ang II in the central nervous system involve excitation of catecholaminergic neurons and stimulation of vasopressin release. Also, it is important to note that sympathetic nerves and catecholamine may facilitate the RAS, while Ang II may, in turn, stimulate the sympathetic system, being an important interaction between RAS and sympathetic-adrenal medulla system, creating a positive feedback in the brain [3].

Also contributing by hypertension induced by stress, the cathecholamines regulate the renin synthesis and RAS activity *via* β-adrenergic receptors in the peripheral organs [29] and Ang II promotes the release of noradrenaline and adrenaline by peripheral sympathetic neurons and adrenal medulla. This interaction is also a positive feedback between enhanced catecholaminergic system and RAS. Also, it was showed that Ang II may directly induce glucocorticoids secretion by adrenal glands [3]. The adrenal steroidogenesis is controlled *via* negative feedback loops of HPA axis and the RAS by glucocorticoids and mineralocorticoids respectively. However, it is noteworthy that during chronic stress the cortisol also activates the mineralocorticoid receptor, and this action decreases the feedback loops of HPA axis and RAS, increasing sodium reabsorption and arterial blood pressure [29].

Besides the mechanisms aforementioned, Ang II and Nitric Oxide (NO) interact with each other in the endothelial cells and VSMC [30], contributing in the hypertension pathogenesis. The endothelium-derived NO relaxes the VSMC. The inhibition of endothelial NO production stimulates ACE activity, generation of Ang II and superoxide anion, leading to vasoconstriction, and hypertension [8]. The inhibition of endothelial NO synthase (eNOS) [31], and the decrease of the cofactor for eNOS, tetrahydrobiopterin (BH_4), increase blood pressure in mice and rats [32, 33]. Also, it was showed that high levels of glucocorticoids promoted supersensitivity of thoracic aorta to phenylephrine [34] and diminished relaxation response to acetylcholine in the thoracic aorta rats submitted to chronic mild unpredictable stress [35]. Thus, it is possible that the sustained increase of blood pressure during the chronic stress should be related to the reduction of the expression of guanosine triphosphate cyclohydrolase 1 mRNA induced by glucocorticoids, since this enzyme is necessary for the synthesis of BH_4 [33, 36], essential for stabilizing eNOS. With eNOS destabilized, the NO production is impaired. Thus, as NO down-regulates the AT_1R [8, 30, 37], it is reasonable supposes that lack of NO induced by stress may induce an opposite situation, favorable for the action of Ang II. In VSMC, NO decreased AT_1R mRNA expression [8,38].

Furthermore, Ang II can increase the superoxide production *via* AT_1R in endothelial cells, VSMC, adventitial fibroblasts through activation of NADH/NADPH oxidase [39]. Superoxide reacts avidly with NO to form peroxynitrite, which oxidizes BH_4, and promotes eNOS uncoupling [40]. High superoxide production impairs the balance between vascular relaxation and contraction, by increasing the expression of endothelium-dependent vasoconstrictors and decreasing the production of endothelium-dependent vasorelaxating factors. This imbalance increases the tone of the underlying VSMC [41], contributing to hypertension.

And in endothelial cells, Ang II increases the production of endothelin-1, a power vasoconstrictor that may be inhibited by NO. On the other hand, the Ang II effects can be inhibited by antagonists of angiotensin II and endothelin receptors. In situations of stress, it has been proposed that a feedback mechanism involving Ang II, endothelin, and NO synthesis could act to regulate vascular tone [8].

Stress, Cardiac Hypertrophy and Atherosclerosis.

Clinical observations indicate a possible participation of the psychological stress on development of cardiac hypertrophy, since the level of stress may influences the geometric heart remodeling in hypertensive individuals. However, evidences of the impact of stress on pathological left ventricular hypertrophy are complicated by absence of fidelity and simple methods to quantify the psychological load [42]. In patients analyzed during their works, Devereux and colleagues [43] showed that regular and recurrent stress increase the impact of the blood pressure responses in the heart. In a case-control study of 191 men employed in New York City, evaluating both clinical and ambulatory blood pressures and using psychometric questionnaires, Schnall and colleagues [44] showed that those workers that were underwent to a high-strain jobs have a significantly greater left ventricle mass than those in low-strain jobs. Human and animals studies have shown that chronic exposure to adrenocortical hormones contributes to the occurrence of cardiac hypertrophy [45]. Also, a recent study correlating cardiac hypertrophy with social defeat and isolation stress, showed interstitial collagen accumulation in left ventricle of stressed rats as compared with control group without significative left ventricle hypertrophy between the groups, but there was right ventricle hypertrophy in stressed rats as compared with control group [46]. Bruder-Nascimento and colleagues [47] also showed cardiac hypertrophy followed by high blood pressure in rats submitted to chronic stress as compared with control group. However, the studies abovementioned not make any relationship among stress, RAS and cardiac hypertrophy.

In the pathological left ventricular hypertrophy it has been observed the following changes in cardiac morphology and function: hypertrophy of cardiac myocytes with high levels of extracellular collagen accumulation, interstitial fibrosis, impairment of the diastolic and systolic function [48]. In this process, the involvement of RAS is evidenced by the actions of Ang II in the myocytes, inducing growth factors, fibroblast proliferation, and collagen synthesis, as well as fibronectin expression *via* AT_1R. Associated to this, the high activity of sympathetic nervous system during stress reaction may contribute to cardiac hypertrophy [28].

Stress may induce hypertension during the presence of the stressor, and this resultant hypertension has special pathologic relevance on the development of left ventricle hypertrophy [49]. In this way, as hypertension may induces structural changes in the arteries, the hypertensive individuals prone to high levels of stress might also develops left ventricle hypertrophy as consequence of increased cardiac overload. Hypertension induces cardiac hypertrophy in up 50% of the patients evaluates by echocardiography [50]. The RAS – induced peripheral vasoconstriction and renal sodium reabsorption increase the blood pressure and this effect causes left ventricle wall tension, activating adaptive changes in creatine kinase isoenzymes and isomyosin patterns [51, 52].

Despite all that exist in the literature about psychological stress and cardiac hypertrophy, further studies need be carried to show more direct relations among psychological stress, RAS, and cardiac hypertrophy. Thus, we postulate that the association of various factors related to RAS might contribute to cardiac hypertrophy generated by psychological stress. During chronic stress, besides increased blood pressure, the high levels of Ang II stimulates the positive inotropism, cardiac protein synthesis, mitogenesis, and stimulates increased sympathetic nervous system activity. And the circulating Ang II has a permissive action in the hypertrophic effects of noradrenaline in the cardiac muscle [52]. Although the hypothesis abovementioned may be plausible, studies are still necessary to highlight as stress really may induce pathological cardiac hypertrophy *via* RAS.

Besides cardiac hypertrophy, stress may be also a co-factor in the etiology of the atherosclerosis. In the cases without any other known causal co-factor, stress may be only risk factor for development of this disease. Structural changes in arteries have been correlated with increased vascular reactivity to stress and occur in asymptomatic young men. Exaggerated responsiveness of atherosclerotic vessels to sympathetic arousal with elevations in blood pressure may serve to enhance the atherosclerotic process [26].

During the stress reaction, RAS is activated by SNS, resulting in the production of renin from kidney, which initiates a series of reactions whereby renin and ACE produce Ang II, which induces vasoconstriction, and chronotropic positive effects, increasing the blood pressure. However, the Ang II can accelerate atherosclerosis independently of any pressor effect [53]. Ang II increases the superoxide production, acting as a pro-inflammatory molecule [28]. Also, Ang II can modify low-density lipoprotein (LDL) and stimulates the foam cells formation in blood vessels [54]. Beside this, it may increase the VSMC proliferation by acting on growth factor-beta, platelet-derived growth factor, and fibroblast growth factor [26].

Besides the aforementioned mechanisms, the inactivation of NO by the increased reactive oxygen species, mainly superoxide anion, is intimately involved with atherogenesis. Peroxynitrite is involved in the oxidation of LDL, and both superoxide and peroxynitrite may oxidize BH_4, leading to uncoupling eNOS. In turn, uncoupling eNOS may produce superoxide anion, in a vicious cycle that accelerates the atherogenesis [8]. In this way, inhibition of ACE or blockade of AT_1R may retard the atherogenesis [7].

Furthermore, in endothelial cells Ang II activates AT_1R which mediates proinflammatory cytokine production and the expression of lectin-like oxidized LDL receptor-1 (LOX-1), which is the major receptor for oxidized LDL [56]. This way, Ang II may contribute for atherosclerosis by increasing the uptake oxidized LDL into endothelial cells, VSMC, and macrophages [8]. Stress can induce dyslipidemia [27, 34, 35], and the accumulation of lipids in blood vessels enhances the expression of RAS components [55], accelerating the atherogenesis. According Nickenig and colleagues [57], activation of AT_1R accelerates the LDL-cholesterol accumulation in VSMC, and Ang II increases LDL uptake by arterial wall macrophages [54]. The hypercholesterolemia induced by stress promotes up-regulation of AT_1R and increases the responsiveness of this receptor to vasoconstrictors, and increases plasma angiotensinogen and angiotensin levels [56]. Moreover, considering the presence of ACE in atherosclerotic lesions, it seems that Ang II may be involved in the local generation of proinflammatory substances [56]. The role of RAS in the atherogenesis is also supported by the effects of AT_1R antagonists that prevent the hypercholesterolemia and endothelial dysfunction [58]. Thus, the chronic stress in conjunction with RAS may interact with each other to promote atherosclerosis.

Then, if will be possible block or reduce the stress components that induces cardiac hypertrophy and atherosclerosis *via* RAS, it will be possible to reduce substantially the morbidity and mortality related to cardiovascular illness.

The putative mechanisms of hypertension, atherosclerosis, and cardiac hypertrophy induced by stress are shown in the Fig. **1**.

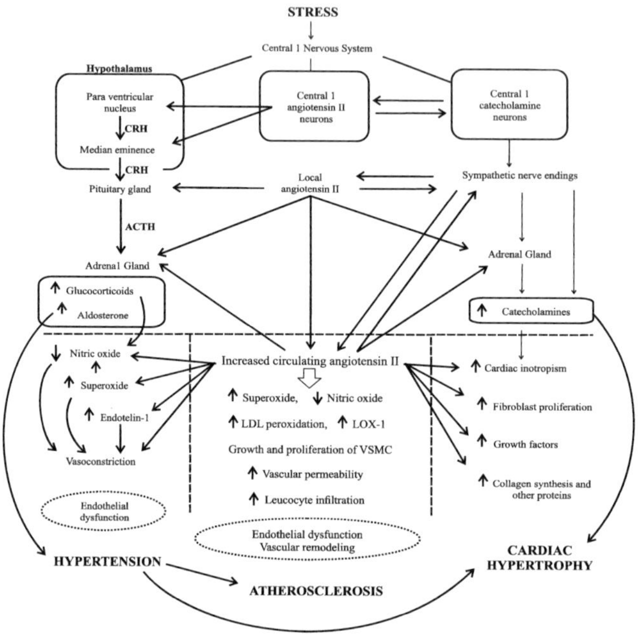

Fig. (1). Putative mechanisms involved in the association among stress, hypertension, atherosclerosis, and cardiac hypertrophy. Corticotropin hormone (CRH), adrenocorticotropic hormone (ACTH), low-density lipoprotein (LDL), lectin-like oxidized LDL receptor-1 (LOX-1), vascular smooth muscle cells (VSMC). The arrows indicates stimulatory effects.

Stress, Renin Angiotensin System, Emotional and Cognitive Effects

There is a link between depression and dysfunction of stress response systems [6]. Sustained presence of stressors or high intensity of stressors may avoid the adaptation and have been associated with depressive signs and symptoms [17].

In this context, chronic stress or hypothalamic-pituitary-adrenal axis dysfunctions are also related with the activation of SRA [17]. And because of this association, it has been proposed that some components of SRA could be markers of depression. Authors suggested that increased levels of aldosterone could be a marker of depression [59], while others [60] have shown that there seems to be a relationship between high plasma concentrations of renin and depression.

It has been reported that stressful events increase the circulating and local Ang II levels and Ang II may participate in the stress reaction [1,61]. This hypothesis is supported by the effects of the peripheral administration of candesartan (an AT_1R receptors antagonist) corticosterone in Wistar Kyoto rats. Candesartan prevented AT_1R binding in anterior pituitary, adrenal and paraventricular nucleus (PVN), and decreased the production of pituitary adrenocorticotropic hormone (ACTH) and corticosterone by adrenal glands [62]. In spontaneously hypertensive rats submitted to cold stress, it has been observed that chronic candesartan in drinking water increased central AT2 receptor expression and this effect has been associated with a decrease in gastric ulceration [63, 64]. In other study, animals treated with AT_1R antagonists did not present the peripheral and central sympathetic activation to stress [65] These findings suggest that AT_1R antagonists could be used in the treatment of stress related disorders [66].

In addition, there is a relationship between antidepressant and RAS inhibitors drugs. The blockade of actions of Ang II by desipramine and fluoxetine, and antidepressant effects of angiotensin-converting enzyme inhibitors (ACEi) have been reported [67]. Antidepressant effects of RAS blocking were evidenced in hypertensive patients, which had also depression. When they were treated with inhibitors of angiotensin-converting enzyme, they presented improvement in mental state and mood [12, 68]. Antidepressive effects of SRA were also reported in laboratory animals submitted to force swimming test, a validated model of human depression [69]. In this behavioral paradigm, immobility is interpreted as learned helplessness which is analogous to depression symptoms. After the treatment with captopril or antidepressants, mice [70] and rats [71] presented reduced immobility during the forced swimming test. Gard *et al.* [67] suggests that the antidepressant-like effects of captopril may involve the reduction of angiotensin II function, as opposed to inhibition of any other actions of ACE, since the AT_1R antagonist losartan has also been shown to give positive antidepressant-like results.

Besides the relationship between RAS inhibition and depressive behavior improvement, some studies have been shown an association of RAS gene polymorphisms, HPA axis activity and depressive illness. Baghai *et al.* [72] have studied the effect of the angiotensin converting enzyme gene insertion (I)/deletion (D) polymorphism, on HPA system. The depressive patients with the DD genotype presented higher basal and stimulated cortisol levels. The treatment with antidepressants and the attenuation of HPA system overdrive have cancelled the cortisol increase.

In addition, the participation of brain RAS in learning and memory has also been studied. Besides to improving mood, well-being and quality of life [68], the treatment with inhibitors of ACE improve cognition and memory [73]. Aged normotensive Dahl rats chronically treated with ACE inhibitor showed an improvement in cognitive function compared to the control animals. It seems that this effect may be related to the inhibition of vasoconstrictor action of Ang II which consequently improves the brain blood perfusion resulting in preservation of neuronal cells and capillaries in the hippocampal region [74].

However, other studies suggest that this effect is independent of the cardiovascular effects, since patients treated with diuretics and β-blockers do not exhibit this improvement in memory and cognition [73]. In laboratory animals, it was described that spontaneously hypertensive rats and Wistar–Kyoto rats, treated with captopril, but not with hydralazine, presented a decrease in age-related memory impairment [75]. Moreover, in animal model of streptozotocin-diabetic rats, which present impaired memory, the treatment with enalapril improved the responses in the water maze test. And this effect was related to the improvement of hippocampal long-term potentiation (LTP), an eletrophysical mechanism involved in learning and memory [76]. Additionally, the treatment with perindopril reduced ACE activity and improved memory in another model of memory deficit in rats. The authors suggested that this memory improvement could be related to effects in the cerebral metabolism and blood flow [77].

It has been also proposed that in the brain, high levels of angiotensin decrease acetylcholine release, and this effect could impair cognition and memory [78, 79]. Perindopril, and inhibitor of ACE, improved the performance of mice in Morris water maze test [80], in the scopolamine-induced amnesia model [80].

Although is already known that the ACEi effect on cognition may be due to modification of the RAS, the role of the Ang II in memory has not yet been clarified. While some studies have shown that Ang II may improve cognition and memory [81, 82], other studies show that angiotensin II has amnesic effects associated with inhibition of the hippocampal LTP [83]. Moreover, the angiotensin II infusion-induced LTP inhibition is prevented by saralasin or losartan treatment, suggesting that these effects occur *via* AT1 receptor activation [84]. In this context, it has been also considered that some effects on memory could be due to Ang II conversion to Ang IV. Therefore, Ang IV has been proposed to be the RAS component responsible for cognitive facilitation by acting in central AT_4 receptors [85].

Clinical study showed that the use of losartan (50mg) improved the memory in healthy young adults treated with scopolamine [86]. However, it has not been clarified if this effect of AT1R blockade is associated with the conversion of Ang II to Ang IV which then activates the AT4 receptor. The treatment with ACE inhibitors enhances cognition and increases Ang I levels. Ang I may be converted to Ang 1-9 and then to Ang III, Ang IV, and Ang 3-7. Ang IV and Ang 3-7 activate the AT_4R subtype [87]. The Ang IV is a component of RAS, a metabolic product of angiotensin II, and actives AT_4R found in large quantities in the hippocampus [88]. It has been shown that Ang IV has positive effects on learning and memory in a range of rodent model [89]. The Ang IV can improve spatial memory and may be involved with synaptic plasticity and memory formation *via* modulation of LTP, by activation of AT_4R in hippocampus [90]. The intracerebroventricular infusion of Ang IV in rats increases performance in the passive avoidance test [91] and reverses memory deficits induced by scopolamine [92], while intracerebroventricular infusion of AT_4R antagonist resulted in reduction of learning and memory [89]. *In vitro*, application of the AT_4R agonist, Nle1-AngIV (Ang IV analogues), enhances synaptic transmission and LTP, whereas the application of AT_4R antagonist, Nle1-Leual3-AngIV, causes inhibition of LTP in the CA1 region of the hippocampus of rats [90].

This potential involvement of brain RAS in learning and memory promotes the investigation of brain RAS components to the identification of substances which could be used for the treatment of Alzheimer's disease [93]. Chronic adverse stress contributes to the onset and progress of Alzheimer's disease and stress responses may be impaired in Alzheimer's patients [94]. Moreover, higher activity of the brain RAS also has been observed in Alzheimer's patients [95] suggesting a link among stress, RAS, and Alzheimer's disease.

The chronic stress can promote plastic and adaptive changes in hippocampal structure, an important brain region for cognitive function like learn and memory [96]. High levels of glucocorticoids can result in dendritic remodeling caused by retraction and simplification of neurons' dendrites in the hippocampal CA3 region [97], inhibition of neurogenesis in the dentate gyrus [98], and LTP impairment [99]. In Alzheimer's disease, these neuronal changes also occurred and it could increase the vulnerability to the negative effects of chronic stress. In a clinical study the patients with Alzheimer's disease treated with brain-penetrating ACE inhibitors presented a slow the rate of cognitive impairment in comparison with the patients treated with non-brain-penetrating ACE inhibitors or calcium channel blockers [100]. Moreover, in an experimental Alzheimer's disease model, the mice treated with the brain-penetrating ACE inhibitor perindopril had better improvement of cognition and brain injury, in comparison with the group treated with non-brainpenetrating ACE inhibitors [101]. The incidence and progression of Alzheimer's disease and dementia is reduced in hypertensive men treated with blockers of AT_1R in comparison to men treated with ACEIs and other anti-hypertensive drugs [102].

In the Alzheimer's disease, there are cerebral accumulations of extracellular amyloid-β protein (Aβ) (both Aβ1–40 and Aβ1–42) deposits and the ratio between Aβ1–40 and Aβ1–42 is relevant to be studied, since Aβ1–40 seems to be neuroprotective, and Aβ1–42 may be neurotoxic [93]. High levels of glucocorticoids may increase Aβ production and decrease Aβ degradation in Alzheimer's disease [103]. In this context, it important to study and develop drugs which could decrease or block the production of Aβ [104]. In Alzheimer's disease animal models, the treatment of mice with antagonists of AngII receptors, valsartan [105] and telmisartan [106], reduced the deposition of Aβ in the brain, and improved the cognitive deficits in comparison with non- treated animals or animals treated with other antihypertensive medications. Moreover, the intranasal administration of losartan had direct neuroprotective effects by reduction of Aβ

[107]. However the mechanisms involved on the association between Aβ metabolism and renin-angiotensin systems are still being investigated.

CONCLUSION

During chronic stress, the sustained activation of sympathetic nervous system, hypothalamic-pituitary - adrenal axis and renin-angiotensin system contribute to the development of cardiovascular and emotional diseases. Both circulating and local RAS are involved in this process. Some of the mechanisms involved in the association among stress, RAS, cardiovascular and emotional diseases have been described, and others are still been investigated in animal models and clinical studies. The results of these studies show that some components of RAS are already been used in the treatment of pathologies associated to stress. Other components of RAS are potential targets for future medications that could be used in the treatment of depression and Alzheimer's disease, among the stress-induced diseases.

CONFLICT OF INTEREST

The authors confirm that they have no conflict of interest to declare for this publication.

ACKNOWLEDGEMENTS

The authors thank FAPESP, CNPq, CAPES and FAEPEX – UNICAMP for research grants.

REFERENCES

[1] Saavedra JM, Benicky J. Brain and peripheral angiotensin II play a major role in stress. Stress 2007; 10(2): 185-93.
[http://dx.doi.org/10.1080/10253890701350735] [PMID: 17514587]

[2] Yang G, Wan Y, Zhu Y. Angiotensin II--an important stress hormone. Biol Signals 1996; 5(1): 1-8.
[http://dx.doi.org/10.1159/000109168] [PMID: 8739318]

[3] Phillips MI, de Oliveira EM. Brain renin angiotensin in disease. J Mol Med 2008; 86(6): 715-22.
[http://dx.doi.org/10.1007/s00109-008-0331-5] [PMID: 18385968]

[4] Krantz DS, Manuck SB. Acute psychophysiologic reactivity and risk of cardiovascular disease: a review and methodologic critique. Psychol Bull 1984; 96(3): 435-64.
[http://dx.doi.org/10.1037/0033-2909.96.3.435] [PMID: 6393178]

[5] Johnson AK, Grippo AJ. Sadness and broken hearts: neurohumoral mechanisms and co-morbidity of ischemic heart disease and psychological depression. J Physiol Pharmacol 2006; 57 (Suppl. 11): 5-29. [PMID: 17244936]

[6] Claes S. Glucocorticoid receptor polymorphisms in major depression. Ann N Y Acad Sci 2009; 1179: 216-28. [http://dx.doi.org/10.1111/j.1749-6632.2009.05012.x] [PMID: 19906242]

[7] Brosnan MJ, Hamilton CA, Graham D, Lygate CA, Jardine E, Dominiczak AF. Irbesartan lowers superoxide levels and increases nitric oxide bioavailability in blood vessels from spontaneously hypertensive stroke-prone rats. J Hypertens 2002; 20(2): 281-6. [http://dx.doi.org/10.1097/00004872-200202000-00018] [PMID: 11821713]

[8] Schulman IH, Zhou MS, Raij L. Interaction between nitric oxide and angiotensin II in the endothelium: role in atherosclerosis and hypertension. J Hypertens Suppl 2006; 24(1): S45-50. [http://dx.doi.org/10.1097/01.hjh.0000220406.46246.f2] [PMID: 16601573]

[9] Weber MA. Angiotensin-II receptor blockers for hypertension and heart failure: quality of life and outcomes. Manag Care Interface 2005; 18(2): 47-54. [PMID: 15766065]

[10] Pavlatou MG, Mastorakos G, Lekakis I, *et al.* Chronic administration of an angiotensin II receptor antagonist resets the hypothalamic-pituitary-adrenal (HPA) axis and improves the affect of patients with diabetes mellitus type 2: preliminary results. Stress 2008; 11(1): 62-72. [http://dx.doi.org/10.1080/10253890701476621] [PMID: 17853061]

[11] Dahlöf B, Lindholm LH, Carney S, Pentikäinen PJ, Ostergren J. Main results of the losartan *versus* amlodipine (LOA) study on drug tolerability and psychological general well-being. J Hypertens 1997; 15(11): 1327-35. [http://dx.doi.org/10.1097/00004872-199715110-00018] [PMID: 9383183]

[12] Etienne PE, Zubensko GS. Does captopril elevate mood? Trends Pharmacol Sci 1987; 8: 329-30. [http://dx.doi.org/10.1016/0165-6147(87)90135-0]

[13] Hertzman M, Adler LW, Arling B, Kern M. Lisinopril may augment antidepressant response. J Clin Psychopharmacol 2005; 25(6): 618-20. [http://dx.doi.org/10.1097/01.jcp.0000186736.99523.1d] [PMID: 16282855]

[14] Braszko JJ, Karwowska-Polecka W, Halicka D, Gard PR. Captopril and enalapril improve cognition and depressed mood in hypertensive patients. J Basic Clin Physiol Pharmacol 2003; 14(4): 323-43. [http://dx.doi.org/10.1515/JBCPP.2003.14.4.323] [PMID: 15198305]

[15] Stier CT Jr, Chander PN, Rocha R. Aldosterone as a mediator in cardiovascular injury. Cardiol Rev 2002; 10(2): 97-107. [http://dx.doi.org/10.1097/00045415-200203000-00008] [PMID: 11895576]

[16] Gomez-Sanchez EP. Brain mineralocorticoid receptors: orchestrators of hypertension and end-organ disease. Curr Opin Nephrol Hypertens 2004; 13(2): 191-6. [http://dx.doi.org/10.1097/00041552-200403000-00007] [PMID: 15202613]

[17] Grippo AJ, Johnson AK. Stress, depression and cardiovascular dysregulation: a review of neurobiological mechanisms and the integration of research from preclinical disease models. Stress

2009; 12(1): 1-21.
[http://dx.doi.org/10.1080/10253890802046281] [PMID: 19116888]

[18] Grippo AJ, Francis J, Beltz TG, Felder RB, Johnson AK. Neuroendocrine and cytokine profile of chronic mild stress-induced anhedonia. Physiol Behav 2005; 84(5): 697-706.
[http://dx.doi.org/10.1016/j.physbeh.2005.02.011] [PMID: 15885245]

[19] Baltatu O, Bader M. Angiotensin. In: Fink G, Ed. Encyclopedia of Stress. San Diego, CA, USA: ELSEVIER 2007; pp. 182-6.
[http://dx.doi.org/10.1016/B978-012373947-6.00034-9]

[20] Leong DS, Terrón JA, Falcón-Neri A, *et al.* Restraint stress modulates brain, pituitary and adrenal expression of angiotensin II AT(1A), AT(1B) and AT(2) receptors. Neuroendocrinology 2002; 75(4): 227-40.
[http://dx.doi.org/10.1159/000054714] [PMID: 11979053]

[21] Dzau VJ, Re RN. Evidence for the existence of renin in the heart. Circulation 1987; 75(1 Pt 2): I134-6.
[PMID: 3539402]

[22] Dzau VJ. Circulating *versus* local renin-angiotensin system in cardiovascular homeostasis. Circulation 1988; 77(6 Pt 2): I4-I13.
[PMID: 3286045]

[23] Touyz RM, Schiffrin EL. Signal transduction mechanisms mediating the physiological and pathophysiological actions of angiotensin II in vascular smooth muscle cells. Pharmacol Rev 2000; 52(4): 639-72.
[PMID: 11121512]

[24] Liang M, Liu Y, Mladinov D, *et al.* MicroRNA: a new frontier in kidney and blood pressure research. Am J Physiol Renal Physiol 2009; 297(3): F553-8.
[http://dx.doi.org/10.1152/ajprenal.00045.2009] [PMID: 19339633]

[25] Linz W, Schölkens BA, Han YF. Beneficial effects of the converting enzyme inhibitor, ramipril, in ischemic rat hearts. J Cardiovasc Pharmacol 1986; 8 (Suppl. 10): S91-9.
[http://dx.doi.org/10.1097/00005344-198600101-00017] [PMID: 2438498]

[26] Black PH, Garbutt LD. Stress, inflammation and cardiovascular disease. J Psychosom Res 2002; 52(1): 1-23.
[http://dx.doi.org/10.1016/S0022-3999(01)00302-6] [PMID: 11801260]

[27] Marcondes FK, Neves VJ, Costa R, *et al.* Dyslipidemia induced by stress. In: Kelishadi R, Ed. Dyslipidemia - From Prevention to Treatment. Rijeka, Croatia: InTech 2012; pp. 367-90.

[28] Jenkins TA, Mendelsohn FA. Angiotensin receptors. In: Fink G, Ed. Encyclopedia of Stress. San Diego, CA, USA: ELSEVIER 2007; pp. 186-90.
[http://dx.doi.org/10.1016/B978-012373947-6.00410-4]

[29] Willenberg HS, Schinner S, Ansurudeen I. New mechanisms to control aldosterone synthesis. Horm Metab Res 2008; 40(7): 435-41.
[http://dx.doi.org/10.1055/s-2008-1065336] [PMID: 18493881]

[30] Yan C, Kim D, Aizawa T, Berk BC. Functional interplay between angiotensin II and nitric oxide: cyclic GMP as a key mediator. Arterioscler Thromb Vasc Biol 2003; 23(1): 26-36.

[http://dx.doi.org/10.1161/01.ATV.0000046231.17365.9D] [PMID: 12524221]

[31] Kashiwagi M, Shinozaki M, Hirakata H, *et al.* Locally activated renin-angiotensin system associated with TGF-beta1 as a major factor for renal injury induced by chronic inhibition of nitric oxide synthase in rats. J Am Soc Nephrol 2000; 11(4): 616-24.
[PMID: 10752520]

[32] Cosentino F, Barker JE, Brand MP, *et al.* Reactive oxygen species mediate endothelium-dependent relaxations in tetrahydrobiopterin-deficient mice. Arterioscler Thromb Vasc Biol 2001; 21(4): 496-502.
[http://dx.doi.org/10.1161/01.ATV.21.4.496] [PMID: 11304463]

[33] Mitchell BM, Dorrance AM, Webb RC. GTP cyclohydrolase 1 inhibition attenuates vasodilation and increases blood pressure in rats. Am J Physiol Heart Circ Physiol 2003; 285(5): H2165-70.
[http://dx.doi.org/10.1152/ajpheart.00253.2003] [PMID: 12855421]

[34] Neves VJ, Moura MJ, Tamascia ML, *et al.* Proatherosclerotic effects of chronic stress in male rats: altered phenylephrine sensitivity and nitric oxide synthase activity of aorta and circulating lipids. Stress 2009; 12(4): 320-7.
[http://dx.doi.org/10.1080/10253890802437779] [PMID: 19085621]

[35] Neves VJ, Moura MJ, Almeida BS, *et al.* Chronic stress, but not hypercaloric diet, impairs vascular function in rats. Stress 2012; 15(2): 138-48.
[http://dx.doi.org/10.3109/10253890.2011.601369] [PMID: 21801080]

[36] Mitchell BM, Dorrance AM, Mack EA, Webb RC. Glucocorticoids decrease GTP cyclohydrolase and tetrahydrobiopterin-dependent vasorelaxation through glucocorticoid receptors. J Cardiovasc Pharmacol 2004; 43(1): 8-13.
[http://dx.doi.org/10.1097/00005344-200401000-00002] [PMID: 14668561]

[37] Watanabe T, Barker TA, Berk BC. Angiotensin II and the endothelium: diverse signals and effects. Hypertension 2005; 45(2): 163-9.
[http://dx.doi.org/10.1161/01.HYP.0000153321.13792.b9] [PMID: 15630047]

[38] Ichiki T, Usui M, Kato M, *et al.* Downregulation of angiotensin II type 1 receptor gene transcription by nitric oxide. Hypertension 1998; 31(1 Pt 2): 342-8.
[http://dx.doi.org/10.1161/01.HYP.31.1.342] [PMID: 9453326]

[39] Lassègue B, Clempus RE. Vascular NAD(P)H oxidases: specific features, expression, and regulation. Am J Physiol Regul Integr Comp Physiol 2003; 285(2): R277-97.
[http://dx.doi.org/10.1152/ajpregu.00758.2002] [PMID: 12855411]

[40] Förstermann U, Münzel T. Endothelial nitric oxide synthase in vascular disease: from marvel to menace. Circulation 2006; 113(13): 1708-14.
[http://dx.doi.org/10.1161/CIRCULATIONAHA.105.602532] [PMID: 16585403]

[41] Guzik TJ, West NE, Black E, *et al.* Vascular superoxide production by NAD(P)H oxidase: association with endothelial dysfunction and clinical risk factors. Circ Res 2000; 86(9): E85-90.
[http://dx.doi.org/10.1161/01.RES.86.9.e85] [PMID: 10807876]

[42] Junior WN, Franchini KG. Influência de fatores ambientais e genéticos na hipertrofia e remodelamento cardíacos na hipertensão arterial. Rev Bras Hipertens 2001; 8: 414-24.

[43] Devereux RB, Pickering TG, Harshfield GA, *et al.* Left ventricular hypertrophy in patients with hypertension: importance of blood pressure response to regularly recurring stress. Circulation 1983; 68(3): 470-6.
[http://dx.doi.org/10.1161/01.CIR.68.3.470] [PMID: 6223721]

[44] Schnall PL, Pieper C, Schwartz JE, *et al.* The relationship between 'job strain,' workplace diastolic blood pressure, and left ventricular mass index. Results of a case-control study. JAMA 1990; 263(14): 1929-35.
[http://dx.doi.org/10.1001/jama.1990.03440140055031] [PMID: 2138234]

[45] Lumbers ER, Boyce AC, Joulianos G, *et al.* Effects of cortisol on cardiac myocytes and on expression of cardiac genes in fetal sheep. Am J Physiol Regul Integr Comp Physiol 2005; 288(3): R567-74.
[http://dx.doi.org/10.1152/ajpregu.00556.2004] [PMID: 15576665]

[46] Carnevali L, Mastorci F, Graiani G, *et al.* Social defeat and isolation induce clear signs of a depression-like state, but modest cardiac alterations in wild-type rats. Physiol Behav 2012; 106(2): 142-50.
[http://dx.doi.org/10.1016/j.physbeh.2012.01.022] [PMID: 22330326]

[47] Bruder-Nascimento T, Campos DH, Leopoldo AS, *et al.* Chronic stress improves the myocardial function without altering L-type Ca+2 channel activity in rats. Arq Bras Cardiol 2012; 99(4): 907-14.
[http://dx.doi.org/10.1590/S0066-782X2012005000082] [PMID: 22936032]

[48] Tanno AP, das Neves VJ, Rosa KT, *et al.* Nandrolone and resistance training induce heart remodeling: role of fetal genes and implications for cardiac pathophysiology. Life Sci 2011; 89(17-18): 631-7.
[http://dx.doi.org/10.1016/j.lfs.2011.08.004] [PMID: 21889516]

[49] Pickering TG. Does psychological stress contribute to the development of hypertension and coronary heart disease? Eur J Clin Pharmacol 1990; 39 (Suppl. 1): S1-7.
[http://dx.doi.org/10.1007/BF03216267] [PMID: 2261940]

[50] Savage DD, Drayer JI, Henry WL, *et al.* Echocardiographic assessment of cardiac anatomy and function in hypertensive subjects. Circulation 1979; 59(4): 623-32.
[http://dx.doi.org/10.1161/01.CIR.59.4.623] [PMID: 421302]

[51] Pauletto P, Nascimben L, Piccolo D, *et al.* Ventricular myosin and creatine-kinase isoenzymes in hypertensive rats treated with captopril. Hypertension 1989; 14(5): 556-62.
[http://dx.doi.org/10.1161/01.HYP.14.5.556] [PMID: 2680963]

[52] Gavras I, Gavras H. Angiotensin II as a cardiovascular risk factor. J Hum Hypertens 2002; 16 (Suppl. 2): S2-6.
[http://dx.doi.org/10.1038/sj.jhh.1001392] [PMID: 11967726]

[53] Black PH. Stress and the inflammatory response: a review of neurogenic inflammation. Brain Behav Immun 2002; 16(6): 622-53.
[http://dx.doi.org/10.1016/S0889-1591(02)00021-1] [PMID: 12480495]

[54] Keidar S, Kaplan M, Aviram M. Angiotensin II-modified LDL is taken up by macrophages *via* the scavenger receptor, leading to cellular cholesterol accumulation. Arterioscler Thromb Vasc Biol 1996; 16(1): 97-105.
[http://dx.doi.org/10.1161/01.ATV.16.1.97] [PMID: 8548433]

[55] Singh BM, Mehta JL. Interactions between the renin-angiotensin system and dyslipidemia: relevance in the therapy of hypertension and coronary heart disease. Arch Intern Med 2003; 163(11): 1296-304. [http://dx.doi.org/10.1001/archinte.163.11.1296] [PMID: 12796065]

[56] Sitia S, Tomasoni L, Atzeni F, *et al.* From endothelial dysfunction to atherosclerosis. Autoimmun Rev 2010; 9(12): 830-4. [http://dx.doi.org/10.1016/j.autrev.2010.07.016] [PMID: 20678595]

[57] Nickenig G, Bäumer AT, Temur Y, Kebben D, Jockenhövel F, Böhm M. Statin-sensitive dysregulated AT1 receptor function and density in hypercholesterolemic men. Circulation 1999; 100(21): 2131-4. [http://dx.doi.org/10.1161/01.CIR.100.21.2131] [PMID: 10571970]

[58] Taguchi I, Inoue T, Kikuchi M, *et al.* Pleiotropic effects of ARB on dyslipidemia. Curr Vasc Pharmacol 2011; 9(2): 129-35. [http://dx.doi.org/10.2174/157016111794519336] [PMID: 21143172]

[59] Murck H, Held K, Ziegenbein M, Künzel H, Koch K, Steiger A. The renin-angiotensin-aldosterone system in patients with depression compared to controls--a sleep endocrine study. BMC Psychiatry 2003; 3(1): 15. [http://dx.doi.org/10.1186/1471-244X-3-15] [PMID: 14585110]

[60] Emanuele E, Geroldi D, Minoretti P, Coen E, Politi P. Increased plasma aldosterone in patients with clinical depression. Arch Med Res 2005; 36(5): 544-8. [http://dx.doi.org/10.1016/j.arcmed.2005.03.046] [PMID: 16099336]

[61] Chung IM, Kim YM, Yoo MH, Shin MK, Kim CK, Suh SH. Immobilization stress induces endothelial dysfunction by oxidative stress *via* the activation of the angiotensin II/its type I receptor pathway. Atherosclerosis 2010; 213(1): 109-14. [http://dx.doi.org/10.1016/j.atherosclerosis.2010.08.052] [PMID: 20850747]

[62] Nishimura Y, Ito T, Hoe K, Saavedra JM. Chronic peripheral administration of the angiotensin II AT(1) receptor antagonist candesartan blocks brain AT(1) receptors. Brain Res 2000; 871(1): 29-38. [http://dx.doi.org/10.1016/S0006-8993(00)02377-5] [PMID: 10882779]

[63] Bregonzio C, Armando I, Ando H, Jezova M, Baiardi G, Saavedra JM. Anti-inflammatory effects of angiotensin II AT1 receptor antagonism prevent stress-induced gastric injury. Am J Physiol Gastrointest Liver Physiol 2003; 285(2): G414-23. [http://dx.doi.org/10.1152/ajpgi.00058.2003] [PMID: 12686508]

[64] Bregonzio C, Seltzer A, Armando I, Pavel J, Saavedra JM. Angiotensin II AT(1) receptor blockade selectively enhances brain AT(2) receptor expression, and abolishes the cold-restraint stress-induced increase in tyrosine hydroxylase mRNA in the locus coeruleus of spontaneously hypertensive rats. Stress 2008; 11(6): 457-66. [http://dx.doi.org/10.1080/10253890801892040] [PMID: 18609298]

[65] Müller H, Kröger J, Jöhren O, *et al.* Stress sensitivity is increased in transgenic rats with low brain angiotensinogen. J Endocrinol 2010; 204(1): 85-92. [http://dx.doi.org/10.1677/JOE-09-0363] [PMID: 19808775]

[66] Pavel J, Benicky J, Murakami Y, Sanchez-Lemus E, Saavedra JM. Peripherally administered angiotensin II AT1 receptor antagonists are anti-stress compounds *in vivo.* Ann N Y Acad Sci 2008;

1148: 360-6.
[http://dx.doi.org/10.1196/annals.1410.006] [PMID: 19120129]

[67] Gard PR. The role of angiotensin II in cognition and behaviour. Eur J Pharmacol 2002; 438(1-2): 1-14. [http://dx.doi.org/10.1016/S0014-2999(02)01283-9] [PMID: 11906704]

[68] Germain L, Chouinard G. Treatment of recurrent unipolar major depression with captopril. Biol Psychiatry 1988; 23(6): 637-41. [http://dx.doi.org/10.1016/0006-3223(88)90010-8] [PMID: 3281718]

[69] Porsolt RD, Le Pichon M, Jalfre M. Depression: a new animal model sensitive to antidepressant treatments. Nature 1977; 266(5604): 730-2. [http://dx.doi.org/10.1038/266730a0] [PMID: 559941]

[70] Giardina WJ, Ebert DM. Positive effects of captopril in the behavioral despair swim test. Biol Psychiatry 1989; 25(6): 697-702. [http://dx.doi.org/10.1016/0006-3223(89)90240-0] [PMID: 2647155]

[71] Martin P, Massol J, Puech AJ. Captopril as an antidepressant? Effects on the learned helplessness paradigm in rats. Biol Psychiatry 1990; 27(9): 968-74.

[72] Baghai TC, Schule C, Zwanzger P, *et al.* Hypothalamic-pituitary-adrenocortical axis dysregulation in patients with major depression is influenced by the insertion/deletion polymorphism in the angiotensin I-converting enzyme gene. Neurosci Lett 2002; 328(3): 299-303. [http://dx.doi.org/10.1016/S0304-3940(02)00527-X] [PMID: 12147330]

[73] Amenta F, Di Tullio MA, Tomassoni D. The cholinergic approach for the treatment of vascular dementia: evidence from pre-clinical and clinical studies. Clin Exp Hypertens 2002; 24(7): 697-713.

[74] Hirawa N, Uehara Y, Kawabata Y, *et al.* Long-term inhibition of renin-angiotensin system sustains memory function in aged Dahl rats. Hypertension 1999; 34(3): 496-502. [http://dx.doi.org/10.1161/01.HYP.34.3.496] [PMID: 10489400]

[75] Wyss JM, Kadish I, van Groen T. Age-related decline in spatial learning and memory: attenuation by captopril. Clin Exp Hypertens 2003; 25(7): 455-74. [http://dx.doi.org/10.1081/CEH-120024988] [PMID: 14596369]

[76] Manschot SM, Biessels GJ, Cameron NE, *et al.* Angiotensin converting enzyme inhibition partially prevents deficits in water maze performance, hippocampal synaptic plasticity and cerebral blood flow in streptozotocin-diabetic rats. Brain Res 2003; 966(2): 274-82. [http://dx.doi.org/10.1016/S0006-8993(02)04211-7] [PMID: 12618350]

[77] Tota S, Kamat PK, Saxena G, Hanif K, Najmi AK, Nath C. Central angiotensin converting enzyme facilitates memory impairment in intracerebroventricular streptozotocin treated rats. Behav Brain Res 2012; 226(1): 317-30. [http://dx.doi.org/10.1016/j.bbr.2011.07.047] [PMID: 21864581]

[78] Barnes JM, Barnes NM, Costall B, *et al.* Angiotensin-converting enzyme inhibition, angiotensin, and cognition. J Cardiovasc Pharmacol 1992; 19 (Suppl. 6): S63-71. [http://dx.doi.org/10.1097/00005344-199219006-00011] [PMID: 1382167]

[79] Barnes JM, Barnes NM, Costall B, *et al.* Angiotensin II inhibits cortical cholinergic function: implications for cognition. J Cardiovasc Pharmacol 1990; 16(2): 234-8.

[http://dx.doi.org/10.1097/00005344-199008000-00009] [PMID: 1697379]

[80] Tota S, Nath C, Najmi AK, Shukla R, Hanif K. Inhibition of central angiotensin converting enzyme ameliorates scopolamine induced memory impairment in mice: role of cholinergic neurotransmission, cerebral blood flow and brain energy metabolism. Behav Brain Res 2012; 232(1): 66-76. [http://dx.doi.org/10.1016/j.bbr.2012.03.015] [PMID: 22460064]

[81] Belcheva I, Ternianov A, Georgiev V. Lateralized learning and memory effects of angiotensin II microinjected into the rat CA1 hippocampal area. Peptides 2000; 21(3): 407-11. [http://dx.doi.org/10.1016/S0196-9781(00)00163-7] [PMID: 10793224]

[82] Braszko JJ. AT(2) but not AT(1) receptor antagonism abolishes angiotensin II increase of the acquisition of conditioned avoidance responses in rats. Behav Brain Res 2002; 131(1-2): 79-86. [http://dx.doi.org/10.1016/S0166-4328(01)00349-7] [PMID: 11844574]

[83] Denny JB, Polan-Curtain J, Wayner MJ, Armstrong DL. Angiotensin II blocks hippocampal long-term potentiation. Brain Res 1991; 567(2): 321-4. [http://dx.doi.org/10.1016/0006-8993(91)90812-A] [PMID: 1817736]

[84] Wayner MJ, Armstrong DL, Polan-Curtain JL, Denny JB. Role of angiotensin II and AT1 receptors in hippocampal LTP. Pharmacol Biochem Behav 1993; 45(2): 455-64. [http://dx.doi.org/10.1016/0091-3057(93)90265-U} [PMID: 8327552]

[85] Braszko JJ, Walesiuk A, Wielgat P. Cognitive effects attributed to angiotensin II may result from its conversion to angiotensin IV. J Renin Angiotensin Aldosterone Syst 2006; 7(3): 168-74. [http://dx.doi.org/10.3317/jraas.2006.027] [PMID: 17094054]

[86] Mechaeil R, Gard P, Jackson A, Rusted J. Cognitive enhancement following acute losartan in normotensive young adults. Psychopharmacology (Berl) 2011; 217(1): 51-60. [http://dx.doi.org/10.1007/s00213-011-2257-9] [PMID: 21484242]

[87] Wright JW, Harding JW. The brain renin-angiotensin system: a diversity of functions and implications for CNS diseases. Pflugers Arch 2013; 465(1): 133-51. [http://dx.doi.org/10.1007/s00424-012-1102-2] [PMID: 22535332]

[88] Wright JW, Krebs LT, Stobb JW, Harding JW. The angiotensin IV system: functional implications. Front Neuroendocrinol 1995; 16(1): 23-52. [http://dx.doi.org/10.1006/frne.1995.1002] [PMID: 7768321]

[89] Wright JW, Stubley L, Pederson ES, Kramár EA, Hanesworth JM, Harding JW. Contributions of the brain angiotensin IV-AT4 receptor subtype system to spatial learning. J Neurosci 1999; 19(10): 3952-61. [PMID: 10234025]

[90] Kramár EA, Armstrong DL, Ikeda S, Wayner MJ, Harding JW, Wright JW. The effects of angiotensin IV analogs on long-term potentiation within the CA1 region of the hippocampus *in vitro*. Brain Res 2001; 897(1-2): 114-21. [http://dx.doi.org/10.1016/S0006-8993(01)02100-X] [PMID: 11282364]

[91] Wright JW, Miller-Wing AV, Shaffer MJ, *et al.* Angiotensin II(3-8) (ANG IV) hippocampal binding: potential role in the facilitation of memory. Brain Res Bull 1993; 32(5): 497-502. [http://dx.doi.org/10.1016/0361-9230(93)90297-O] [PMID: 8221142]

[92] Pederson ES, Harding JW, Wright JW. Attenuation of scopolamine-induced spatial learning impairments by an angiotensin IV analog. Regul Pept 1998; 74(2-3): 97-103. [http://dx.doi.org/10.1016/S0167-0115(98)00028-7] [PMID: 9712169]

[93] Wright JW, Harding JW. The brain RAS and Alzheimer's disease. Exp Neurol 2010; 223(2): 326-33. [http://dx.doi.org/10.1016/j.expneurol.2009.09.012] [PMID: 19782074]

[94] Rothman SM, Mattson MP. Adverse stress, hippocampal networks, and Alzheimer's disease. Neuromolecular Med 2010; 12(1): 56-70. [http://dx.doi.org/10.1007/s12017-009-8107-9] [PMID: 19943124]

[95] Duron E, Hanon O. Antihypertensive treatments, cognitive decline, and dementia. J Alzheimers Dis 2010; 20(3): 903-14. [PMID: 20182022]

[96] Conrad CD. A critical review of chronic stress effects on spatial learning and memory. Prog Neuropsychopharmacol Biol Psychiatry 2010; 34(5): 742-55. [http://dx.doi.org/10.1016/j.pnpbp.2009.11.003] [PMID: 19903505]

[97] McEwen BS, Gianaros PJ. Stress- and allostasis-induced brain plasticity. Annu Rev Med 2011; 62: 431-45. [http://dx.doi.org/10.1146/annurev-med-052209-100430] [PMID: 20707675]

[98] Gould E, McEwen BS, Tanapat P, Galea LA, Fuchs E. Neurogenesis in the dentate gyrus of the adult tree shrew is regulated by psychosocial stress and NMDA receptor activation. J Neurosci 1997; 17(7): 2492-8. [PMID: 9065509]

[99] Sousa N, Cerqueira JJ, Almeida OF. Corticosteroid receptors and neuroplasticity. Brain Res Brain Res Rev 2008; 57(2): 561-70. [http://dx.doi.org/10.1016/j.brainresrev.2007.06.007] [PMID: 17692926]

[100] Ohrui T, Tomita N, Sato-Nakagawa T, *et al.* Effects of brain-penetrating ACE inhibitors on Alzheimer disease progression. Neurology 2004; 63(7): 1324-5. [http://dx.doi.org/10.1212/01.WNL.0000140705.23869.E9] [PMID: 15477567]

[101] Dong YF, Kataoka K, Tokutomi Y, *et al.* Perindopril, a centrally active angiotensin-converting enzyme inhibitor, prevents cognitive impairment in mouse models of Alzheimer's disease. FASEB J 2011; 25(9): 2911-20. [http://dx.doi.org/10.1096/fj.11-182873] [PMID: 21593435]

[102] Li NC, Lee A, Whitmer RA, *et al.* Use of angiotensin receptor blockers and risk of dementia in a predominantly male population: prospective cohort analysis. BMJ 2010; 340: b5465. [http://dx.doi.org/10.1136/bmj.b5465] [PMID: 20068258]

[103] Green KN, Billings LM, Roozendaal B, McGaugh JL, LaFerla FM. Glucocorticoids increase amyloid-beta and tau pathology in a mouse model of Alzheimer's disease. J Neurosci 2006; 26(35): 9047-56. [http://dx.doi.org/10.1523/JNEUROSCI.2797-06.2006] [PMID: 16943563]

[104] Zou K, Michikawa M. Angiotensin-converting enzyme as a potential target for treatment of Alzheimer's disease: inhibition or activation? Rev Neurosci 2008; 19(4-5): 203-12. [http://dx.doi.org/10.1515/REVNEURO.2008.19.4-5.203] [PMID: 19145983]

[105] Wang J, Ho L, Chen L, *et al.* Valsartan lowers brain beta-amyloid protein levels and improves spatial learning in a mouse model of Alzheimer disease. J Clin Invest 2007; 117(11): 3393-402. [http://dx.doi.org/10.1172/JCI31547] [PMID: 17965777]

[106] Tsukuda K, Mogi M, Iwanami J, *et al.* Cognitive deficit in amyloid-beta-injected mice was improved by pretreatment with a low dose of telmisartan partly because of peroxisome proliferator-activated receptor-gamma activation. Hypertension 2009; 54(4): 782-7. [http://dx.doi.org/10.1161/HYPERTENSIONAHA.109.136879] [PMID: 19635982]

[107] Danielyan L, Klein R, Hanson LR, *et al.* Protective effects of intranasal losartan in the APP/PS1 transgenic mouse model of Alzheimer disease. Rejuvenation Res 2010; 13(2-3): 195-201. [http://dx.doi.org/10.1089/rej.2009.0944] [PMID: 20370487]

CHAPTER 14

Exercise and Renin Angiotensin System

Tatiana Sousa Cunha[1,*], Kleiton Augusto Santos Silva[2], Andrea Sanches[3], Sebastião Donato Silva Jr.[4], Vanessa Oliveira[2], Lília Firoozmand[1], Fernanda Klein Marcondes[3] and **Lisete C. Michelini[4]**

[1] *Science and Technology Institute, Federal University of Sao Paulo, Sao Jose dos Campos, Brazil*

[2] *Nephrology Division, Department of Medicine, Federal University of Sao Paulo, Sao Paulo, Brazil*

[3] *Department of Physiological Sciences, Piracicaba Dental School, University of Campinas, Piracicaba, Brazil*

[4] *Department of Physiology & Biophysics, Institute of Biomedical Sciences - University of Sao Paulo, Brazil*

Abstract: The number of people affected by cardiovascular disease is increasing in the Western world, and it is partially explained by urbanization, industrialization, work condition and inadequate diet. Cardiovascular disease killed nearly 17 million people in 2011, and of these, 7 million died of ischaemic heart disease and 6.2 million from stroke [1]. This chapter will focus on the contribution of regular physical exercise for prevention and reversal of cardiovascular disease, and on the role of renin angiotensin system (RAS) in these processes. Experimental and clinical studies show that exercise training is efficient to block RAS overactivity, thus preventing and/or reversing cardiac dysfunction and deleterious remodeling of the heart in pathological conditions such as hypertension, myocardial infarction, heart failure and obesity. Indeed, studies show that the association between RAS inhibition and exercise training can bring major benefits to individuals with heart disease (especially those with mild, moderate or severe heart failure) and also cardiometabolic alterations, acting synergically as a successful combination to the recovery and maintenance of health of these patients.

* **Corresponding author Lisete C. Michelini:** Department of Physiology & Biophysics, Institute of Biomedical Sciences - University of Sao Paulo Av. Prof. Lineu Prestes, 1524 05508-000 Sao Paulo, SP, Brazil; E-mail: michelin@usp.br

Dulce Elena Casarini, Danielle Yuri Arita, Tatiana Sousa Cunha & Juliana Almada Colucci (Eds.)

Keywords: ACE polymorphism, Angiotensin receptors, Barorreflex, Cardiovascular disease, Central nervous system, Endothelium, Exercise, Hypertension, Hypothalamus, Nephropathy, Obesity, Oxidative stress, Renin angiotensin system, VO_2.

INTRODUCTION

The number of people affected with cardiovascular and renal disease is increasing in the Western world, and it is partially explained by urbanization, industrialization, work condition and inadequate diet. Cardiovascular disease killed nearly 17 million people in 2011, and of these, 7 million died of ischaemic heart disease and 6.2 million from stroke [1]. This chapter will focus on the contribution of regular physical exercise to prevention and reversal of cardiovascular disease, and on the role of renin angiotensin system (RAS) on these processes.

Role of RAS on Central and Peripheral Responses to Exercise

Brain

After the original demonstration that angiotensin II (Ang II)increased blood pressure by a direct action on the central nervous system [2] it became clear that this peptide had several central effects [3]. Subsequent studies demonstrated that angiotensin receptors were located in circumventricular organs as well in areas inside the blood-brain barrier [3, 4]. Since Ang II does not cross blood-brain barrier, it seemed unlikely that effects, other than those mediated by the circumventricular organs, were due to the circulating peptide. These observations raised the possibility that Ang II could be synthesized within the central nervous system. Indeed in the seventies, Ganten *et al.* [5] using refined biochemical techniques, highly sensitive radioimmunoassay and immunohistochemical methods, showed that the components required for the generation of Ang II are present within the brain [5, 6]. The brain was the first extrarenal tissue in which all components of the RAS were systematically demonstrated and confirmed by the local expression of its mRNA message [7]. These findings led to new hypothesis and functional concept of a 'local' RAS actions based on brain synthesis of Ang II and other biologically active angiotensins.

Renin activity in the brain was first reported by Ganten *et al.* [5] and confirmed by subsequent molecular biology techniques and transgenic and knock-out animal models [7]. Levels of renin expression in the brain are low, but renin activity is high and present in many brain areas as the hypothalamus, pituitary, pineal gland of different species, although decreasing with ageing [7]. It has been suggested that renin might be taken up from circulation [8]. Indeed a high prorenin receptor (it binds the inactive precursor prorenin and renders it active) expression was detected in the brain [9]. mRNA and protein for the angiotensin converting enzyme isoforms (ACE and ACE2) are largely expressed in several brain areas, with high levels found in the choroid plexus, circumventricular organs, caudate putamen, brain stem, cerebellum, hippocampus and intermediate levels in the hypothalamus, thalamus, pituitary and basal ganglia [7, 10]. Other angiotensin-forming enzymes as tonin, cathepsin, chymase, aminopeptidadese A and N were also present in the brain [11].

Besides the enzymatic machinery, the precursor - angiotensinogen (Aogen) - is highly expressed in the brain. Aogen mRNA is mainly localized in cells stained for glial fibrillary acid protein, suggesting the glia as the main source for Aogen synthesis in the brain, although it was also found in pure neuronal cultures, indicating the possibility of intraneuronal synthesis as well. Following synthesis, Aogen is secreted into the extracellular since high concentration of the precursor was detected in the cerebrospinal fluid in dogs and rats [7]. It is also possible that part of the intraneuronal Aogen content could be taken from the cerebrospinal fluid pool. Aogen mRNA and Aogen immunoreactivity were found in the basal ganglia, preoptic region, hypothalamus, midbrain, pons, medulla oblongata and cerebellum, the highest levels being observed in the hypothalamus and brain stem [12].

In the presence of Aogen and biosynthetic enzymes all components of angiotensin family (Ang I, Ang II, Ang (1-7), Ang III, Ang IV) are synthesized in the brain. Highest levels of Ang II (the active peptide of the vasoconstrictor, trophic, pro-fibrotic and pro-inflammatory ACE-Ang II-AT_1R axis of RAS) were found in the paraventricular and supraoptic nuclei of the hypothalamus, pituitary and cortex, with high content being observed in the brain stem, superior colliculus, amygdala, cerebellum, hippocampus and olfactory bulb [7, 11]. Brain Ang II effects are widespread in the brain, including a variety of functions such as blood pressure, body fluid balance and food intake regulation, the control of reproduction, anxiety and memory. Ang (1-7), the active peptide of the counter regulatory, vasodilator, atrophic, anti-fibrotic and anti-inflammatory ACE2-Ang (1-7)-Mas receptor axis of RAS, was also found in the paraventricular and supraoptic nuclei of hypothalamus, medulla oblongata and amygdala. In the brain Ang (1-7) was shown to participate in blood pressure control, circadian rhythms and hippocampus' long-term potentiation [10, 13].

High densities of angiotensin receptors are detected in the brain. They are receptors for Ang II and Ang III (AT_1 and AT_2), Ang IV AT_4 and Ang (1-7) (Mas receptor). AT_1 receptors are densely distributed in brain regions with (mediating effects of blood-borne Ang II) and without blood-brain barrier (effects of locally synthesized angiotensins). AT_1 receptors show a dominant presence in brain nuclei involved in body fluid, neuroendocrine and cardiovascular control and are mainly found in the subfornical organ, organum vasculosum of the lamina terminalis, median preoptic nucleus, anterior pituitary, hypothalamic periventricular and paraventricular nuclei, nucleus of tractus solitarii and area postrema [14]. AT_2 receptors are highly expressed in the fetal, with reduced expression in the adult life. In the adult brain AT_2 receptors participate in sensory and limbic functions and are found in several thalamic and geniculate nuclei, optic tract, cerebellum and inferior olive [14]. AT_4 receptors, the ligands of Ang IV, are located in areas implicated in memory acquisition and retrieval, stress and spatial learning, being found in the cortex, hippocampus, amygdala, thalamus and hypothalamus [7]. AT_4 receptor was also shown to be an insulin-regulated aminopeptidase (IRAP), whose physiological function in the brain is still unknown [11]. The Mas protooncogene, a heptahelical orphan receptor, has been proposed as the endogenous receptor for Ang (1-7) [15, 16]. In the brain Mas receptor was found in the endothelial cells of the vasculature, in the cortex, cardiovascular-related areas, hippocampus and olfactory bulb. Upon stimulation Mas elicits numerous protective actions such as local nitric oxide generation, anti-inflammatory and anti-oxidative stress [10, 16]. Mas receptor can also heterodimerize with the AT_1 receptor, thereby antagonizing the effects of the ACE-Ang II- AT_1 receptor axis of RAS.

As summarized above, RAS components are widely distributed throughout all levels of the brain. However, studies attempting to correlate the expression of precursor, biosynthetic enzymes, peptides and receptors in specific brain areas showed areas where all components are found (no mismatch), but in many others there are marked distribution mismatches (presence of one or two components, but absence of others) [12]. These observations lead to the proposition brain RAS may function in 2 different ways: as a neurohormone and/or as neurotransmitter. The neurohormonal system presupposes that Aogen, released from the glial cells into the cerebrospinal fluid, is processed to Ang II and other active angiotensins by the different biosynthetic enzymes (also present in the extracellular space). The formed peptides, Ang II, Ang III, Ang IV and Ang (1-7) diffuse into the cerebrospinal fluid to gain access to their specific receptors localized on neurons or glia where they exert their actions. This action mechanism is called "Volume transmission" and is responsible for almost [90% - 95%] of RAS effects in the brain. Angiotensinergic neurons (synthesizing and storing Ang II intracellularly) were identified by immunocytochemical probes direct against Ang II in restricted brain areas *e.g.* subfornical organ, organum vasculosum of lamina terminalis, paraventricular and supra-optic nuclei of the hypothalamus, nucleus tractus solitarii, ventrolateral medulla that play a significant role in the control of fluid balance [12, 16]. Upon stimulation, angiotensinergic neurons release Ang II at nerve endings to act at receptors located on postsynaptic cells. This mode of brain RAS operation, called "Wiring transmission", is responsible for a small percentage of RAS effects within the brain.

By his widespread actions within the brain, RAS (through his ACE-Ang II-AT_1 receptor and ACE2-Ang (1-7)-Mas receptor axes), is a crucial modulator of central and peripheral regulatory functions as fluid and electrolyte homeostasis, blood pressure, sympathetic and parasympathetic outflow to all peripheral tissues controlling their endogenous functions, behavior and cognition. However, imbalances between RAS axes, with the predominance of Ang II synthesis and AT_1 receptor effects cause vasoconstriction, hypertrophy, volume retention, increased blood pressure, tissue inflammation, anxiety, depression and other dysfunctions, which predispose to the appearance of several pathologies. In the last decades it has been shown that pharmacological blockade of the vasoconstrictor axis and/or the improvement of the contra-regulatory axis (*e.g.* converting enzyme and renin inhibitors, AT_1 receptor blockers, administration of Ang (1-7), compounds to activate AT_2 receptors) are largely efficient to improve homeostasis in different diseases as hypertension, heart failure, stroke, kidney ischemia, dementia, tissue inflammation and autoimmune disorders for review see [10, 17, 18]. More recently exercise training, a non-pharmacological tool, starts been employed as adjuvant of pharmacological therapies to improve RAS imbalance in several tissues, including the brain.

Two original studies published in 2007 demonstrated the ability of exercise training to downregulate the expression of RAS in the brain of spontaneously hypertensive rats (SHR) and to prevent arterial baroreflex dysfunction in normotensive rats infused with Ang II into the cerebrospinal fluid [19, 20]. Trained SHR exhibited a large decrease in Aogen expression within brain stem areas involved in cardiovascular control, which was positively correlated with training-induced blood pressure fall, without any change in the expression of both precursor and blood pressure in normotensive rats submitted to a similar protocol [19]. Interestingly, functional response and training-induced reduction on Aogen expression were quite similar to pressure fall and Aogen downregulation observed in cardiovascular areas after chronic AT_1 receptor blockade with losartan [21] suggesting that both treatments are acting on similar brain mechanisms. It was also shown that exercise training and losartan as well as apocynin were able to restore the decreased baroreflex sensitivity in rats centrally infused with Ang II [20]. In addition, training downregulated both AT_1 receptor and NADPH oxidase protein expression in the paraventricular nucleus of the hypothalamus of Ang II-infused rats [20]. Together these results indicated that training-induced improvements on cardiovascular control in hypertension (characterized by high brain Ang II expression) are mediated by reduced expression of AT_1 receptor and associated with reduced oxidative stress in brain areas involved in cardiovascular control. A recent study confirmed the above results showing that chronic exercise prevented ACE and AT_1 receptor, upregulated ACE2 and Mas receptor, while reducing NADPH oxidase, inducible nitric oxide synthase expression within the paraventricular hypothalamus and rostroventrolateral medulla of the SHR [22]. It was also confirmed that training disrupted pro-inflammatory and upregulated anti-inflammatory profile [22] and caused sympathoinhibition *via* reduced oxidative stress [23] in brain cardiovascular areas of hypertensive rats, linking the beneficial effects of training with the restoration of RAS axes' balance and a low degree of both inflammation and oxidative stress.

Exercise has also been shown to enhance depressed baroreflex sensitivity by an Ang II-dependent mechanism in chronic heart failure [24]. In this study, heart failure rabbits were trained with and without simultaneous Ang II infusion. Interestingly, exercise training reduced plasma Ang II, downregulated gene and protein expression of AT_1 receptors in the rostroventrolateral medulla, improved baroreflex gain and reduced renal sympathetic nerve activity, these effects being blocked when plasma Ang II was restored to levels similar to those observed in non-exercised heart failure rabbits [24]. In heart failure AT_1 receptor expression was correlated with increased oxidative stress, increased both sympathetic nerve activity and left ventricular end diastolic pressure, all these effects being corrected by exercise training, which is capable to enhance the quality of life and survival of patients with chronic heart failure [25]. It should be noted that heart failure rats treated with losartan exhibited similar reductions of left ventricular end diastolic pressure and sympathetic nerve activity as those heart failure animals submitted to exercise training, reinforcing again that both therapeutic strategies should be acting through the brain RAS [25 - 27]. In accordance, Kar *et al.* [28] showed that ACE mRNA and protein expression were upregulated in several brain nuclei as the paraventricular in the hypothalamus, solitary tract and rostroventrolateral in the brain stem, while local ACE2 expression was decreased in heart failure rabbits. After exercise training, however, ACE expression was largely reduced and ACE2 expression markedly increased, thus restoring RAS balance (reduced ACE/ACE2 ratio in trained heart failure rabbits) in brain areas that regulate autonomic function [28].

Although some studies have shown the involvement of brain RAS in the pathogenesis of hypertension and heart failure (predominance of ACE-Ang II-AT_1 receptor axis), as well as in exercise-induced amelioration of hypertension and heart failure consequences (reduction of the vasoconstrictor axis and/or improvement of counter-regulatory axis), the underlying mechanisms are largely unknown. Other studies are necessary to confirm and expand our knowledge on the effects of exercise training on brain RAS expression/activity and its interaction with circulating Ang II and local RAS modulating the control of heart, kidney, vasculature, skeletal muscle and adrenal gland.

Heart

In the last decades, all components of the RAS within the heart have been cloned. Gene expression studies demonstrated the local synthesis of the precursor, biosynthetic enzymes and receptors of biologically active angiotensins, confirming the local synthesis of the biologically active RAS peptides in the heart [7].

Preliminary evidence for cardiac RAS expression was obtained several years ago. Aogen was shown to be produced in all parts of the heart as well as in cultured cardiac myocytes and fibroblasts [29]. On the other hand, renin expression in the heart is controversial. Although renin mRNA has been found in atria, ventricles and isolated cardiomyocytes, it was rather low [30, 31]. Recently, however, it was shown that the classical full-length renin mRNA was not expressed, but the truncated renin mRNA (also known as exxon 1A renin) was detected in the heart [7]. Although the controversy for the local synthesis, there is no doubt concerning the presence of renin within the heart, which has been attributed to diffusion into the interstitial space [a non-specific uptake], to the presence of specific binding sites or to pro-renin- and/or renin-receptor mediated uptake [7, 32]. Regarding the ACE and its homologue ACE2, their mRNA and protein expression have been consistently demonstrated in cardiomyocytes [31, 33, 34]. Interestingly, the chymase, an alternative pathway to convert Ang I to Ang II that is not blocked by the ACE inhibitors, was also highly expressed in the heart [35].

The presence in the heart of RAS precursor, Aogen, as well as the enzymes renin, ACE, and ACE2, indicates that both Ang II [36, 37] and Ang (1-7), the main biologically active components of RAS can be locally synthesized in the heart. Ang II exerts its biological actions by binding with the AT_1 and AT_2 receptors. On the other hand Ang (1-7) exerts its effects by binding with the Mas receptor [15].

The importance of RAS as a regulator of heart function and structure has been studied for over a century. RAS is involved in the control of cardiac contractility, hypertrophy, fibrosis, collagen and extracellular matrix deposition [38, 39]. This control is provided primarily by the integrated actions of two opposing RAS axis: ACE–AngII–AT_1 receptor and ACE2–Ang (1-7)–Mas receptor [7, 40].

Although the ACE–AngII–AT_1 receptor axis is important for normal heart function, its overactivation causes deleterious cardiac remodeling characterized by cardiomyocytes' hypertrophy, interstitial and perivascular fibrosis, microvascular rarefaction, all these effects leading to cardiac dysfunction, as demonstrated in rats with experimental left ventricular hypertrophy and in transgenic rats overexpressing mouse renin, human Aogen, renin, ACE and/or AT_1 receptor [7, 41 - 46]. Overactivation of the vasoconstrictor axis may also alters diastolic function of the heart [41]. On the other hand the activation of the ACE2–Ang (1-7)–Mas receptor axis may reduce cardiomyocytes' growth and inhibit collagen synthesis, which are beneficial to the heart function [40, 47]. Indeed the deletion of Mas receptor in the heart of the mice increased collagen I, collagen III and fibronectin and decreased collagen type VI (a pro-fibrotic profile), which was accompanied by cardiac dysfunction [38]. It should be noted that ACE2, by metabolizing Ang II to Ang (1-7), also counteracts the effects of the vasoconstrictor axis, which is a positive effect in the hypertrophied heart [48]. On the other hand, the reduction of ACE2 levels and/or its inability to metabolize Ang II to Ang (1-7) perpetuates the actions of Ang II after biomechanical stress and exacerbates the adverse myocardial remodeling [49].

It has also been suggested that AT_2 receptor activation could counteract the effects of AT_1 receptor and improve heart function [50]. Although highly expressed in fetal tissues, AT_2 receptor expression is low in the adult life and restricted to certain tissues as the limbic system, kidney and heart, which minimizes its importance on cardiac dynamics [16]. Recently, however, newly described anti-proliferative and anti-inflammatory effects of the AT_2R, contributing to cardiac repair in cardiovascular diseases, increased its importance in the control of heart homeostasis [51].

In hypertension, as other disease states, there is an imbalance between vasoconstrictor and vasodilator axis of the RAS, with the predominance of the ACE–AngII–AT_1 receptor axis which leads to hypertrophy, fibrosis and cardiac dysfunction. As stressed by previous excellent reviews, pharmacological blockade of the RAS is highly effective to reduce/correct several cardiac dysfunctions [52, 53] .In recent years, non-pharmacological tools as life style changes have been successfully employed to reduce RAS overactivation [54, 55]. In this regard, exercise training has emerged as an important therapy to blunt/normalize heart function while reducing plasma and tissue RAS expression [55, 56].

Physical training encompasses both static (resistance training) and aerobic exercises (dynamic training). Both types of training induce chronic intermittent workload to the heart, which causes cardiac remodeling. The resistance training imposes a large pressure overload to the heart with a marked elevation of blood pressure, which leads to the addition of parallel sarcomeres in the left ventricle, resulting in the development of *concentric hypertrophy*, also known as pathological hypertrophy [57 - 59]. On the other hand, the aerobic training induces volume overload with smaller pressure changes, leading to the addition of sarcomeres in series in the ventricles, thus causing the development of *eccentric* or *physiological hypertrophy*. Eccentric hypertrophy by allowing higher stroke volume and increased cardiac output with smaller heart rate increase is beneficial to the trained individuals [55].

The involvement of RAS in physiological cardiac remodeling has been demonstrated. Although the responsible mechanism(s) is(are) not completely clear, Ang II might be an important regulator of myocardial growth in response to aerobic training. Swimming training causes cardiac hypertrophy and leads the activation of local RAS, the magnitude of the responses being influenced by training intensity [60]. Training-induced cardiac hypertrophy increased AT_1 receptor expression without alteration in other RAS components [61]. Interestingly it was observed that mechanical stretch caused a counterclockwise rotation of the AT_1 receptor 7-transmembrane domain, which might activate intracellular signaling pathways independently of Ang II [62]. It was also shown that left ventricle growth in athletes might be influenced by ACE polymorphism since DD athletes exhibited higher cardiac ACE activity and increased LV mass when compared to II athletes after 10 weeks of endurance training [63, 64].

Exercise training was also efficient to block RAS overactivity, thus preventing and/or reversing cardiac dysfunction and deleterious remodeling of the heart in pathological conditions such as hypertension, myocardial infarction, heart failure and obesity [65, 66]. Indeed clinical and experimental studies confirmed the beneficial effects of training on cardiovascular function in both normotensive and hypertensive humans and other mammals [24, 25, 54, 55]. RAS was also highly activated in acute heart failure in order to maintain blood pressure and preserve organ perfusion. In the long term, however, RAS hyperactivity has deleterious effects upon the heart [67]. Similar to the effects observed in hypertensive patients, exercise training was shown to be an important strategy to reduce RAS overactivity in heart failure patients. It is important to note that humans with chronic heart failure exhibited decreased plasma Ang II levels when submitted to low intensity aerobic training [68]. Similar effects were observed in sympathetic hyperactivity-induced heart failure in mice: training decreased cardiac Ang II levels and ACE activity and increased ACE2 expression and prevented both exercise intolerance and ventricular dysfunction, with little impact on cardiac remodeling [69]. It was also observed that Sprague Dawley rats exercising after post-myocardial infarct showed low circulating RAS and preserved cardiac function [70].

Obesity is another risk factor for RAS hyperactivity and the development of cardiac diseases. Huang *et al.* [71] described in Zucker rats (a genetic model of obesity) increased gene expression and cardiac ACE activity, high Ang II levels, higher expression of AT_1 and AT_2 receptors and heart hypertrophy. On the other hand, trained Zucker rats exhibited reduced cardiac ACE, Ang II and AT_2 receptor, increased protein expression and ACE2 activity, which were associated with the prevention of cardiac hypertrophy [65].

An important point to be considered when exercise is used as a non pharmacological therapeutic strategy is the intensity or volume of exercise. High-intensity training in old SHR (a long-term established hypertension) produced a pro-fibrotic phenotype with unfavorable expression patterns of calcium handling proteins, which were linked to RAS hyperactivity, since ACE inhibition attenuated training-dependent effect on pro-fibrotic markers [72]. On the other hand low to moderate exercise intensity in 21-month old SHR reversed left ventricle hypertrophy, collagen content and blood pressure without worsen the inflammatory profile associated with hypertension [73]. Indeed many scientific publications show that low to moderate training intensity confers beneficial adaptations in the cardiovascular system such as blood pressure reduction in humans and animals models of hypertension [19, 54, 55, 74]. Blood pressure fall reduces heart overload and improved cardiac function. It was also observed in SHR that, independent of blood pressure changes, exercise-training for 8 weeks increased the expression of Ang (1–7) and Mas receptor in the heart and causes left ventricle remodeling, suggesting the involvement of the vasodilator axis in training-induced changes on cardiac structure and function [56]. Although the exact mechanism involved in training-induced cardiac remodeling (concentric and eccentric hypertrophy) is still unclear, experimental evidence suggest that low to moderate exercise training is highly efficient to counterbalance and/or reverse cardiac hypertrophy observed in hypertension, myocardial infarction, heart failure and obesity. Beneficial cardiac remodeling is accompanied by changes in local RAS expression and activity, characterized by blunting of ACE–Ang II–AT_1 receptor axis effects and/or improvement of ACE2–Ang (1-7)–Mas receptor axis. Therefore, in the treatment of cardiovascular diseases, exercise training is an important non-pharmacological strategy to minimize and/or avoid heart deleterious effects.

Vasculature

The identification of mRNA expression of RAS components in the vasculature is a solid evidence for a local synthesis, independent of the systemic RAS [75]. The presence of Aogen mRNA was demonstrated in the rat aorta many years ago [76]. Subsequent studies detected the presence of Aogen mRNA [77] and protein in different layers of the vessel wall, confirming its local expression and suggesting that secreted Aogen may diffuse through the vascular wall to be accessible to the vascular renin [7]. Renin mRNA is hardly detected in the vasculature due to the small sample size, often requiring pooling of the samples and the use of very sensitive assays [7, 78]. Although renin mRNA expression had been detected in conductance and resistance vessels of human beings [31], rats [79, 80] and in pathological situations such as neointima formation [81], the majority of the renin found in the vasculature is probably due its uptake from the circulation *via* the pro-renin receptor [78].

Some studies described the expression of ACE mRNA in the vessel wall, but its local expression has been questioned. ACE was present predominantly in the surface of endothelial cells [82, 83]. Rats exhibited strong and homogeneous ACE expression in the endothelium of all vessels – aorta, large and small arteries, arterioles, venules and veins [84]. The mRNA expression of ACE2 was also detected in the endothelial cells of arteries and veins but also in the smooth muscle cells of the vascular wall and other organs [85]. The detection of the precursor (Aogen) and the enzymes (renin, ACE, ACE2) in vessels confirm the capacity of the vascular wall to synthesize Ang II and Ang (1-7) locally.

Ang II binds to its G-protein-coupled receptors (GPCRs), AT_1 and AT2 receptors present on vascular smooth muscle and endothelial cells, to mediate his vascular effects [86]. In vascular smooth muscle cells the activation of AT_1 receptor by Ang II enhances intracellular calcium and induces vasoconstriction, thereby increasing vascular tone and blood pressure [87]. Ang II binding to AT_1 receptor also activates downstream signaling pathways involved in inflammation, atherosclerosis, hypertrophy, remodeling and angiogenesis [88, 89]. On the other hand Ang II binding to AT_2 receptor (mainly present on endothelial cells) activates the kallikrein-kinin system and stimulates nitric oxide generation to cause vasodilatation [90]. Since AT_2 receptor expression, abundant in the fetus, is largely reduced in the adult life, the effects of Ang II binding to AT_1receptor predominate.

Ang (1-7) is also synthesized in the endothelium and vascular wall. It is primarily generated from Ang II by ACE2 action and interacts with the Mas receptor, mainly present on endothelial cells. Ang (1-7) mediates vasodilatation, anti-inflammatory anti-arrhythmogenic and anti-thrombotic responses, thus opposing Ang II effects [91, 92].

As observed in other tissues the 2 RAS axes, ACE–AngII–AT_1R and ACE2–Ang (1-7)–Mas receptor, are active in the vasculature and maintain vascular homeostasis. An unbalance between them, with the predominance of ACE–AngII–AT_1R axis, causes marked vasoconstriction, inflammatory and fibrotic responses, remodeling and vessel hypertrophy. Initially the functional and structural changes, mediated by Ang II *via* AT_1 receptor, are adaptive; subsequently, however, they become maladaptive resulting in vascular dysfunction [93]. Predominance of Ang II effects on ACE–AngII–AT_1 receptor axis are characteristic features of hypertension, heart failure, atherosclerosis and other diseases. In contrast, activation of the ACE2–Ang (1-7)–Mas receptor axis, causes vasodilation, anti-hypertrophy and anti-inflammatory responses, thereby blunting vascular dysfunction.

Vascular remodeling (with increased vessel wall/lumen ratio) and increased peripheral resistance are important hallmarks of hypertension [94]. In primary or essential hypertension, increased wall/lumen ratio of arteries/arterioles was caused by the rearrangement of smooth muscle cells around a smaller lumen, without net growth of the vascular wall, a phenomenon termed 'inward eutrophic remodeling'. In secondary hypertension, a 'hypertrophic remodeling' was detected, with net growth of the vessel wall [94]. Vascular remodeling in hypertensive rats is attributed to the hyperactivity of vascular RAS [95]. Therapeutic tools to reduce the activity of ACE–AngII–AT_1 receptor axis, to improve the activity of the ACE2–Ang (1-7)–Mas receptor axis and/or to overexpress AT_2 receptor in vascular smooth muscle cells are currently tested in order to prevent hypertension-induced vascular hypertrophy [96, 97]. Besides the pharmacological approach, exercise training, a non-pharmacological therapeutic tool was shown to be able to revert or reduce hypertension-induced vascular remodeling. Indeed SHR submitted to low-intensity aerobic training exhibited normalized arterioles wall/lumen ratio ('outward eutrophic remodeling') in the myocardium, diaphragm, soleus, gastrocnemius, gracilis and temporalis muscles, with local resistance reduction, which was correlated with the observed pressure fall [98 - 100].

While the involvement of RAS in the beneficial vascular remodeling induced by exercise is not clear, some pharmacological studies suggest a closed link. In hypertensive patients a long-term RAS blockade (ACE inhibitors and Ang II receptor blockers) reduced the wall/lumen ratio of small resistance vessels, while β-blockers and diuretics were devoid of effects, despite similar decreases on blood pressure [101, 102]. There is also experimental evidence showing in coarcted hypertensive rats similar reduction on RAS expression and blood pressure following AT_1 receptor blockade or exercise training [19, 103, 104]. An interesting study associating AT_1 receptor blockade and exercise training in SHR showed no additional effect after one or other treatment, suggesting that both are acting through the same pathways to reduce pressure [105].

The use of exercise training in the treatment/prevention of hypertension, as well as heart failure, metabolic syndrome, diabetes and obesity increased in the last decade [25, 54, 55]. Indeed exercise, activating on neural, local and/or circulating factors, has a great influence on vascular homeostasis. *In vivo* and *in vitro* studies demonstrate that exercise-mediated shear stress induces local release of vasodilator agents (nitric oxide, bradykinin) and alters gene expression in endothelial and vascular smooth muscle cells [106, 107] which impacts vascular function and structure. Although the precise mechanisms underlying these effects remain unclear, it was suggested the involvement of the RAS.

The ability of exercise to change RAS expression has been observed in several tissues as the brain, heart and plasma. However, the interaction between exercise and vascular RAS still remains unclear. Silva *et al.* [108] observed an increase in Mas receptor expression in SHR aortas after 8 weeks of swimming training, which was accompanied by an improvement of endothelium-dependent vasodilatation in response to Ang (1-7). Ang (1-7)-induced vasodilatation depended on nitric oxide and/or prostaglandin production [109, 110]. Indeed in Mas-deficient mice these responses are absent. Since Ang (1-7) is able to attenuate Ang II-induced reactive oxygen species generation in endothelial cells, exercise-induced Mas expression increase could be involved in the balance between nitric oxide and reactive oxygen species generation, being, therefore, an important mediator in cardiovascular homeostasis [92].

RAS activation was present in coronary artery disease and a marked endothelium-dependent vasodilatation was observed after exercise-training. Regular exercise was also able to reduce AT_1 receptor and NADPH oxidase expression in mammary artery rings of coronary artery disease patients resulting in decreased local ROS generation and improvement of endothelial function [111]. Ongoing experiments in our laboratory are showing that SHR *vs.* WKY exhibited higher

Ang II content in the renal, iliac and carotid arteries; Ang (1-7) content was also higher iliac and carotid arteries, but lower in the renal artery. Our experiments are also showing that low-intensity training caused a prompt Ang II content reduction in all arteries studied from both SHR and WKY rats. Although Ang (1-7) reductions were also observed, the ratio Ang II/Ang (1-7) was reduced on renal SHR arteries at the end of training, indicating higher training-induced activation of ACE2-Ang (1-7)-Mas receptor axis in this arterial segment [112].

Although some studies have shown the impact of the exercise upon vascular RAS, many questions need to be clarified. New studies in the future in experimental models and humans would clarify this scenario and confirm the importance of exercise training to correct local RAS dysfunctions, thus improving vascular homeostasis.

Adipose Tissue

All of the main RAS components are present in the adipose tissue. The adipose RAS is responsible for promoting adipocyte triglyceride storage (by inhibiting lipolysis and increasing lipogenesis) and in this context, the adipose tissue is able to secrete Aogen, ACE, ACE2, AT_1 receptor, Mas receptor, among other components [113, 114] Giacchetti *et al.* [115] showed that there are different levels of expression of the various components of the RAS in subcutaneous adipose tissue and visceral adipose tissue, suggesting a different role and regulation of this system in the both tissues [115]. Furthermore, the fed state seems to interfere in this process, considering that feeding increases adipose Aogen expression in rodents, while fasting decreases it [116]. The fact of the Aogen produced by adipose tissue may be released into the bloodstream suggests that high circulating Aogen levels may be partially attributed to increased fat mass and obesity [117]. On the other hand, weight loss leads to reduction in Aogen expression in adipose tissue [118] and thus, non-pharmacological measures which promote weight reduction produce hemodynamic, metabolic, and neuroendocrine effects that improve the cardiovascular risk of obese subjects [119].

In this sense, the practice of aerobic exercise of moderate intensity associated with the controlled diet decreases the body weight of obese individuals. Both obese men and women (BMI > 30 kg/m^2) that have achieved a 5% or greater weight reduction have reduced by 40% plasma renin activity. Weight and renin reduction have also been accompanied by a 6-mmHg reduction in diastolic blood pressure [119].

Central angiotensinergic pathways that mediate metabolic responses to exercise are not well established, although it is known that the central angiotensinergic system is involved in metabolic adjustments during graded exercise [120]. Brain hypothalamic regions expressing Ang II or AT_1 receptor such as hypothalamic paraventricular nucleus and preoptic area are possible control sites [11], which are related to fat weight, lipid mobilization, and maintaining metabolism [121 - 123].

Leite *et al.* [120] showed that central AT_1 receptor blockade with intracerebroventricular injection of losartan produces marked hyperglycemia and increased mobilization of free fatty acids from adipose tissue in rats. The high levels of plasma free fatty acids in losartan treated animals was evident soon after the first three minutes and remained increased until the end of the exercise, at the point of fatigue. As opposed, in control rats the plasma free fat acids was only evident at 60% of maximal work and continued high until fatigue, indicating that, at fatigue point, plasma free fatty acids levels of animals treated with losartan was approximately 28% higher than that of controls.

Several regions of central nervous system make connection to the sympathetic nervous system, which in turn is increased during exercise and leads to rises in blood pressure and heart rate, besides redirection energy substrates such as increased free fatty acids in the process of activation of lipolysis by adipose tissue [124 - 126]. Ang II acts directly on the modulation of the sympathetic outflow of the adipose tissue [127] and the central AT_1 blockade may induce a faster activation of the sympathetic nervous system at a lower level of exercise intensity [120], although the brain RAS may increases sympathetic stimulation [114].

Peripherally, the sympathetic nervous system activated in response to exercise may contribute to activation of the RAS and this, seems to be more prominent in obese individuals, considering that adipose Aogen expression and its release during sympathetic stimulation are increased in obesity. It can be partially explained by the fact that acute exercise promotes intense release of lipolytic hormones and increases the responsiveness of beta-adrenergic receptors from adipocytes to catecholamines [128]. In animal models, the Zucker fatty rat (a genetic model of obesity), an intermittent aerobic moderate exercise lasting for 10 weeks did not influence the body weight and the adiposity index of epididymal and retroperitoneal adipose tissues. Furthermore, the exercise also did not affect the transcription of Aogen, ACE, and AT_1 receptor genes in the epididymal adipose tissue. On the other hand, the leptin and adiponectin gene expression were found increased in the epididymal and retroperitoneal adipose tissue after exercise, respectively [129].

Wang *et al.* [130] observed that exercise training of moderate intensity may significantly suppress body weight and epididymal fat weight gain in male rats F344/NSlc treated with high-fat diet [130]. These findings are also observed after treatment with candesartan cilexetil (AT_1 receptor blocker, with anti-inflammatory properties which plays an important role in adipose tissue metabolism) [131]. Thus, in this study, was shown that the RAS may modulate the gain of adipose tissue in rats treated with high-fat diet and both exercise and candesartan cilexetil suppressed fat weight gain [130].

Despite already being well established in clinical and experimental studies the effective participation of the RAS in adipose tissue, there are few studies that deal on the role of the adipose RAS on central and peripheral responses to exercise. Moreover, there is still no consensus on this relationship, which requires the development of additional studies.

Cross Talk Between Angiotensin II and Oxidative Stress in Health and Disease: How May Exercise Affect these Pathways?

The oxidative stress was first defined as the imbalance between production and removal of oxidants agents [132]. Recently, however, oxidative stress has been considered as an imbalance between oxidants and antioxidants, with the predominance of oxidants causing a redox signaling disorder and/or molecular damage [133]. Reactive oxygen species (ROS) are part of the normal metabolism - their crucial role has been demonstrated in many physiological processes, such as ATP production, gene activation and defense mechanisms against infection [134 - 138]. In contrast, the excessive ROS production is responsible, at least in part, for the oxidative damage in different organs and tissues, with serious implications in the etiology of several chronic diseases. Indeed, it is well established the involvement of ROS in cardiovascular diseases including hypertension, stroke, coronary artery disease, atherosclerosis and other vascular dysfunctions [139 - 141].

ROS can be generated by many enzymatic systems such as cytochrome P 450, xanthine oxidase, uncoupling endothelial nitric oxide synthase, as well as nicotinamide adenine dinucleotide phosphate-oxidase or NADPH oxidase [142 - 144]. NADPH oxidase by catalyzing the reduction of molecular oxygen to the superoxide anion is a unique enzyme that produces ROS as its primary function [145]. NADPH oxidase was first described in phagocytic cells, being a multimeric protein complex with membrane and cytoplasmic components. The cytochrome b558 oxidase is the component associated with the cellular membrane – it is formed by a large ($gp91^{phox}$) and a small subunit ($p22^{phox}$). NADPH oxidase also comprises three cytoplasmic subunits: $p47^{phox}$, $p67^{phox}$ and $p40^{phox}$, and RAC, a small regulatory G protein [146]. Later, other subunits homologues to the $gp91^{phox}$ and active in non-phagocytic cells were also identified and designed as the NOX family of NADPH oxidases. This family consists of seven members including Nox1, Nox2 (formerly termed $gp91^{phox}$), Nox3, Nox4, Nox5, Duox1 and Duox2, which are expressed in several tissues mediating diverse biological actions [147]. Although the specific regulation and function of each Nox remains to be elucidated, all the Noxes appear to interact with the $p22^{phox}$ component. Nox2 needs the $p47^{phox}$ and $p67^{phox}$ for its activation, whereas Nox1 interacts with the homologues of $p47^{phox}$ (NOXO1) and $p67^{phox}$ (NOXA1) [148 - 150].

NADPH oxidases are activated and regulated by many factors such as mechanical forces, cytokines, genetics variants, and metabolic factors [151]. Among the metabolic factors great emphasis has been given to the Ang II [152, 153]. It is known that Ang II, *via* AT_1 receptors, is a key regulator of cardiovascular NADPH oxidase [154, 155]. The signaling by which Ang II stimulates NADPH oxidase has not been completely elucidated, but phospholipase D, protein kinase C, phospholipase A, phosphatidylinositol 3-kinase appear to be involved [156 -

158]. Furthermore, the tyrosine kinase Src is essential for the effects of Ang II, not only in the synthesis of NADPH oxidase subunits by stimulating increased expression of $gp91^{phox}$, $p22^{phox}$, $p47^{phox}$, $p67^{phox}$ and $p40^{phox}$, but also by inducing phosphorylation of the $p47^{phox}$ subunit, the crucial event for the activation of NADPH oxidase [88, 153, 159]. Subsequently to its phosphorylation, $p47^{phox}$ interacts with $p67^{phox}$ translocated to the membrane, where it associates with cytochrome b 558. This association allows the transfer of electrons from the molecular oxygen to form the superoxide anion – an important ROS component.

Clinical studies showing increased plasma biomarkers of lipid peroxidation and oxidative stress in cardiovascular diseases have suggested a close relationship between them [160 - 162]. Moreover, Ang II and AT_1 receptor are involved in the up-regulation of NADPH oxidase and increased ROS production in vascular smooth muscle cells of arteries/arterioles in hypertensive individuals [163, 164]. In fact, human endothelial cells treated with Ang II, showed overproduction of superoxide anion due to an up-regulation of $gp91^{phox}$ subunit, while AT_1 receptor blockade downregulates $gp91^{phox}$ expression, leading to lower superoxide anion production [165]. AT_1 receptor blockade in hypertensive patients also inhibited the increased oxidative stress by normalizing the expression of $p22^{phox}$ subunit of the NADPH oxidase [140].

Animal models support the clinical data. For example, in stroke-prone SHR it was shown that AT_1 receptor blockade blunted ROS overproduction in the brain [166] and improves vascular function by reducing NADPH oxidase expression and the oxidative stress [167]. In rats with miocarditis, AT_1 receptor blockade decreased oxidative stress simultaneously with reduced $p47^{phox}$, $p67^{phox}$ and $gp91^{phox}$ protein expression in the heart [168]. On the other hand, Ang II infusion in rats and mice increased both the expression of NADPH oxidase subunits and ROS production while increasing pressure levels [169, 170]. Apocynin (a specific inhibitor of NADPH oxidase) treatment in Ang II-infused animals caused blood pressure reduction [169] or no change [170], suggesting that Ang II infusion increased blood pressure by activating NADPH oxidase as well as other independent pathways. The role of Ang II in ROS generation *via* NADPH oxidase has been confirmed in knockout models: Nox2 and $p47^{phox}$ knockout mice exhibited less vascular dysfunction and Ang II infusion did not increase superoxide production and blood pressure [171 - 173]. On the other hand mice overexpressing $p22^{phox}$ showed high ROS content and pronounced vascular dysfunction, but no blood pressure change [174]. Together, these results confirmed that Ang II-activated NADPH oxidase pathway is a crucial source for superoxide production in vessels leading to vascular dysfunction that may contribute to [but is not the only cause] hypertension.

Based on experimental evidence showing that ROS reduction is an efficient tool to avoid cardiovascular diseases, therapeutic approaches have been proposed. In particular, aerobic training has been shown to be a powerful tool against excessive ROS production. For example, patients with coronary artery disease submitted to aerobic training had lower expression of both AT_1 receptor and NADPH oxidase, resulting in decreased ROS production in the mammary arteries [111]. This effect can be attributed, at least in part, to the training-induced reduction in AT_1 receptor signaling pathway, since Ang II-induced contraction in these vessels was lower in trained individuals [111]. It was shown that old active (*versus* old inactive) men exhibited lower $p47^{phox}$ expression in endothelial cells, which was associated with smaller oxidative stress markers and a better flow-mediated vasodilatation in the brachial artery [175]. Young active men also showed lower levels of $gp91^{phox}$ in circulating endothelial progenitor cells after a single bout of aerobic exercise, suggesting that exercise can modulate the redox profile in young as well as old active men [176].

Aerobic training attenuated $gp91^{phox}$ expression and ROS production in the heart of the SHR [177]. It also prevented hypertension-induced increases in ACE and AT_1 receptor protein expression and up-regulated ACE2 and Mas receptor expression. These changes were associated with lower levels of plasma Ang II and reduced expression of $gp91^{phox}$ subunit, suggesting reduced NADPH oxidase activity and smaller oxidative stress [22]. Furthermore, training, by reducing plasma Ang II and AT_1 receptor expression in the kidney, decreased ROS levels and prevented deleterious changes in renal the structures of the young SHR [178].

It was also observed that exercise training prevented arterial baroreflex dysfunction in rats treated with central Ang II. In trained Ang II-infused rats, the levels of AT_1 receptor, $p47^{phox}$ and $gp91^{phox}$ were similar to untrained rats infused with vehicle, suggesting that trained-induced normalization of superoxide anion production could contribute to the beneficial effects observed [20]. In mice, Ang II infusion caused a significant reduction in exercise capacity simultaneously with increased NADPH oxidase activity and high superoxide anion production in the skeletal muscles [179] confirming the negative relationship between exercise capacity and Ang II-induced ROS production. The mechanisms underlying the effects of aerobic training on NADPH oxidase and Ang II cross talk are not completely understood. Future investigations are still necessary to clarify training-induced effects in different pathological conditions.

The Impact of Association Between RAS Inhibition and Exercise Training: When and How to Use?

Several randomized controlled trials and review studies have clearly demonstrated that ACE inhibitors and AT_1 receptor blockade provide significant improvement in morbidity and mortality in patients with heart disease and metabolic disorders [127, 180 - 185]. It is also known that physical training has beneficial effects in patients with these cardiometabolic alterations [186 - 188]. Although the practice of regular physical exercise is responsible for modulating the components of the RAS [19, 56, 189], decreasing the expression of AT1 receptors [111] and down-regulating ACE, Ang II and AT_2 receptor in Zucker rat strain [65], it remains unclear whether the therapeutic effects of the exercise training associated with RAS inhibition therapy is indeed effective.

In SHR it is believed that exercise-induced reduction in blood pressure may be mediated in part by improvement in central vasodilatory RAS components [9]. Regarding the process of muscle contraction associated with inhibition of brain RAS, in the central nervous system, different responses are observed depending on the area in which receptors are located. Patel *et al.* [190] observed that the inhibition of AT_1 receptors within the rostral ventrolateral medulla reduced glutamate and raised g-amino butyric acid (GABA) concentrations, attenuating the cardiovascular responses during static muscle contraction of the left triceps surae muscle in anesthetized Sprague-Dawley rats. However, the inhibition of AT_1 receptors within the caudal ventrolateral medulla increased glutamate and decreased GABA levels within the ventrolateral medulla [190]. Furthermore, the intracerebroventricular infusion of losartan may worse the thermoregulation and running performance in rats. In trained rats, the intracerebroventricular infusion of losartan increased the oxygen consumption and the metabolic cost and promoted a decrease in the mechanical efficiency and precipitation of fatigue in rats submitted to running exercise until fatigue when compared with control group [191].

In the peripheral system, captopril treatment (30mg/kg per day in drinking water) associated to the practice of aerobic voluntary exercise in old female SHR by free wheel running during 26 weeks increased the decorin expression (proteoglycan known to improve adverse remodelling by inhibiting TGF-β_1 (transforming growth factor beta 1)) and attenuated the training intensity-dependent expression of TGF-β_1, collagen III, showing that captopril attenuated the high intensity training-dependent effect on fibrotic markers. It is worth mentioning that these results were not accompanied by any significant differences in blood pressure, although heart rate significantly decreased in trained SHR treated compared to sedentary SHR treated. This study also showed that all rats treated with captopril survived during the trial period, compared to the others non treated groups in which were observed decompensated heart failure and sudden death. Thus, it was demonstrated that in the presence of effective inhibition of RAS in combination with voluntary aerobic, exercise significantly contributed to reverse cardiac remodeling and to heart health maintenance in SHR rats [72]. In OLETF rats (model of type 2 diabetes) the combination between temocapril (2 mg/kg per day) and exercise training by wheel running during 4 weeks significantly decreased more the fasting level of plasma glucose than either treatment alone [192]. Positive results were observed during RAS inhibition and exercise in another study using OLETF rats. The combination between losartan (1 mg/Kg per day, added to the diet) and exercise training by wheel running during 4 weeks significantly decreased systolic blood pressure and improved insulin resistance compared with losartan alone [193].

Despite the lack of data on the role of AT_1 blockade in normal myocardial, it is known that losartan (10 mg/Kg per day in drinking water) may prevent resistance training-induced hypertrophy in non-infarcted male Wistar rats [61]. In addition, in non-infarcted male Wistar rats, treadmill exercise training (5 days/week, 60min/day, for 6 weeks) plus losartan (10 mg/Kg per day, as drinking water) treatment decreased systolic pressure compared with losartan treatment alone, suggesting that exercise training may improve the systolic function in association with AT_1 receptor blockade [194].

In postmyocardial infarction rats, the practice of aerobic exercise alone has been shown to improve aerobic capacity and cardiac function and the same result was observed when physical training was associated with losartan treatment [195]. In postmyocardial infarction exercise training and losartan have been shown to attenuate ventricular remodelling compared to exercise training alone [196, 197]. However, despite the high-intensity exercise training (5 days/week for 8 weeks) alone and either losartan treatment (2 g/L *ad libitum* in drinking water) alone have been promoted improvement vasorelaxation and reversed endothelial dysfunction (in the abdominal aorta) in a model of experimentally-induced heart failure in female Sprague-Dawley rats, when losartan and exercise training were combined, no additional vasorelaxation occurred [198].

Considering experimental nephropathy, moderate treadmill exercise alone or in combination with exercise and losartan treatment (5 mg/Kg per day using osmotic minipump) for 12-weeks, improved the capillarization as well as the proportion of type I fibre in extensor digitorum longus muscle and also enhances renoprotective and peripheral effects in spontaneously type 2 diabetes mellitus rats with nephropathy. Thus, the combination of losartan and exercise may provide a new therapeutic approach to ideal renoprotection in diabetic nephropathy [199]. Moreover, both losartan (5 mg/ per day, i.p.) or enalapril (2 mg/kg per day, i.p.), associated with moderate treadmill exercise for 4-weeks, significantly and similarly decreased blood pressure and the index of glomerular sclerosis in a model of experimentally-induced renal failure in SHR rats compared with exercise alone [200]. However, in both studies, antihypertensive drugs plus exercise could only slightly decrease proteinuria, without difference between their respective groups [199, 200].

In some cases the inhibition of AT_1 receptors may be more efficient than ACE inhibitor treatment. Oliveira *et al.* [60] observed that losartan (20 mg/kg per day in drinking water) was more effective than enalapril (60 mg/kg per day in drinking water) to prevent the cardiac hypertrophy induced by low to moderate intensity swimming training in female normotensive Wistar rats. In another case the blockade the inhibition of AT_1 receptors may be more effective than the exercise. Liu *et al.* [201] showed that the blockade of AT_1 receptors enhanced baroreflex sensitivity in nontrained experimental chronic heart failure rabbits, but had not effect in the trained experimental chronic heart failure group [201].

In clinical trials, chronic blockade of the RAS has increased exercise capacity in patients with asymptomatic or symptomatic heart failure [202, 203]. In individuals with chronic heart failure, moderate physical training plus lisinopril (10 mg daily, for 12 weeks), achieved the most significant improvements in symptoms compared with with lisinopril treatment alone or training alone [186]. However, Di Marco *et al.* [204] have not seen difference in the ventilator response to exercise in chronic obstructive pulmonary disease patients during 4 weeks treatment with enalapril (10 mg daily).

With respect to AT_1 receptor blockade, in individuals with asymptomatic left ventricular dysfunction, it enhanced exercise tolerance and reduced the peak systolic blood pressure during treadmill exercise [202]. In patients with atherosclerosis or its risk factors, practice of arm exercise in the supine position before and after AT_1 receptor blockade with intracoronary losartan (5 mg) showed that exercise reduced coronary vascular resistance. However, before losartan, exercise could not alter mean epicardial coronary artery diameter, but after losartan there was significant epicardial coronary artery dilation with exercise, demonstrating that in patients with atherosclerosis or its risk factors the epicardial coronary vasomotion during exercise can be improved by acutely inhibiting AT_1 receptors [205]. Despite the antagonism of the AT_1 receptor may result in increased plasma renin activity and Ang II concentration [206], the combination of AT_1 receptor blockade (valsartan 320 mg daily) and the direct renin inhibitor (aliskiren 300 mg daily) triggered similar effects on lowering blood pressure at rest and during treadmill exercise in hypertensive patients with mild-to-moderate hypertension [207].

Despite no substantial differences were observed between losartan and captopril treatment on exercise capacity in elderly symptomatic patients with chronic heart failure [208], the valsartan proved to be more effective than enalapril in improving impaired left ventricular diastolic function of patients with mild or moderate essential hypertension (without left ventricular hypertrophy and normal systolic performance) in response to upright bicycle exercise testing [209]. The combination of both therapies may also be a successful alternative for patients with heart failure. Addition of AT_1 receptor blockade (losartan) to the ACE inhibitor treatment improved the peak exercise performance and functional capacity in patients with chronic heart failure [210]. Hamroff *et al.* [211] also showed that AT_1 receptor blockade to optimal ACE inhibition therapy improves peak exercise capacity and relieves symptoms in individuals with severe symptomatic congestive heart failure (still under treatment with optimal doses of ACE inhibitors, digoxin, and diuretics), demonstrating that addition of AT_1 receptor blockade to maximal ACE inhibition enhanced exercise capacity in patients with severe heart failure. The benefits of the combination of both drug therapies have also been observed by Avanza *et al.* [212] which demonstrated that blocking of the RAS activity by the use of losartan and enalapril is more efficient in the reduction of the left ventricular hypertrophy than physical exercise or the use of drugs which block sympathetic nervous system in normotensive individuals with blood pressure hyperactivity during the treadmill stress test [212].

With respect to the association between the RAS inhibition and other drug therapies for blood pressure control, the first alternative may be better to promote greater exercise capacity. ACE inhibition (ivabradine up to 7.5 mg twice a day) alone or in combination with beta-blocker (carvedilol/ivabradine up to 12.5/5 mg twice a day) is more effective than beta-blocker (carvedilol up to 25 mg twice a day) alone in improving exercise capacity and quality of life in heart failure patients during 6-min walking test distance [213].

Genetic Variations in The Renin-Angiotensin System and Response to Exercise

The ACE gene polymorphism is characterized by the presence (I, insertion) or absence (D, deletion) of a 288 pair-base *Alu* repeated sequence within intron 16. Based on this, 3 genotypes are expressed from ACE polymorphism: II, DD and I/D. Homozygous individuals for the ACE DD genotype are likely to increased plasmatic and tissue of ACE [214], and compared with the presence of ACE DD genotype, presence of ACE II or I/D genotype has been associated with a better physical capacity of endurance exercise [63]. In Caucasians, ACE I/D was associated with swimmer status, and the presence of allele D had more frequency in short-middle distance swimmers under both additive and I-allele dominant models. ACE I/D was also associated with swimmer status in East Asians. However, the presence of allele I was overrepresented in the Short distance swimmer group [130].

Regarding cardiac environment, D allele has been associated with increased cardiac muscle mass. In some pathological conditions, such as hypertension, it seems that the presence of ACE DD genotype promotes a hypertrophic phenotype. The involvement of ACE levels and smooth muscle cell proliferation and vasoconstriction prompt researchers to evaluate the association between ACE genotype and these pathological conditions. High level of ACE increases plasminogen activator inhibitor-1 that is a risk for developing coronary thrombosis. However, there is no consistent evidence regarding the association between ACE polymorphism and myocardial disease [215]. In addition, these individuals are more likely to develop diabetes, multivessel disease and unstable angina. It has also been showed that ACE I/D genotype is associated with coronary arterial disease [216].

Numerous studies have been demonstrated the influence of genetic variation of the ACE polymorphism on athletic performance [217, 218], for example, incidence of D allele in ACE DD or ACE I/D genotype has been associated with different profile of physical performance [power and sprint], as well as, pathological conditions (cardiac hypertrophy) associated to high response to cardiac overload, and increased production of Ang II, consequently, increases in vascular smooth muscle growth is evident [63, 214, 217, 219 - 222].

VO_{2max} is the gold standard to measure cardiovascular capacity and skeletal muscle efficiency regarding to endurance exercise training. Since, ACE genotypes are related to different response to exercise and cardiac adaptation, the relationship between VO_{2max} and ACE polymorphism could be possible. However, several studies have shown that there is no association between different levels of VO_{2max} and ACE polymorphism, at least when no disease condition is implied.

However, the studies used a small number of participants and no longer period of exercise was applied. In COPD, was found different levels of VO_{2max} and ACE II and DD genotype [223, 224].

ACE genotype is also related to skeletal muscle adaptation to exercise training and atrophy process. Although the presence of local RAS into skeletal muscle is controversial and clearly needs further investigations, several studies have been implicated the important role of ACE polymorphism in skeletal muscle growth and the particular response to exercise training [225]. As previously described ACE D allele is related to strength and power, and in fact, individuals who have more incidence of ACE I allele is more adapted to learning exercise movement when performing resistance exercise training.

Although the association among genetic variation of ACE I/D and physical performance has been described by several studies, some outcomes are controversial, and it is possible that some or all of the associations reported between physical performance and the ACE gene polymorphism could be due to linkage disequilibrium with other gene or genes in close proximity to the ACE locus and not to the ACE gene *per se*.

CONCLUSION

Experimental and clinical studies show that exercise training is efficient to block RAS overactivity, thus preventing and/or reversing cardiac dysfunction and deleterious remodeling of the heart in pathological conditions such as hypertension, myocardial infarction, heart failure and obesity. Indeed, studies show that the association between RAS inhibition and exercise training can bring major benefits to individuals with heart disease especially those with mild, moderate or severe heart failure and also cardiometabolic alterations, acting synergically as a successful combination to the recovery and maintenance of health of these patients.

CONFLICT OF INTEREST

The authors confirm that they have no conflict of interest to declare for this publication.

ACKNOWLEDGEMENTS

The authors thank FAPESP, CNPq, CAPES for research grants.

REFERENCES

[1] Organization WH. A global brief on Hypertension: Silent killer, global public health crisis. Switzerland: World Health Organization 2013.

[2] Bickerton RB. Evidence for a central mechanism of angiotensin induced hypertension. Proc Soc Exp Biol Med 1961; (106): 834-7. [http://dx.doi.org/10.3181/00379727-106-26492]

[3] Ferrario CM, Gildenberg PL, McCubbin JW. Cardiovascular effects of angiotensin mediated by the central nervous system. Circ Res 1972; 30(3): 257-62. [http://dx.doi.org/10.1161/01.RES.30.3.257] [PMID: 4334162]

[4] Reid IA. Is there a brain renin-angiotensin system? Circ Res 1977; 41(2): 147-53. [http://dx.doi.org/10.1161/01.RES.41.2.147] [PMID: 194727]

[5] Ganten D, Minnich JL, Granger P, *et al.* Angiotensin-forming enzyme in brain tissue. Science 1971; 173(3991): 64-5. [http://dx.doi.org/10.1126/science.173.3991.64] [PMID: 4325865]

[6] Ganten D, Speck G. The brain renin-angiotensin system: a model for the synthesis of peptides in the brain. Biochem Pharmacol 1978; 27(20): 2379-89. [http://dx.doi.org/10.1016/0006-2952(78)90348-9] [PMID: 365183]

[7] Paul M, Poyan Mehr A, Kreutz R. Physiology of local renin-angiotensin systems. Physiol Rev 2006; 86(3): 747-803. [http://dx.doi.org/10.1152/physrev.00036.2005] [PMID: 16816138]

[8] Danser AH. Local renin-angiotensin systems: the unanswered questions. Int J Biochem Cell Biol 2003; 35(6): 759-68. [http://dx.doi.org/10.1016/S1357-2725(02)00178-4] [PMID: 12676161]

[9] Nguyen G, Burcklé CA, Sraer JD. Renin/prorenin-receptor biochemistry and functional significance. Curr Hypertens Rep 2004; 6(2): 129-32. [http://dx.doi.org/10.1007/s11906-004-0088-3] [PMID: 15010017]

[10] Xu P, Sriramula S, Lazartigues E. ACE2/ANG-(1-7)/Mas pathway in the brain: the axis of good. Am J Physiol Regul Integr Comp Physiol 2011; 300(4): R804-17. [http://dx.doi.org/10.1152/ajpregu.00222.2010] [PMID: 21178125]

[11] McKinley MJ, Albiston AL, Allen AM, *et al.* The brain renin-angiotensin system: location and physiological roles. Int J Biochem Cell Biol 2003; 35(6): 901-18. [http://dx.doi.org/10.1016/S1357-2725(02)00306-0] [PMID: 12676175]

[12] Bunnemann B, Fuxe K, Ganten D. The brain renin-angiotensin system: localization and general significance. J Cardiovasc Pharmacol 1992; 19 (Suppl. 6): S51-62. [http://dx.doi.org/10.1097/00005344-199219006-00010] [PMID: 1382166]

[13] Santos RA, Campagnole-Santos MJ, Andrade SP. Angiotensin-(1-7): an update. Regul Pept 2000; 91(1-3): 45-62.
[http://dx.doi.org/10.1016/S0167-0115(00)00138-5] [PMID: 10967201]

[14] Lenkei Z, Palkovits M, Corvol P, Llorens-Cortes C. Distribution of angiotensin type-1 receptor messenger RNA expression in the adult rat brain. Neuroscience 1998; 82(3): 827-41.
[http://dx.doi.org/10.1016/S0306-4522(97)00328-X] [PMID: 9483539]

[15] Santos RA, Simoes e Silva AC, Maric C, *et al.* Angiotensin-(1-7) is an endogenous ligand for the G protein-coupled receptor Mas. Proc Natl Acad Sci USA 2003; 100(14): 8258-63.
[http://dx.doi.org/10.1073/pnas.1432869100] [PMID: 12829792]

[16] Bader M. Tissue renin-angiotensin-aldosterone systems: Targets for pharmacological therapy. Annu Rev Pharmacol Toxicol 2010; 50: 439-65.
[http://dx.doi.org/10.1146/annurev.pharmtox.010909.105610] [PMID: 20055710]

[17] Ferrario CM. ACE2: more of Ang-(1-7) or less Ang II? Curr Opin Nephrol Hypertens 2011; 20(1): 1-6.
[http://dx.doi.org/10.1097/MNH.0b013e3283406f57] [PMID: 21045683]

[18] Saavedra JM. Angiotensin II AT(1) receptor blockers as treatments for inflammatory brain disorders. Clin Sci 2012; 123(10): 567-90.
[http://dx.doi.org/10.1042/CS20120078] [PMID: 22827472]

[19] Felix JV, Michelini LC. Training-induced pressure fall in spontaneously hypertensive rats is associated with reduced angiotensinogen mRNA expression within the nucleus tractus solitarii. Hypertension 2007; 50(4): 780-5.
[http://dx.doi.org/10.1161/HYPERTENSIONAHA.107.094474] [PMID: 17646572]

[20] Pan YX, Gao L, Wang WZ, *et al.* Exercise training prevents arterial baroreflex dysfunction in rats treated with central angiotensin II. Hypertension 2007; 49(3): 519-27.
[http://dx.doi.org/10.1161/01.HYP.0000256955.74461.93] [PMID: 17224469]

[21] Sangaleti CT, Crescenzi A, Michelini LC. Endogenous angiotensin and pressure modulate brain angiotensinogen and AT1A mRNA expression. Hypertension 2004; 43(2): 317-23.
[http://dx.doi.org/10.1161/01.HYP.0000112030.79692.21] [PMID: 14732738]

[22] Agarwal D, Welsch MA, Keller JN, Francis J. Chronic exercise modulates RAS components and improves balance between pro- and anti-inflammatory cytokines in the brain of SHR. Basic Res Cardiol 2011; 106(6): 1069-85.
[http://dx.doi.org/10.1007/s00395-011-0231-7] [PMID: 22124756]

[23] Kishi T, Hirooka Y, Katsuki M, *et al.* Exercise training causes sympathoinhibition through antioxidant effect in the rostral ventrolateral medulla of hypertensive rats. Clin Exp Hypertens 2012; 34(4): 278-83.
[http://dx.doi.org/10.3109/10641963.2012.681084] [PMID: 22578069]

[24] Mousa TM, Liu D, Cornish KG, Zucker IH. Exercise training enhances baroreflex sensitivity by an angiotensin II-dependent mechanism in chronic heart failure. J Appl Physiol 2008; 104(3): 616-24.

[25] Zucker IH, Schultz HD, Patel KP, Wang W, Gao L. Regulation of central angiotensin type 1 receptors and sympathetic outflow in heart failure. Am J Physiol Heart Circ Physiol 2009; 297(5): H1557-66.

[http://dx.doi.org/10.1152/ajpheart.00073.2009] [PMID: 19717736]

[26] Kleiber AC, Zheng H, Sharma NM, Patel KP. Chronic AT1 receptor blockade normalizes NMDA-mediated changes in renal sympathetic nerve activity and NR1 expression within the PVN in rats with heart failure. Am J Physiol Heart Circ Physiol 2010; 298(5): H1546-55. [http://dx.doi.org/10.1152/ajpheart.01006.2009] [PMID: 20173042]

[27] Zheng H, Sharma NM, Liu X, Patel KP. Exercise training normalizes enhanced sympathetic activation from the paraventricular nucleus in chronic heart failure: role of angiotensin II. Am J Physiol Regul Integr Comp Physiol 2012; 303(4): R387-94. [http://dx.doi.org/10.1152/ajpregu.00046.2012] [PMID: 22718804]

[28] Kar S, Gao L, Zucker IH. Exercise training normalizes ACE and ACE2 in the brain of rabbits with pacing-induced heart failure. J Appl Physiol 2010; 108(4): 923-32.

[29] Campbell DJ, Habener JF. Angiotensinogen gene is expressed and differentially regulated in multiple tissues of the rat. J Clin Invest 1986; 78(1): 31-9. [http://dx.doi.org/10.1172/JCI112566] [PMID: 3013940]

[30] Paul M, Wagner D, Metzger R, *et al.* Quantification of renin mRNA in various mouse tissues by a novel solution hybridization assay. J Hypertens 1988; 6(3): 247-52. [http://dx.doi.org/10.1097/00004872-198803000-00010] [PMID: 3283228]

[31] Paul M, Wagner J, Dzau VJ. Gene expression of the renin-angiotensin system in human tissues. Quantitative analysis by the polymerase chain reaction. J Clin Invest 1993; 91(5): 2058-64. [http://dx.doi.org/10.1172/JCI116428] [PMID: 8387539]

[32] Peters J, Farrenkopf R, Clausmeyer S, *et al.* Functional significance of prorenin internalization in the rat heart. Circ Res 2002; 90(10): 1135-41. [http://dx.doi.org/10.1161/01.RES.0000019242.51541.99] [PMID: 12039805]

[33] Crackower MA, Sarao R, Oudit GY, *et al.* Angiotensin-converting enzyme 2 is an essential regulator of heart function. Nature 2002; 417(6891): 822-8. [http://dx.doi.org/10.1038/nature00786] [PMID: 12075344]

[34] Burrell LM, Risvanis J, Kubota E, *et al.* Myocardial infarction increases ACE2 expression in rat and humans. Eur Heart J 2005; 26(4): 369-75. [http://dx.doi.org/10.1093/eurheartj/ehi114] [PMID: 15671045]

[35] Urata H, Nishimura H, Ganten D. Chymase-dependent angiotensin II forming systems in humans. Am J Hypertens 1996; 9(3): 277-84. [http://dx.doi.org/10.1016/0895-7061(95)00349-5] [PMID: 8695029]

[36] Dzau VJ. Implications of local angiotensin production in cardiovascular physiology and pharmacology. Am J Cardiol 1987; 59(2): 59A-65A. [http://dx.doi.org/10.1016/0002-9149(87)90178-0] [PMID: 3028117]

[37] Lindpaintner K, Jin M, Wilhelm MJ, *et al.* Intracardiac generation of angiotensin and its physiologic role. Circulation 1988; 77(6 Pt 2): I18-23. [PMID: 3286043]

[38] Santos RA, Castro CH, Gava E, *et al.* Impairment of *in vitro* and *in vivo* heart function in angiotensin-(1-7) receptor MAS knockout mice. Hypertension 2006; 47(5): 996-1002.

[http://dx.doi.org/10.1161/01.HYP.0000215289.51180.5c] [PMID: 16567589]

[39] Yamamoto K, Ohishi M, Katsuya T, *et al.* Deletion of angiotensin-converting enzyme 2 accelerates pressure overload-induced cardiac dysfunction by increasing local angiotensin II. Hypertension 2006; 47(4): 718-26.
[http://dx.doi.org/10.1161/01.HYP.0000205833.89478.5b] [PMID: 16505206]

[40] Iwai M, Horiuchi M. Devil and angel in the renin angiotensin system: ACE angiotensin II AT1 receptor axis *vs.* ACE2 angiotensin-(1 7) Mas receptor axis. Hypertension Research 2009; 32(7): 533-6.

[41] Schunkert H, Jackson B, Tang SS, *et al.* Distribution and functional significance of cardiac angiotensin converting enzyme in hypertrophied rat hearts. Circulation 1993; 87(4): 1328-39.
[http://dx.doi.org/10.1161/01.CIR.87.4.1328] [PMID: 8384939]

[42] Pinto YM, Buikema H, van Gilst WH, *et al.* Cardiovascular end-organ damage in Ren-2 transgenic rats compared to spontaneously hypertensive rats. J Mol Med 1997; 75(5): 371-7.
[http://dx.doi.org/10.1007/s001090050123] [PMID: 9181479]

[43] Tian XL, Pinto YM, Costerousse O, *et al.* Overexpression of angiotensin converting enzyme-1 augments cardiac hypertrophy in transgenic rats. Hum Mol Genet 2004; 13(14): 1441-50.
[http://dx.doi.org/10.1093/hmg/ddh147] [PMID: 15128700]

[44] Hoffmann S. Cardiac-specific overexpression of angiotensin II type 1 receptor in transgenic rats. Methods Mol Med 2005; 112: 389-403.
[PMID: 16010032]

[45] Hoffmann S, Krause T, van Geel PP, *et al.* Overexpression of the human angiotensin II type 1 receptor in the rat heart augments load induced cardiac hypertrophy. J Mol Med 2001; 79(10): 601-8.
[http://dx.doi.org/10.1007/s001090100246] [PMID: 11692158]

[46] Müller DN, Fischli W, Clozel JP, *et al.* Local angiotensin II generation in the rat heart: role of renin uptake. Circ Res 1998; 82(1): 13-20.
[http://dx.doi.org/10.1161/01.RES.82.1.13] [PMID: 9440700]

[47] McCollum LT, Gallagher PE, Ann Tallant E. Angiotensin-(1-7) attenuates angiotensin II-induced cardiac remodeling associated with upregulation of dual-specificity phosphatase 1. Am J Physiol Heart Circ Physiol 2012; 302(3): H801-10.
[http://dx.doi.org/10.1152/ajpheart.00908.2011] [PMID: 22140049]

[48] Zhong J, Basu R, Guo D, Chow FL, Byrns S, Schuster M, *et al.* Angiotensin-converting enzyme 2 suppresses pathological hypertrophy, myocardial fibrosis, and cardiac dysfunction. Circulation 2010; 122(7): 717-28.
[http://dx.doi.org/10.1161/CIRCULATIONAHA.110.955369]

[49] Patel VB, Bodiga S, Fan D, *et al.* Cardioprotective effects mediated by angiotensin II type 1 receptor blockade and enhancing angiotensin 1-7 in experimental heart failure in angiotensin-converting enzyme 2-null mice. Hypertension 2012; 59(6): 1195-203.
[http://dx.doi.org/10.1161/HYPERTENSIONAHA.112.191650] [PMID: 22508831]

[50] Navar LG, Inscho EW, Majid SA, Imig JD, Harrison-Bernard LM, Mitchell KD. Paracrine regulation of the renal microcirculation. Physiol Rev 1996; 76(2): 425-536.

[PMID: 8618962]

[51] Ludwig M, Steinhoff G, Li J. The regenerative potential of angiotensin AT2 receptor in cardiac repair. Can J Physiol Pharmacol 2012; 90(3): 287-93.
[http://dx.doi.org/10.1139/y11-108] [PMID: 22364522]

[52] Yusuf S, Sleight P, Pogue J, Bosch J, Davies R, Dagenais G. Effects of an angiotensin-convertin--enzyme inhibitor, ramipril, on cardiovascular events in high-risk patients. N Engl J Med 2000; 342(3): 145-53.
[http://dx.doi.org/10.1056/NEJM200001203420301] [PMID: 10639539]

[53] Dahlöf B, Devereux RB, Kjeldsen SE, *et al.* Cardiovascular morbidity and mortality in the Losartan Intervention For Endpoint reduction in hypertension study (LIFE): a randomised trial against atenolol. Lancet 2002; 359(9311): 995-1003.
[http://dx.doi.org/10.1016/S0140-6736(02)08089-3] [PMID: 11937178]

[54] Chobanian AV, Bakris GL, Black HR, *et al.* The Seventh Report of the Joint National Committee on Prevention, Detection, Evaluation, and Treatment of High Blood Pressure: the JNC 7 report. JAMA 2003; 289(19): 2560-72.
[http://dx.doi.org/10.1001/jama.289.19.2560] [PMID: 12748199]

[55] Pescatello LS, Franklin BA, Fagard R, Farquhar WB, Kelley GA, Ray CA. American College of Sports Medicine position stand. Exercise and hypertension. Med Sci Sports Exerc 2004; 36(3): 533-53.
[http://dx.doi.org/10.1249/01.MSS.0000115224.88514.3A] [PMID: 15076798]

[56] Filho AG, Ferreira AJ, Santos SH, *et al.* Selective increase of angiotensin(1-7) and its receptor in hearts of spontaneously hypertensive rats subjected to physical training. Exp Physiol 2008; 93(5): 589-98.
[PMID: 18448664]

[57] Longhurst JC, Kelly AR, Gonyea WJ, Mitchell JH. Echocardiographic left ventricular masses in distance runners and weight lifters. J Appl Physiol 1980; 48(1): 154-62.
[PMID: 7353968]

[58] American College of Sports Medicine position stand. Progression models in resistance training for healthy adults. Med Sci Sports Exerc 2009; 41(3): 687-708.
[http://dx.doi.org/10.1249/MSS.0b013e3181915670] [PMID: 19204579]

[59] Grossman W, Jones D, McLaurin LP. Wall stress and patterns of hypertrophy in the human left ventricle. J Clin Invest 1975; 56(1): 56-64.
[http://dx.doi.org/10.1172/JCI108079] [PMID: 124746]

[60] Oliveira EM, Sasaki MS, Cerêncio M, Baraúna VG, Krieger JE. Local renin-angiotensin system regulates left ventricular hypertrophy induced by swimming training independent of circulating renin: a pharmacological study. J Renin Angiotensin Aldosterone Syst 2009; 10(1): 15-23.
[http://dx.doi.org/10.1177/1470320309102304] [PMID: 19286754]

[61] Barauna VG, Magalhaes FC, Krieger JE, Oliveira EM. AT1 receptor participates in the cardiac hypertrophy induced by resistance training in rats. Am J Physiol Regul Integr Comp Physiol 2008; 295(2): R381-7.
[http://dx.doi.org/10.1152/ajpregu.00933.2007] [PMID: 18495827]

[62] Yasuda N, Miura S, Akazawa H, *et al.* Conformational switch of angiotensin II type 1 receptor underlying mechanical stress-induced activation. EMBO Rep 2008; 9(2): 179-86. [http://dx.doi.org/10.1038/sj.embor.7401157] [PMID: 18202720]

[63] Montgomery HE, Marshall R, Hemingway H, *et al.* Human gene for physical performance. Nature 1998; 393(6682): 221-2. [http://dx.doi.org/10.1038/30374] [PMID: 9607758]

[64] Myerson SG, Montgomery HE, Whittingham M, *et al.* Left ventricular hypertrophy with exercise and ACE gene insertion/deletion polymorphism: a randomized controlled trial with losartan. Circulation 2001; 103(2): 226-30. [http://dx.doi.org/10.1161/01.CIR.103.2.226] [PMID: 11208681]

[65] Barretti DL, Magalhães FdeC, Fernandes T, *et al.* Effects of aerobic exercise training on cardiac renin-angiotensin system in an obese Zucker rat strain. PLoS One 2012; 7(10): e46114. [http://dx.doi.org/10.1371/journal.pone.0046114] [PMID: 23077501]

[66] Wienbergen H, Hambrecht R. [Physical exercise training for cardiovascular diseases]. Herz 2012; 37(5): 486-92. [Physical exercise training for cardiovascular diseases]. [http://dx.doi.org/10.1007/s00059-012-3624-y] [PMID: 22760599]

[67] Georgiopoulou VV, Kalogeropoulos AP, Butler J. Heart failure in hypertension: prevention and treatment. Drugs 2012; 72(10): 1373-98. [http://dx.doi.org/10.2165/11631100-000000000-00000] [PMID: 22747449]

[68] Braith RW, Welsch MA, Feigenbaum MS, Kluess HA, Pepine CJ. Neuroendocrine activation in heart failure is modified by endurance exercise training. J Am Coll Cardiol 1999; 34(4): 1170-5. [http://dx.doi.org/10.1016/S0735-1097(99)00339-3] [PMID: 10520808]

[69] Pereira MG, Ferreira JC, Bueno CR Jr, *et al.* Exercise training reduces cardiac angiotensin II levels and prevents cardiac dysfunction in a genetic model of sympathetic hyperactivity-induced heart failure in mice. Eur J Appl Physiol 2009; 105(6): 843-50. [http://dx.doi.org/10.1007/s00421-008-0967-4] [PMID: 19125280]

[70] Wan W, Powers AS, Li J, Ji L, Erikson JM, Zhang JQ. Effect of post-myocardial infarction exercise training on the renin-angiotensin-aldosterone system and cardiac function. Am J Med Sci 2007; 334(4): 265-73. [http://dx.doi.org/10.1097/MAJ.0b013e318068b5ed] [PMID: 18030183]

[71] Huang TH, He L, Qin Q, *et al.* Salacia oblonga root decreases cardiac hypertrophy in Zucker diabetic fatty rats: inhibition of cardiac expression of angiotensin II type 1 receptor. Diabetes Obes Metab 2008; 10(7): 574-85. [http://dx.doi.org/10.1111/j.1463-1326.2007.00750.x] [PMID: 17645561]

[72] da Costa Rebelo RM, Schreckenberg R, Schlüter KD. Adverse cardiac remodelling in spontaneously hypertensive rats: acceleration by high aerobic exercise intensity. J Physiol 2012; 590(21): 5389-400. [http://dx.doi.org/10.1113/jphysiol.2012.241141] [PMID: 22930266]

[73] Rossoni LV, Oliveira RA, Caffaro RR, *et al.* Cardiac benefits of exercise training in aging spontaneously hypertensive rats. J Hypertens 2011; 29(12): 2349-58. [http://dx.doi.org/10.1097/HJH.0b013e32834d2532] [PMID: 22045123]

[74] Ceroni A, Chaar LJ, Bombein RL, Michelini LC. Chronic absence of baroreceptor inputs prevents training-induced cardiovascular adjustments in normotensive and spontaneously hypertensive rats. Exp Physiol 2009; 94(6): 630-40.
[http://dx.doi.org/10.1113/expphysiol.2008.046128] [PMID: 19251981]

[75] Nguyen Dinh Cat A, Touyz RM. A new look at the renin-angiotensin system--focusing on the vascular system. Peptides 2011; 32(10): 2141-50.
[http://dx.doi.org/10.1016/j.peptides.2011.09.010] [PMID: 21945916]

[76] Ohkubo H, Nakayama K, Tanaka T, Nakanishi S. Tissue distribution of rat angiotensinogen mRNA and structural analysis of its heterogeneity. J Biol Chem 1986; 261(1): 319-23.
[PMID: 3753601]

[77] Cassis LA, Lynch KR, Peach MJ. Localization of angiotensinogen messenger RNA in rat aorta. Circ Res 1988; 62(6): 1259-62.
[http://dx.doi.org/10.1161/01.RES.62.6.1259] [PMID: 3383369]

[78] Müller DN, Hilgers KF, Bohlender J, *et al.* Effects of human renin in the vasculature of rats transgenic for human angiotensinogen. Hypertension 1995; 26(2): 272-8.
[http://dx.doi.org/10.1161/01.HYP.26.2.272] [PMID: 7635534]

[79] Samani NJ, Morgan K, Brammar WJ, Swales JD. Detection of renin messenger RNA in rat tissues: increased sensitivity using an RNAse protection technique. J of Hypertension 1987; 5(2): S19-21.
[http://dx.doi.org/10.1097/00004872-198707002-00005]

[80] Neubauer B, Machura K, Schnermann J, Wagner C. Renin expression in large renal vessels during fetal development depends on functional beta1/beta2-adrenergic receptors. Am J Physiol Renal Physiol 2011; 301(1): F71-7.
[http://dx.doi.org/10.1152/ajprenal.00443.2010] [PMID: 21389089]

[81] Fernandez-Alfonso MS, Martorana PA, Licka I, *et al.* Early induction of angiotensin I-converting enzyme in rat carotid artery after balloon injury. Hypertension 1997; 30(2 Pt 1): 272-7.
[http://dx.doi.org/10.1161/01.HYP.30.2.272] [PMID: 9260992]

[82] Falkenhahn M, Franke F, Bohle RM, *et al.* Cellular distribution of angiotensin-converting enzyme after myocardial infarction. Hypertension 1995; 25(2): 219-26.
[http://dx.doi.org/10.1161/01.HYP.25.2.219] [PMID: 7531176]

[83] Zhuo J, Moeller I, Jenkins T, *et al.* Mapping tissue angiotensin-converting enzyme and angiotensin AT1, AT2 and AT4 receptors. J Hypertens 1998; 16(12 Pt 2): 2027-37.
[http://dx.doi.org/10.1097/00004872-199816121-00026] [PMID: 9886893]

[84] Metzger R, Franke FE, Bohle RM, Alhenc-Gelas F, Danilov SM. Heterogeneous distribution of angiotensin I-converting enzyme (CD143) in the human and rat vascular systems: vessel, organ and species specificity. Microvasc Res 2011; 81(2): 206-15.
[http://dx.doi.org/10.1016/j.mvr.2010.12.003] [PMID: 21167844]

[85] Hamming I, Timens W, Bulthuis ML, Lely AT, Navis G, van Goor H. Tissue distribution of ACE2 protein, the functional receptor for SARS coronavirus. A first step in understanding SARS pathogenesis. J Pathol 2004; 203(2): 631-7.
[http://dx.doi.org/10.1002/path.1570] [PMID: 15141377]

[86] Mehta PK, Griendling KK. Angiotensin II cell signaling: physiological and pathological effects in the cardiovascular system. Am J Physiol Cell Physiol 2007; 292(1): C82-97. [http://dx.doi.org/10.1152/ajpcell.00287.2006] [PMID: 16870827]

[87] Allen AM, Zhuo J, Mendelsohn FA. Localization and function of angiotensin AT1 receptors. Am J Hypertens 2000; 13(1 Pt 2): 31S-8S. [http://dx.doi.org/10.1016/S0895-7061(99)00249-6] [PMID: 10678286]

[88] Cai H, Griendling KK, Harrison DG. The vascular NAD(P)H oxidases as therapeutic targets in cardiovascular diseases. Trends Pharmacol Sci 2003; 24(9): 471-8. [http://dx.doi.org/10.1016/S0165-6147(03)00233-5] [PMID: 12967772]

[89] Schulman IH, Zhou MS, Raij L. Nitric oxide, angiotensin II, and reactive oxygen species in hypertension and atherogenesis. Curr Hypertens Rep 2005; 7(1): 61-7. [http://dx.doi.org/10.1007/s11906-005-0056-6] [PMID: 15683588]

[90] Yayama K, Okamoto H. Angiotensin II-induced vasodilation *via* type 2 receptor: role of bradykinin and nitric oxide. Int Immunopharmacol 2008; 8(2): 312-8. [http://dx.doi.org/10.1016/j.intimp.2007.06.012] [PMID: 18182246]

[91] Sampaio WO, Souza dos Santos RA, Faria-Silva R, da Mata Machado LT, Schiffrin EL, Touyz RM. Angiotensin-(1-7) through receptor Mas mediates endothelial nitric oxide synthase activation *via* Akt-dependent pathways. Hypertension 2007; 49(1): 185-92. [http://dx.doi.org/10.1161/01.HYP.0000251865.35728.2f] [PMID: 17116756]

[92] Sampaio WO, Henrique de Castro C, Santos RA, Schiffrin EL, Touyz RM. Angiotensin-(1-7) counter regulates angiotensin II signaling in human endothelial cells. Hypertension 2007; 50(6): 1093- 8. [http://dx.doi.org/10.1161/HYPERTENSIONAHA.106.084848] [PMID: 17984366]

[93] Gibbons GH, Dzau VJ. The emerging concept of vascular remodeling. N Engl J Med 1994; 330(20): 1431-8. [http://dx.doi.org/10.1056/NEJM199405193302008] [PMID: 8159199]

[94] Mulvany MJ. Small artery remodeling and significance in the development of hypertension. j of Physiology 2002; 17(3): 105-9.

[95] Okamura T, Miyazaki M, Inagami T, Toda N. Vascular renin-angiotensin system in two-kidney, one clip hypertensive rats. Hypertension 1986; 8(7): 560-5. [http://dx.doi.org/10.1161/01.HYP.8.7.560] [PMID: 3013774]

[96] Lazartigues E, Feng Y, Lavoie JL. The two fACEs of the tissue renin-angiotensin systems: implication in cardiovascular diseases. Curr Pharm Des 2007; 13(12): 1231-45. [http://dx.doi.org/10.2174/138161207780618911] [PMID: 17504232]

[97] Tsutsumi Y, Matsubara H, Masaki H, *et al.* Angiotensin II type 2 receptor overexpression activates the vascular kinin system and causes vasodilation. J Clin Invest 1999; 104(7): 925-35. [http://dx.doi.org/10.1172/JCI7886] [PMID: 10510333]

[98] Amaral SL, Zorn TM, Michelini LC. Exercise training normalizes wall-to-lumen ratio of the gracilis muscle arterioles and reduces pressure in spontaneously hypertensive rats. J Hypertens 2000; 18(11): 1563-72.

[http://dx.doi.org/10.1097/00004872-200018110-00006] [PMID: 11081768]

[99] Melo RM, Martinho E Jr, Michelini LC. Training-induced, pressure-lowering effect in SHR: wide effects on circulatory profile of exercised and non exercised muscles. Hypertension 2003; 42(4): 851-7. [http://dx.doi.org/10.1161/01.HYP.0000086201.27420.33] [PMID: 12913057]

[100] Coimbra R, Sanchez LS, Potenza JM, Rossoni LV, Amaral SL, Michelini LC. Is gender crucial for cardiovascular adjustments induced by exercise training in female spontaneously hypertensive rats? Hypertension 2008; 52(3): 514-21. [http://dx.doi.org/10.1161/HYPERTENSIONAHA.108.114744] [PMID: 18695147]

[101] Schiffrin EL. Remodeling of resistance arteries in essential hypertension and effects of antihypertensive treatment. Am J Hypertens 2004; 17(12 Pt 1): 1192-200. [http://dx.doi.org/10.1016/j.amjhyper.2004.05.023] [PMID: 15607629]

[102] Agabiti-Rosei E, Heagerty AM, Rizzoni D. Effects of antihypertensive treatment on small artery remodelling. J Hypertens 2009; 27(6): 1107-14. [http://dx.doi.org/10.1097/HJH.0b013e328329272e] [PMID: 19293726]

[103] Santos CM, Pontieri V, Leomil Neto M, Michelini LC. Losartan improves baroreflex control of heart rate of coarcted hypertensive rats. Am J Physiol 1995; 269(3 Pt 2): H812-8. [PMID: 7573522]

[104] Bezerra SM, dos Santos CM, Moreira ED, Krieger EM, Michelini LC. Chronic AT(1) receptor blockade alters autonomic balance and sympathetic responses in hypertension. Hypertension 2001; 38(3 Pt 2): 569-75. [http://dx.doi.org/10.1161/hy09t1.095393] [PMID: 11566933]

[105] Azevedo LF, Brum PC, Mattos KC, Junqueira CM, Rondon MU, Barretto AC, *et al.* Effects of losartan combined with exercise training in spontaneously hypertensive rats. Brazilian journal of medical and biological research 2003; 36(11): 1595-603. [http://dx.doi.org/10.1590/S0100-879X2003001100018]

[106] Tinken TM, Thijssen DH, Hopkins N, *et al.* Impact of shear rate modulation on vascular function in humans. Hypertension 2009; 54(2): 278-85. [http://dx.doi.org/10.1161/HYPERTENSIONAHA.109.134361] [PMID: 19546374]

[107] Laughlin MH, Pollock JS, Amann JF, Hollis ML, Woodman CR, Price EM. Training induces nonuniform increases in eNOS content along the coronary arterial tree. J Appl Physiol 2001; 90(2): 501-10.

[108] Silva J. Efeitos sequenciais do treinamento aerobio sobre o conteudo de Ang I, Ang II e Ang (1-7) em diferentes segmentos arteriais de WKY e SHR. 2011.

[109] Feterik K, Smith L, Katusic ZS. Angiotensin-(1-7) causes endothelium-dependent relaxation in canine middle cerebral artery. Brain Res 2000; 873(1): 75-82. [http://dx.doi.org/10.1016/S0006-8993(00)02482-3] [PMID: 10915812]

[110] Ren Y, Garvin J, Carretero OA. Mechanism involved in bradykinin-induced efferent arteriole dilation. Kidney Int 2002; 62(2): 544-9. [http://dx.doi.org/10.1046/j.1523-1755.2002.00482.x] [PMID: 12110016]

[111] Adams V, Linke A, Kränkel N, *et al.* Impact of regular physical activity on the NAD(P)H oxidase and

angiotensin receptor system in patients with coronary artery disease. Circulation 2005; 111(5): 555-62. [http://dx.doi.org/10.1161/01.CIR.0000154560.88933.7E] [PMID: 15699275]

[112] Silva Jr SD, Zampieri TT, Ruggeri A, *et al.* Down regulation of the vascular renin-angiotensin system by aerobic training – Focus on the balance between vasoconstrictor and vasodilator axes. Circ J 2015; 79: 1372-80.
[http://dx.doi.org/10.1253/circj.CJ-14-1179] [PMID: 25808225]

[113] Muñoz MC, Giani JF, Dominici FP. Angiotensin-(1-7) stimulates the phosphorylation of Akt in rat extracardiac tissues *in vivo via* receptor Mas. Regul Pept 2010; 161(1-3): 1-7.
[http://dx.doi.org/10.1016/j.regpep.2010.02.001] [PMID: 20188769]

[114] Kalupahana NS, Moustaid-Moussa N. The adipose tissue renin-angiotensin system and metabolic disorders: a review of molecular mechanisms. Crit Rev Biochem Mol Biol 2012; 47(4): 379-90.
[http://dx.doi.org/10.3109/10409238.2012.694843] [PMID: 22720713]

[115] Giacchetti G, Faloia E, Mariniello B, *et al.* Overexpression of the renin-angiotensin system in human visceral adipose tissue in normal and overweight subjects. Am J Hypertens 2002; 15(5): 381-8.
[http://dx.doi.org/10.1016/S0895-7061(02)02257-4] [PMID: 12022238]

[116] Frederich RC Jr, Kahn BB, Peach MJ, Flier JS. Tissue-specific nutritional regulation of angiotensinogen in adipose tissue. Hypertension 1992; 19(4): 339-44.
[http://dx.doi.org/10.1161/01.HYP.19.4.339] [PMID: 1555865]

[117] Rahmouni K, Correia ML, Haynes WG, Mark AL. Obesity-associated hypertension: new insights into mechanisms. Hypertension 2005; 45(1): 9-14.
[http://dx.doi.org/10.1161/01.HYP.0000151325.83008.b4] [PMID: 15583075]

[118] Engeli S, Böhnke J, Gorzelniak K, *et al.* Weight loss and the renin-angiotensin-aldosterone system. Hypertension 2005; 45(3): 356-62.
[http://dx.doi.org/10.1161/01.HYP.0000154361.47683.d3] [PMID: 15630041]

[119] Barbato KB, Martins RdeC, Rodrigues MdeL, Braga JU, Francischetti EA, Genelhu V. [Effects of greater-than-5% weight reduction on hemodynamic, metabolic and neuroendocrine profiles of grade I obese subjects]. Arq Bras Cardiol 2006; 87(1): 12-21.
[PMID: 16906265]

[120] Leite LH, Lacerda AC, Balthazar CH, Marubayashi U, Coimbra CC. Central angiotensin AT1 receptors are involved in metabolic adjustments in response to graded exercise in rats. Peptides 2009; 30(10): 1931-5.
[http://dx.doi.org/10.1016/j.peptides.2009.07.018] [PMID: 19647773]

[121] Yoshida T, Semprun-Prieto L, Wainford RD, Sukhanov S, Kapusta DR, Delafontaine P. Angiotensin II reduces food intake by altering orexigenic neuropeptide expression in the mouse hypothalamus. Endocrinology 2012; 153(3): 1411-20.
[http://dx.doi.org/10.1210/en.2011-1764] [PMID: 22234465]

[122] Foster MT, Song CK, Bartness TJ. Hypothalamic paraventricular nucleus lesion involvement in the sympathetic control of lipid mobilization. Obesity (Silver Spring) 2010; 18(4): 682-9.
[http://dx.doi.org/10.1038/oby.2009.345] [PMID: 19851310]

[123] Bagnasco M, Dube MG, Kalra PS, Kalra SP. Evidence for the existence of distinct central appetite,

energy expenditure, and ghrelin stimulation pathways as revealed by hypothalamic site-specific leptin gene therapy. Endocrinology 2002; 143(11): 4409-21.
[http://dx.doi.org/10.1210/en.2002-220505] [PMID: 12399438]

[124] Yeo WK, Carey AL, Burke L, Spriet LL, Hawley JA. Fat adaptation in well-trained athletes: effects on cell metabolism. Applied physiology, nutrition, and metabolism 2011; 36(1): 12-22.
[http://dx.doi.org/10.1139/H10-089]

[125] Kitaoka R, Fujikawa T, Miyaki T, Matsumura S, Fushiki T, Inoue K. Increased noradrenergic activity in the ventromedial hypothalamus during treadmill running in rats. J Nutr Sci Vitaminol (Tokyo) 2010; 56(3): 185-90.
[http://dx.doi.org/10.3177/jnsv.56.185] [PMID: 20651459]

[126] Guyenet PG. The sympathetic control of blood pressure. Nat Rev Neurosci 2006; 7(5): 335-46.
[http://dx.doi.org/10.1038/nrn1902] [PMID: 16760914]

[127] de Kloet AD, Krause EG, Scott KA, *et al.* Central angiotensin II has catabolic action at white and brown adipose tissue. Am J Physiol Endocrinol Metab 2011; 301(6): E1081-91.
[http://dx.doi.org/10.1152/ajpendo.00307.2011] [PMID: 21862725]

[128] Arner P, Kriegholm E, Engfeldt P, Bolinder J. Adrenergic regulation of lipolysis *in situ* at rest and during exercise. J Clin Invest 1990; 85(3): 893-8.
[http://dx.doi.org/10.1172/JCI114516] [PMID: 2312732]

[129] Krskova K, Eckertova M, Kukan M, *et al.* Aerobic training lasting for 10 weeks elevates the adipose tissue FABP4, Giα, and adiponectin expression associated by a reduced protein oxidation. Endocr Regul 2012; 46(3): 137-46.
[http://dx.doi.org/10.4149/endo_2012_03_137] [PMID: 22808905]

[130] Wang G, Mikami E, Chiu LL, de Perini A, Deason M, Fuku N, *et al.* Association analysis of ACE and ACTN3 in Elite Caucasian and East Asian Swimmers. Med Sci Sports Exerc 2012.
[PMID: 23190598]

[131] Zorad S, Dou JT, Benicky J, *et al.* Long-term angiotensin II AT1 receptor inhibition produces adipose tissue hypotrophy accompanied by increased expression of adiponectin and PPARgamma. Eur J Pharmacol 2006; 552(1-3): 112-22.
[http://dx.doi.org/10.1016/j.ejphar.2006.08.062] [PMID: 17064684]

[132] Cadenas E, Sies H. Oxidative stress: excited oxygen species and enzyme activity. Adv Enzyme Regul 1985; 23: 217-37.
[http://dx.doi.org/10.1016/0065-2571(85)90049-4] [PMID: 3907304]

[133] Sies H. Biological redox systems and oxidative stress. Cell Mol Life Sci 2007; 64(17): 2181-8.
[http://dx.doi.org/10.1007/s00018-007-7230-8] [PMID: 17565441]

[134] Dröge W. Free radicals in the physiological control of cell function. Physiol Rev 2002; 82(1): 47-95.
[http://dx.doi.org/10.1152/physrev.00018.2001] [PMID: 11773609]

[135] Cakir Y, Ballinger SW. Reactive species-mediated regulation of cell signaling and the cell cycle: the role of MAPK. Antioxidants & redox signaling 2005; 7(5-6): 726-40.
[http://dx.doi.org/10.1089/ars.2005.7.726]

[136] Lyle AN, Griendling KK. Modulation of vascular smooth muscle signaling by reactive oxygen

species. Physiology (Bethesda) 2006; 21: 269-80.
[http://dx.doi.org/10.1152/physiol.00004.2006] [PMID: 16868316]

[137] Powers SK, Jackson MJ. Exercise-induced oxidative stress: cellular mechanisms and impact on muscle force production. Physiol Rev 2008; 88(4): 1243-76.
[http://dx.doi.org/10.1152/physrev.00031.2007] [PMID: 18923182]

[138] Lassègue B, Griendling KK. NADPH oxidases: functions and pathologies in the vasculature. Arterioscler Thromb Vasc Biol 2010; 30(4): 653-61.
[http://dx.doi.org/10.1161/ATVBAHA.108.181610] [PMID: 19910640]

[139] Houston MC. Nutraceuticals, vitamins, antioxidants, and minerals in the prevention and treatment of hypertension. Prog Cardiovasc Dis 2005; 47(6): 396-449.
[http://dx.doi.org/10.1016/j.pcad.2005.01.004] [PMID: 16115519]

[140] Cal LA, Maso LD, Caielli P, *et al.* Effect of olmesartan on oxidative stress in hypertensive patients: mechanistic support to clinical trials derived evidence. Blood Press 2011; 20(6): 376-82.
[http://dx.doi.org/10.3109/08037051.2011.575570] [PMID: 21504378]

[141] Higashi Y, Sasaki S, Nakagawa K, Matsuura H, Oshima T, Chayama K. Endothelial function and oxidative stress in renovascular hypertension. N Engl J Med 2002; 346(25): 1954-62.
[http://dx.doi.org/10.1056/NEJMoa013591] [PMID: 12075056]

[142] McNally JS, Davis ME, Giddens DP, *et al.* Role of xanthine oxidoreductase and NAD(P)H oxidase in endothelial superoxide production in response to oscillatory shear stress. Am J Physiol Heart Circ Physiol 2003; 285(6): H2290-7.
[http://dx.doi.org/10.1152/ajpheart.00515.2003] [PMID: 12958034]

[143] Adlam D, Bendall JK, De Bono JP, *et al.* Relationships between nitric oxide-mediated endothelial function, eNOS coupling and blood pressure revealed by eNOS-GTP cyclohydrolase 1 double transgenic mice. Exp Physiol 2007; 92(1): 119-26.
[http://dx.doi.org/10.1113/expphysiol.2006.035113] [PMID: 17012144]

[144] Vásquez-Vivar J, Kalyanaraman B, Martásek P, *et al.* Superoxide generation by endothelial nitric oxide synthase: the influence of cofactors. Proc Natl Acad Sci USA 1998; 95(16): 9220-5.
[http://dx.doi.org/10.1073/pnas.95.16.9220] [PMID: 9689061]

[145] Lambeth JD. NOX enzymes and the biology of reactive oxygen. Nat Rev Immunol 2004; 4(3): 181-9.
[http://dx.doi.org/10.1038/nri1312] [PMID: 15039755]

[146] Bokoch GM, Zhao T. Regulation of the phagocyte NADPH oxidase by Rac GTPase. Antioxidants & redox signaling 2006; 8(9-10): 1533-48.
[http://dx.doi.org/10.1089/ars.2006.8.1533]

[147] Touyz RM, Briones AM, Sedeek M, Burger D, Montezano AC. NOX isoforms and reactive oxygen species in vascular health. Mol Interv 2011; 11(1): 27-35.
[http://dx.doi.org/10.1124/mi.11.1.5] [PMID: 21441119]

[148] Cheng G, Lambeth JD. Alternative mRNA splice forms of NOXO1: differential tissue expression and regulation of Nox1 and Nox3. Gene 2005; 356: 118-26.
[http://dx.doi.org/10.1016/j.gene.2005.03.008] [PMID: 15949904]

[149] Ambasta RK, Schreiber JG, Janiszewski M, Busse R, Brandes RP. Noxa1 is a central component of

the smooth muscle NADPH oxidase in mice. Free Radic Biol Med 2006; 41(2): 193-201. [http://dx.doi.org/10.1016/j.freeradbiomed.2005.12.035] [PMID: 16814099]

[150] Ambasta RK, Kumar P, Griendling KK, Schmidt HH, Busse R, Brandes RP. Direct interaction of the novel Nox proteins with p22phox is required for the formation of a functionally active NADPH oxidase. J Biol Chem 2004; 279(44): 45935-41. [http://dx.doi.org/10.1074/jbc.M406486200] [PMID: 15322091]

[151] Takeya R, Sumimoto H. Regulation of novel superoxide-producing NAD[P]H oxidases. Antioxidants & redox signaling 2006; 8(9-10): 1523-32.2006;

[152] Griendling KK, Minieri CA, Ollerenshaw JD, Alexander RW. Angiotensin II stimulates NADH and NADPH oxidase activity in cultured vascular smooth muscle cells. Circ Res 1994; 74(6): 1141-8. [http://dx.doi.org/10.1161/01.RES.74.6.1141] [PMID: 8187280]

[153] Touyz RM, Yao G, Schiffrin EL. c-Src induces phosphorylation and translocation of p47phox: role in superoxide generation by angiotensin II in human vascular smooth muscle cells. Arterioscler Thromb Vasc Biol 2003; 23(6): 981-7. [http://dx.doi.org/10.1161/01.ATV.0000069236.27911.68] [PMID: 12663375]

[154] Seshiah PN, Weber DS, Rocic P, Valppu L, Taniyama Y, Griendling KK. Angiotensin II stimulation of NAD(P)H oxidase activity: upstream mediators. Circ Res 2002; 91(5): 406-13. [http://dx.doi.org/10.1161/01.RES.0000033523.08033.16] [PMID: 12215489]

[155] Ushio-Fukai M, Alexander RW, Akers M, Griendling KK. p38 Mitogen-activated protein kinase is a critical component of the redox-sensitive signaling pathways activated by angiotensin II. Role in vascular smooth muscle cell hypertrophy. J Biol Chem 1998; 273(24): 15022-9. [http://dx.doi.org/10.1074/jbc.273.24.15022] [PMID: 9614110]

[156] Zafari AM, Ushio-Fukai M, Minieri CA, Akers M, Lassegue B, Griendling KK. Arachidonic acid metabolites mediate angiotensin II-induced NADH/NADPH oxidase activity and hypertrophy in vascular smooth muscle cells. Antioxidants & redox signaling 1999; 1(2): 167-79.

[157] Touyz RM, Schiffrin EL. Signal transduction mechanisms mediating the physiological and pathophysiological actions of angiotensin II in vascular smooth muscle cells. Pharmacol Rev 2000; 52(4): 639-72. [PMID: 11121512]

[158] Janiszewski M, Lopes LR, Carmo AO, *et al.* Regulation of NAD(P)H oxidase by associated protein disulfide isomerase in vascular smooth muscle cells. J Biol Chem 2005; 280(49): 40813-9. [http://dx.doi.org/10.1074/jbc.M509255200] [PMID: 16150729]

[159] Touyz RM, Chen X, Tabet F, *et al.* Expression of a functionally active gp91phox-containing neutrophil-type NAD(P)H oxidase in smooth muscle cells from human resistance arteries: regulation by angiotensin II. Circ Res 2002; 90(11): 1205-13. [http://dx.doi.org/10.1161/01.RES.0000020404.01971.2F] [PMID: 12065324]

[160] Lee VM, Quinn PA, Jennings SC, Ng LL. Neutrophil activation and production of reactive oxygen species in pre-eclampsia. J Hypertens 2003; 21(2): 395-402. [http://dx.doi.org/10.1097/00004872-200302000-00032] [PMID: 12569271]

[161] Minuz P, Patrignani P, Gaino S, *et al.* Determinants of platelet activation in human essential

hypertension. Hypertension 2004; 43(1): 64-70.
[http://dx.doi.org/10.1161/01.HYP.0000105109.44620.1B] [PMID: 14656953]

[162] Fortuño A, Oliván S, Beloqui O, *et al.* Association of increased phagocytic NADPH oxidase-dependent superoxide production with diminished nitric oxide generation in essential hypertension. J Hypertens 2004; 22(11): 2169-75.
[http://dx.doi.org/10.1097/00004872-200411000-00020] [PMID: 15480102]

[163] Touyz RM, Schiffrin EL. Increased generation of superoxide by angiotensin II in smooth muscle cells from resistance arteries of hypertensive patients: role of phospholipase D-dependent NAD(P)H oxidase-sensitive pathways. J Hypertens 2001; 19(7): 1245-54.
[http://dx.doi.org/10.1097/00004872-200107000-00009] [PMID: 11446714]

[164] Touyz RM, Yao G, Quinn MT, Pagano PJ, Schiffrin EL. p47phox associates with the cytoskeleton through cortactin in human vascular smooth muscle cells: role in NAD(P)H oxidase regulation by angiotensin II. Arterioscler Thromb Vasc Biol 2005; 25(3): 512-8.
[http://dx.doi.org/10.1161/01.ATV.0000154141.66879.98] [PMID: 15618548]

[165] Rueckschloss U, Quinn MT, Holtz J, Morawietz H. Dose-dependent regulation of NAD(P)H oxidase expression by angiotensin II in human endothelial cells: protective effect of angiotensin II type 1 receptor blockade in patients with coronary artery disease. Arterioscler Thromb Vasc Biol 2002; 22(11): 1845-51.
[http://dx.doi.org/10.1161/01.ATV.0000035392.38687.65] [PMID: 12426214]

[166] Araki S, Hirooka Y, Kishi T, Yasukawa K, Utsumi H, Sunagawa K. Olmesartan reduces oxidative stress in the brain of stroke-prone spontaneously hypertensive rats assessed by an *in vivo* ESR method. Hypertension research 2009; 32(12): 1091-6.

[167] Takai S, Jin D, Aritomi S, Niinuma K, Miyazaki M. Powerful vascular protection by combining cilnidipine with valsartan in stroke-prone, spontaneously hypertensive rats. Hypertension research 2013; 36(4): 342-8.
[http://dx.doi.org/10.1038/hr.2012.187]

[168] Sukumaran V, Watanabe K, Veeraveedu PT, *et al.* Olmesartan, an AT1 antagonist, attenuates oxidative stress, endoplasmic reticulum stress and cardiac inflammatory mediators in rats with heart failure induced by experimental autoimmune myocarditis. Int J Biol Sci 2011; 7(2): 154-67.
[http://dx.doi.org/10.7150/ijbs.7.154] [PMID: 21383952]

[169] Rey FE, Cifuentes ME, Kiarash A, Quinn MT, Pagano PJ. Novel competitive inhibitor of NAD(P)H oxidase assembly attenuates vascular O(2)(-) and systolic blood pressure in mice. Circ Res 2001; 89(5): 408-14.
[http://dx.doi.org/10.1161/hh1701.096037] [PMID: 11532901]

[170] Ceravolo GS, Fernandes L, Munhoz CD, *et al.* Angiotensin II chronic infusion induces B1 receptor expression in aorta of rats. Hypertension 2007; 50(4): 756-61.
[http://dx.doi.org/10.1161/HYPERTENSIONAHA.107.094706] [PMID: 17664391]

[171] Landmesser U, Cai H, Dikalov S, *et al.* Role of p47(phox) in vascular oxidative stress and hypertension caused by angiotensin II. Hypertension 2002; 40(4): 511-5.
[http://dx.doi.org/10.1161/01.HYP.0000032100.23772.98] [PMID: 12364355]

[172] Li JM, Wheatcroft S, Fan LM, Kearney MT, Shah AM. Opposing roles of p47phox in basal *versus*

angiotensin II-stimulated alterations in vascular O2- production, vascular tone, and mitogen-activated protein kinase activation. Circulation 2004; 109(10): 1307-13.
[http://dx.doi.org/10.1161/01.CIR.0000118463.23388.B9] [PMID: 14993144]

[173] Jung O, Schreiber JG, Geiger H, Pedrazzini T, Busse R, Brandes RP. gp91phox-containing NADPH oxidase mediates endothelial dysfunction in renovascular hypertension. Circulation 2004; 109(14): 1795-801.
[http://dx.doi.org/10.1161/01.CIR.0000124223.00113.A4] [PMID: 15037533]

[174] Laude K, Cai H, Fink B, *et al.* Hemodynamic and biochemical adaptations to vascular smooth muscle overexpression of p22phox in mice. Am J Physiol Heart Circ Physiol 2005; 288(1): H7-H12.
[http://dx.doi.org/10.1152/ajpheart.00637.2004] [PMID: 15471976]

[175] Pierce GL, Donato AJ, LaRocca TJ, Eskurza I, Silver AE, Seals DR. Habitually exercising older men do not demonstrate age-associated vascular endothelial oxidative stress. Aging Cell 2011; 10(6): 1032-7.
[http://dx.doi.org/10.1111/j.1474-9726.2011.00748.x] [PMID: 21943306]

[176] Jenkins NT, Witkowski S, Spangenburg EE, Hagberg JM. Effects of acute and chronic endurance exercise on intracellular nitric oxide in putative endothelial progenitor cells: role of NAPDH oxidase. Am J Physiol Heart Circ Physiol 2009; 297(5): H1798-805.
[http://dx.doi.org/10.1152/ajpheart.00347.2009] [PMID: 19717732]

[177] Agarwal D, Haque M, Sriramula S, Mariappan N, Pariaut R, Francis J. Role of proinflammatory cytokines and redox homeostasis in exercise-induced delayed progression of hypertension in spontaneously hypertensive rats. Hypertension 2009; 54(6): 1393-400.
[http://dx.doi.org/10.1161/HYPERTENSIONAHA.109.135459] [PMID: 19841289]

[178] Agarwal D, Elks CM, Reed SD, Mariappan N, Majid DS, Francis J. Chronic exercise preserves renal structure and hemodynamics in spontaneously hypertensive rats. Antioxidants & redox signaling 2012; 16(2): 139-52.
[http://dx.doi.org/10.1089/ars.2011.3967]

[179] Inoue N, Kinugawa S, Suga T, *et al.* Angiotensin II-induced reduction in exercise capacity is associated with increased oxidative stress in skeletal muscle. Am J Physiol Heart Circ Physiol 2012; 302(5): H1202-10.
[http://dx.doi.org/10.1152/ajpheart.00534.2011] [PMID: 22210751]

[180] Kluger J, Cody RJ, Laragh JH. The contributions of sympathetic tone and the renin-angiotensin system to severe chronic congestive heart failure: response to specific inhibitors (prazosin and captopril). Am J Cardiol 1982; 49(7): 1667-74.
[http://dx.doi.org/10.1016/0002-9149(82)90244-2] [PMID: 7044087]

[181] Tikellis C, Cooper ME, Thomas MC. Role of the renin-angiotensin system in the endocrine pancreas: implications for the development of diabetes. Int J Biochem Cell Biol 2006; 38(5-6): 737-51.
[http://dx.doi.org/10.1016/j.biocel.2005.08.007] [PMID: 16198140]

[182] Harrison-Bernard LM. The renal renin-angiotensin system. Adv Physiol Educ 2009; 33(4): 270-4.
[http://dx.doi.org/10.1152/advan.00049.2009] [PMID: 19948673]

[183] Ma TK, Kam KK, Yan BP, Lam YY. Renin-angiotensin-aldosterone system blockade for cardiovascular diseases: current status. Br J Pharmacol 2010; 160(6): 1273-92.

[http://dx.doi.org/10.1111/j.1476-5381.2010.00750.x] [PMID: 20590619]

[184] Ginelli P, Bella JN. Treatment of diastolic dysfunction in hypertension. Nutr Metab Cardiovasc Dis 2012; 22(8): 613-8.
[http://dx.doi.org/10.1016/j.numecd.2012.04.016] [PMID: 22743209]

[185] Hu DY, Huang J, Cai NS, *et al.* A multi-center, double-blind, randomized, parallel group study to evaluate the effects of two different doses of losartan on morbidity and mortality in Chinese patients with symptomatic heart failure intolerant of angiotensin converting enzyme inhibitor treatment. Chin Med J (Engl) 2012; 125(21): 3868-74.
[PMID: 23106890]

[186] Meyer TE, Casadei B, Coats AJ, *et al.* Angiotensin-converting enzyme inhibition and physical training in heart failure. J Intern Med 1991; 230(5): 407-13.
[http://dx.doi.org/10.1111/j.1365-2796.1991.tb00465.x] [PMID: 1658183]

[187] Martínez de Morentin PB, López M. "Mens sana in corpore sano": exercise and hypothalamic ER stress. PLoS Biol 2010; 8(8): e1000464.
[http://dx.doi.org/10.1371/journal.pbio.1000464] [PMID: 20808779]

[188] Tschentscher M, Niederseer D, Niebauer J. Health benefits of Nordic walking: a systematic review. Am J Prev Med 2013; 44(1): 76-84.
[http://dx.doi.org/10.1016/j.amepre.2012.09.043] [PMID: 23253654]

[189] Zucker IH, Wang W, Pliquett RU, Liu JL, Patel KP. The regulation of sympathetic outflow in heart failure. The roles of angiotensin II, nitric oxide, and exercise training. Ann N Y Acad Sci 2001; 940: 431-43.
[http://dx.doi.org/10.1111/j.1749-6632.2001.tb03696.x] [PMID: 11458699]

[190] Patel D, Böhlke M, Phattanarudee S, Kabadi S, Maher TJ, Ally A. Cardiovascular responses and neurotransmitter changes during blockade of angiotensin II receptors within the ventrolateral medulla. Neurosci Res 2008; 60(3): 340-8.
[http://dx.doi.org/10.1016/j.neures.2007.12.002] [PMID: 18207270]

[191] Leite LH, Lacerda AC, Balthazar CH, Marubayashi U, Coimbra CC. Central AT(1) receptor blockade increases metabolic cost during exercise reducing mechanical efficiency and running performance in rats. Neuropeptides 2007; 41(3): 189-94.
[http://dx.doi.org/10.1016/j.npep.2007.01.002] [PMID: 17350681]

[192] Harada N, Takishita E, Ishimura N, Minami A, Sakamoto S, Nakaya Y. Combined effect of ACE inhibitor and exercise training on insulin resistance in type 2 diabetic rats. Life Sci 2002; 70(15): 1811-20.
[http://dx.doi.org/10.1016/S0024-3205(02)01495-9] [PMID: 12002525]

[193] Ishizawa K, Yoshizumi M, Tsuchiya K, *et al.* Effects of losartan in combination with or without exercise on insulin resistance in Otsuka Long-Evans Tokushima Fatty rats. Eur J Pharmacol 2001; 430(2-3): 359-67.
[http://dx.doi.org/10.1016/S0014-2999(01)01405-4] [PMID: 11711055]

[194] Libonati JR. Cardiac remodeling and function following exercise and angiotensin II receptor antagonism. Eur J Appl Physiol 2012; 112(8): 3149-54.
[http://dx.doi.org/10.1007/s00421-011-2263-y] [PMID: 22143841]

[195] Kemi OJ, Høydal MA, Haram PM, *et al.* Exercise training restores aerobic capacity and energy transfer systems in heart failure treated with losartan. Cardiovasc Res 2007; 76(1): 91-9. [http://dx.doi.org/10.1016/j.cardiores.2007.06.008] [PMID: 17628515]

[196] Jain M, Liao R, Ngoy S, Whittaker P, Apstein CS, Eberli FR. Angiotensin II receptor blockade attenuates the deleterious effects of exercise training on post-MI ventricular remodelling in rats. Cardiovasc Res 2000; 46(1): 66-72. [http://dx.doi.org/10.1016/S0008-6363(99)00429-0] [PMID: 10727654]

[197] Xu X, Wan W, Ji L, *et al.* Exercise training combined with angiotensin II receptor blockade limits post-infarct ventricular remodelling in rats. Cardiovasc Res 2008; 78(3): 523-32. [http://dx.doi.org/10.1093/cvr/cvn028] [PMID: 18252761]

[198] Kemi OJ, Haram PM, Høydal MA, Wisløff U, Ellingsen Ø. Exercise training and losartan improve endothelial function in heart failure rats by different mechanisms. Scand Cardiovasc J 2013; 47(3): 160-7. [http://dx.doi.org/10.3109/14017431.2012.754935] [PMID: 23205578]

[199] Tufescu A, Kanazawa M, Ishida A, *et al.* Combination of exercise and losartan enhances renoprotective and peripheral effects in spontaneously type 2 diabetes mellitus rats with nephropathy. J Hypertens 2008; 26(2): 312-21. [http://dx.doi.org/10.1097/HJH.0b013e3282f2450b] [PMID: 18192846]

[200] Kohzuki M, Kamimoto M, Wu XM, *et al.* Renal protective effects of chronic exercise and antihypertensive therapy in hypertensive rats with chronic renal failure. J Hypertens 2001; 19(10): 1877-82. [http://dx.doi.org/10.1097/00004872-200110000-00024] [PMID: 11593110]

[201] Liu JL, Irvine S, Reid IA, Patel KP, Zucker IH. Chronic exercise reduces sympathetic nerve activity in rabbits with pacing-induced heart failure: A role for angiotensin II. Circulation 2000; 102(15): 1854-62. [http://dx.doi.org/10.1161/01.CIR.102.15.1854] [PMID: 11023943]

[202] Warner JG Jr, Metzger DC, Kitzman DW, Wesley DJ, Little WC. Losartan improves exercise tolerance in patients with diastolic dysfunction and a hypertensive response to exercise. J Am Coll Cardiol 1999; 33(6): 1567-72. [http://dx.doi.org/10.1016/S0735-1097(99)00048-0] [PMID: 10334425]

[203] Tutarel O, Meyer GP, Bertram H, Wessel A, Schieffer B, Westhoff-Bleck M. Safety and efficiency of chronic ACE inhibition in symptomatic heart failure patients with a systemic right ventricle. Int J Cardiol 2012; 154(1): 14-6. [http://dx.doi.org/10.1016/j.ijcard.2010.08.068] [PMID: 20843567]

[204] Di Marco F, Guazzi M, Vicenzi M, *et al.* Effect of enalapril on exercise cardiopulmonary performance in chronic obstructive pulmonary disease: A pilot study. Pulm Pharmacol Ther 2010; 23(3): 159-64. [http://dx.doi.org/10.1016/j.pupt.2010.01.004] [PMID: 20096799]

[205] Prasad A, Halcox JP, Waclawiw MA, Quyyumi AA. Angiotensin type 1 receptor antagonism reverses abnormal coronary vasomotion in atherosclerosis. J Am Coll Cardiol 2001; 38(4): 1089-95. [http://dx.doi.org/10.1016/S0735-1097(01)01511-X] [PMID: 11583887]

[206] Goldberg MR, Tanaka W, Barchowsky A, *et al.* Effects of losartan on blood pressure, plasma renin activity, and angiotensin II in volunteers. Hypertension 1993; 21(5): 704-13. [http://dx.doi.org/10.1161/01.HYP.21.5.704] [PMID: 8491505]

[207] Williams B, Baschiera F, Lacy PS, Botha J, Prescott MF, Brunel P. Blood pressure and plasma renin activity responses to different strategies to inhibit the renin-angiotensin-aldosterone system during exercise. J Renin Angiotensin Aldosterone Syst 2013; 14(1): 56-66. [http://dx.doi.org/10.1177/1470320312454766] [PMID: 22859712]

[208] Houghton AR, Harrison M, Cowley AJ. Haemodynamic, neurohumoral and exercise effects of losartan *vs.* captopril in chronic heart failure: results of an ELITE trial substudy. Evaluation of Losartan in the Elderly. Eur J Heart Fail 1999; 1(4): 385-93. [http://dx.doi.org/10.1016/S1388-9842(99)00038-0] [PMID: 10937952]

[209] Cuocolo A, Storto G, Izzo R, *et al.* Effects of valsartan on left ventricular diastolic function in patients with mild or moderate essential hypertension: comparison with enalapril. J Hypertens 1999; 17(12 Pt 1): 1759-66. [http://dx.doi.org/10.1097/00004872-199917120-00014] [PMID: 10658943]

[210] Dayi SU, Akbulut T, Akgoz H, *et al.* Long-term combined therapy with losartan and an angiotensin-converting enzyme inhibitor improves functional capacity in patients with left ventricular dysfunction. Acta Cardiol 2005; 60(4): 373-7. [http://dx.doi.org/10.2143/AC.60.4.2004985] [PMID: 16128369]

[211] Hamroff G, Katz SD, Mancini D, *et al.* Addition of angiotensin II receptor blockade to maximal angiotensin-converting enzyme inhibition improves exercise capacity in patients with severe congestive heart failure. Circulation 1999; 99(8): 990-2. [http://dx.doi.org/10.1161/01.CIR.99.8.990] [PMID: 10051289]

[212] Avanza AC Jr, Mansur AP, Ramires JA. Efficacy of exercise, losartan, enalapril, atenolol and rilmenidine in subjects with blood pressure hyperreactivity at treadmill stress test and left ventricular hypertrophy. J Hum Hypertens 2009; 23(4): 259-66. [http://dx.doi.org/10.1038/jhh.2008.127] [PMID: 18946484]

[213] Volterrani M, Cice G, Caminiti G, *et al.* Effect of Carvedilol, Ivabradine or their combination on exercise capacity in patients with Heart Failure (the CARVIVA HF trial). Int J Cardiol 2011; 151(2): 218-24. [http://dx.doi.org/10.1016/j.ijcard.2011.06.098] [PMID: 21764469]

[214] Rigat B, Hubert C, Alhenc-Gelas F, Cambien F, Corvol P, Soubrier F. An insertion/deletion polymorphism in the angiotensin I-converting enzyme gene accounting for half the variance of serum enzyme levels. J Clin Invest 1990; 86(4): 1343-6. [http://dx.doi.org/10.1172/JCI114844] [PMID: 1976655]

[215] Koch W, Kastrati A, Mehilli J, Böttiger C, von Beckerath N, Schömig A. Insertion/deletion polymorphism of the angiotensin I-converting enzyme gene is not associated with restenosis after coronary stent placement. Circulation 2000; 102(2): 197-202. [http://dx.doi.org/10.1161/01.CIR.102.2.197] [PMID: 10889131]

[216] Marre M, Bernadet P, Gallois Y, *et al.* Relationships between angiotensin I converting enzyme gene polymorphism, plasma levels, and diabetic retinal and renal complications. Diabetes 1994; 43(3): 384-

8.
[http://dx.doi.org/10.2337/diab.43.3.384] [PMID: 8314010]

[217] Alvarez R, Terrados N, Ortolano R, *et al.* Genetic variation in the renin-angiotensin system and athletic performance. Eur J Appl Physiol 2000; 82(1-2): 117-20.
[http://dx.doi.org/10.1007/s004210050660] [PMID: 10879452]

[218] Rankinen T, Pérusse L, Gagnon J, *et al.* Angiotensin-converting enzyme ID polymorphism and fitness phenotype in the HERITAGE Family Study. J Appl Physiol 2000; 88(3): 1029-35.
[PMID: 10710400]

[219] Gayagay G, Yu B, Hambly B, *et al.* Elite endurance athletes and the ACE I allele--the role of genes in athletic performance. Hum Genet 1998; 103(1): 48-50.
[http://dx.doi.org/10.1007/s004390050781] [PMID: 9737775]

[220] Nazarov IB, Woods DR, Montgomery HE, *et al.* The angiotensin converting enzyme I/D polymorphism in Russian athletes. Eur J Hum Genet 2001; 9(10): 797-801.
[http://dx.doi.org/10.1038/sj.ejhg.5200711] [PMID: 11781693]

[221] Williams AG, Dhamrait SS, Wootton PT, *et al.* Bradykinin receptor gene variant and human physical performance. J Appl Physiol 2004; 96(3): 938-42.
[http://dx.doi.org/10.1152/japplphysiol.00865.2003] [PMID: 14607851]

[222] Pescatello LS, Kostek MA, Gordish-Dressman H, *et al.* ACE ID genotype and the muscle strength and size response to unilateral resistance training. Med Sci Sports Exerc 2006; 38(6): 1074-81.
[http://dx.doi.org/10.1249/01.mss.0000222835.28273.80] [PMID: 16775548]

[223] Puthucheary Z, Skipworth JR, Rawal J, Loosemore M, Van Someren K, Montgomery HE. The ACE gene and human performance: 12 years on. Sports Med 2011; 41(6): 433-48.
[http://dx.doi.org/10.2165/11588720-000000000-00000] [PMID: 21615186]

[224] Zhang X, Wang C, Dai H, Lin Y, Zhang J. Association between angiotensin-converting enzyme gene polymorphisms and exercise performance in patients with COPD. Respirology 2008; 13(5): 683-8.
[http://dx.doi.org/10.1111/j.1440-1843.2008.01325.x] [PMID: 18713090]

[225] Zhang L, Du J, Hu Z, *et al.* IL-6 and serum amyloid A synergy mediates angiotensin II-induced muscle wasting. J Am Soc Nephrol 2009; 20(3): 604-12.
[http://dx.doi.org/10.1681/ASN.2008060628] [PMID: 19158350]

CHAPTER 15

Renin-Angiotensin System in Animal Models of Diabetes and Hypertension

Roseli Peres Moreira[1], **Nádia de Sousa da Cunha Bertoncello**[1,2], **Rodolfo Mattar Rosa**[1], **Isabela Bezerra Loyola**[1], **Juliana Dinéia Perez Brandão**[1] and **Juliana Almada Colucci**[1,3,*]

[1] *Nephrology Division, Department of Medicine, Escola Paulista de Medicina, Universidade Federal de Sao Paulo, Sao Paulo, Brazil*

[2] *Science and Technology Institute, Federal University of Sao Paulo, São José dos Campos, Brazil*

[3] *Pós-Graduação em Ciências da Saúde, Universidade de Santo Amaro – Sao Paulo, Brazil*

Abstract: Translational research has currently become the focus of many ongoing studies. The use of inbred animals represents an advantage to human studies to a certain point because of the elimination of several uncontrollable variables. However, we need to consider the limitation of such approach in the translational potential to humans. Within the field of hypertension and diabetes research, animal models are irreplaceable research tools providing insight into human diseases. These two diseases independently predispose to renal and cardiovascular complications but, more importantly, can aggravate each other. Although some of the best models for diabetes and hypertension are spontaneous, the use of transgenic models provides a better control of the pathological mechanisms to be studied and the combination of the available tools will most likely make a difference in understanding how the RAS is modulated in diabetes and hypertension. Although these animals add a few layers of complexity and are sometimes closer to the human pathological mechanism, there are still many challenges to overcome.

* **Corresponding author Juliana Almada Colucci:** Departamento de Medicina, Disciplina de Nefrologia, Universidade Federal de São Paulo Rua Botucatu, 740 Vila Clementino, São Paulo – SP 04023-900; Phone: +55 11 59041687; E-mail: colucci@nefro.epm.br.

Dulce Elena Casarini, Danielle Yuri Arita, Tatiana Sousa Cunha & Juliana Almada Colucci (Eds.)

Keywords: Animal models, Basic research, Diabetes, Hypertension, *In vivo* studies, Knock out, Mice, Rats, RAS, Renin-angiotensin system, SHR, Spontaneously hypertensive rats, Transgenic, Translational medicine, Type 1 diabetes, Type 2 diabetes.

INTRODUCTION

Diabetes and hypertension are comorbid diseases that independently predispose to renal and cardiovascular complications. Both diseases aggravate each other in terms of subsequent renal and cardiovascular complications [1, 2]. Achieving proper blood pressure control is key in hypertension, although even with a vast choice of antihypertensive drugs it remains a challenge, especially with concomitant diabetes. The metabolic side effects of the most used treatments is an important issue and whether blood pressure reduction *per se* is the most important target of antihypertensive treatment or if there are specific benefits associated with certain antihypertensive regimens, in particular inhibitors of the renin-angiotensin system (RAS) is still controversial. In general, agents that at the same time suspend the RAS and enhance the aldosterone pathway appear to be notably useful in diabetic renal and cardiovascular disease [1, 3, 4]. Most patients with diabetes and hypertension will require more than 2 or 3 antihypertensive drugs as recommended in the latest US, European, and World Health Organization (WHO) guidelines, but there is still no consensus on the most beneficial combination [1].

This chapter describes the use of animal models of diabetes and hypertension in the search for better diagnostic and therapeutical tools.

ANIMAL MODELS IN RAS RESEARCH

Animal models have provided massive data in the growing complexity of the RAS. Ever since Tigerstedt and Bergmann discovered renin in 1898, RAS has been extremely important in the regulation of blood pressure (BP) and volume homeostasis. Subsequently, an aberrant activity of the RAS has been suggested as a pathogenic factor and/or a complicating factor in the context of hypertension and diabetes [5]. Through the course of research history, the use of relevant models to mimic human diseases is certain to have contributed with vast information by allowing us to better understand the cause and progression of the disease and also by giving insights of potential therapeutic interventions [6]. On the other hand their value in predicting the efficiency of treatment strategies in clinical trials is still controversial [7, 8]. Animal models have been used for several reasons. Firstly, animal studies provide unique insights into the pathophysiology and causes of disease and usually unveil unknown targets for directed treatments. Secondly, animal studies provide a genetic manipulation rarely achievable in humans and finally, if preliminary testing on animals show that they do not have a clinical importance, the human testing phase may not be necessary [9].

Animal Models of Hypertension and RAS

The use of relevant models to mimic human cardiovascular disease provides useful information by giving us an overview of the cause and progression of the disease status and also by revealing potential therapeutic interventions, which would not be possible in the context of clinical research [6]. Many animal models have been extensively used in the study of hypertension but it is important to point out that each one has a particular role in the development of the disease [6].

Genetic Models

Spontaneously Hypertensive Rat

Spontaneously hypertensive rats (SHRs) originates from Wistar and non-hypertensive Wistar–Kyoto (WKY) rats inbreeding [10]. These rats spontaneously become hypertense at about 4 to 6 weeks of age but environmental factors can affect the development of hypertension [11]. In 1999, Zicha *et al.* stated that >90% of the papers available in this field of research used this model [11]. In the early stages of hypertension, SHRs have normal total peripheral resistance and increased cardiac output. By the time the cardiac output returns to normal hypertrophied blood vessels promote an increase in peripheral resistance, establishing hypertension [12]. Between 6 and 24 months of age, as the hypertension advances, the SHR develops structural alterations in the heart, which are associated with progressive cardiac hypertrophy [6, 13]. Later, using the SHR background, Okamoto *et al.* developed a stroke-prone spontaneously hypertensive rat (SHRSP) [14].

The extensive use of the SHR has made it the model of choice for a wide range of hypertension/RAS related studies, mainly due to the similarity to human essential hypertension [15].

Dahl Salt-Sensitive Rats

A Sprague-Dawley (SP) originated strain, this is, as the name indicates, a salt sensitive hypertensive rat. Dahl *et al.* described this model by selecting the SP rats on the basis of monitored BP levels after rats were fed a high salt diet (8% NaCl). This experiment originated two different strains: Dahl-sensitive (DS) and Dahl-resistant (DR) rats. The ingestion of a high salt diet leads to systemic arterial hypertension in the DS rats while the DR animals can still maintain normal BP on the same diet. How the BP increases in response to high salt intake in salt-sensitive patients with essential hypertension is complex and only partially understood [16].

Transgenic Hypertension Models

Since HT has a polygenic nature and depends on environmental factors it is challenging to identify the genetic factors that directly increase BP [17].

In 1995, Krege *et al.* published a study in which they had successfully inactivated the angiotensin-converting enzyme (ACE) gene in mice. Although all homozygous female mutants have remained fertile, the fertility of homozygous male mutants suffered great reduction, a problem related to the testicular form of ACE. Although both male and female heterozygotes had reduced serum ACE activity, only heterozygous males had blood pressures that were 15-20 mm Hg less than normal. [18]. Two years later, the same author published new data describing experiments of ACE gene titration. ACE activities in the serum augmented from 62% of normal in the one-copy animals to 144% of normal in the three-copy animals. Interestingly, the blood pressures of the transgenic mice did not change significantly, indicating that adaptations successfully stabilized the blood pressures of mice that have changes in ACE gene function. Therefore, quantitative in ACE expression will affect blood pressures when there is also an additional effect of environmental factors that overcome the accompanied by additional environmental or genetic factors that together with ACE exceed the capacity of compensatory mechanisms [19]. The development of new transgenic techniques has increased the level of complexity to the development of animal models of hypertension, especially in the context of RAS, with many important publications unveiling valuable information about ACE functions on BP regulation as well as on tissue RAS [20 - 23].

The improvement of molecular biology techniques for the rat made possible the manipulation of specific genes, providing novel perspectives on the development of new animal models of hypertension. One good example of this advance is the development of the TGR(mREN2)27 transgenic rat by Mullins [24]. This model brought new insights in the functions of the RAS by harboring the mouse Ren-2 gene and exhibiting fulminant hypertension. The circulating RAS is down-regulated in this animal while the tissue-specific production of AII is activated and the physiological consequence of this stimulation leads to hypertension. In addition, TGR have moderate structural lesions of the nephron [25]. TGR(hREN) and TGR(hAOGEN) were manipulated to carry the human genes for renin and angiotensinogen, respectively, making them valuable tools for the study of the expression pattern of the genes [26]. This model is of particular interest for the study of *in vivo* consequences of severe RAS activation, even though it does not represent human hypertension.

Borderline Hypertensive Rat

The borderline hypertensive rat (BHR) is the first offspring of an SHR and WKY cross. It is an environmentally induced hypertension models that producfiltration. Because AII does not reduce elevation on BP after exposure to stress. Although the mechanism mediating this effect is not fully known, the sympathetic nervous system has been implicated. BHR are characterized by a high plasma concentration of vasopressin, exogenous vasopressin-induced hyperpressor action and cardiac hypertrophy [6].

Hypertension Induced By Ang II

Angiotensin II is recognized as the most potent vasoconstrictor in the human body taking a significant part in the control of vascular tone and BP. Due to its central role, Ang II is also deeply involved in diseases such as hypertension and heart failure. The vasoconstriction of the peripheral vasculature and growth of smooth muscle cells of blood vessels and heart are influenced by Ang II [27]. The Ang II action does not promote instant elevation of systemic BP but it leads to a slow emerging hypertension (taking between 6 to 10 days). Excess of Ang II, causes the pressure natriuretic association to be shifted to greater arterial pressures so that higher arterial pressures are needed to uphold sodium balance. Ang II reduces pressure natriuresis by augmenting tubular reabsorption and/or dropping glomerular filtration. Because Ang II does not reduce glomerular filtration in most situations, the sodium retaining activities of Ang II are typically produced by increased tubular reabsorption [28].

Renovascular Hypertension

In 1934, by partially constricting the renal artery of a dog, Goldblatt *et al.* have successfully established a new hypertension model. The technique involves compressing one or both renal arteries by use of silver clamp [29]. Renal-induced experimental hypertension includes the following combinations: two-kidney one-clip hypertension (2K1C; constriction of one renal artery while the contralateral kidney is left intact); one-kidney one-clip hypertension (1K1C; one renal artery is constricted and the contralateral kidney is removed), and two-kidney two-clip hypertension (2K2C; constriction of aorta or both renal arteries) [6]. Renin synthesis is stimulated by the reduction in renal perfusion thus releasing AII. The octapeptide will have direct vascular effects, acutely increasing BP, but also acting on most organs. Tightening the renal artery of the remaining kidney in uninephrectomized rats produces 1K1C Goldblatt hypertension, a good model for studying volume expansion in the development of hypertension. There is no resulting increase in sodium and water excretion caused by the absence of the non manipulated kidney therefore fluid volume is retained [30]. In the 2K2C model, the severe renal ischaemia leads to activation of RAS and the sympathetic nervous system and the raise of serum vasopressin, with consequent augmented BP [31].

Endocrine Hypertension: Salt and Mineralocorticoids

The renal effects of hyperaldosteronism in humans can be reproduced by this model. Mineralocorticoids cause sodium and water retention of in the body until augmented pressure on the kidneys and suppression of renin secretion promotes escape diuresis [6]. 11-desoxycorticosterone acetate (DOCA) and high-salt diet cause a 30-fold increase in sodium absorption and elevated BP within 3 weeks [32]. DOCA salt models are not appropriate for long-term studies in prolonged, steady disease because they progress quickly to severe hypertension and hypertrophy. Besides, they do not mimic human hypertensive patients in a very realistic way [33].

Neurogenic Hypertension

Neurogenic hypertension occurs when a neural change causes a permanent increase in BP. The central nervous system is likely involved in the genesis of hypertension and the most used model is the denervation of sinoartic baroreceptors (SAD). In rats SAD promotes chronic increase in BP, but the rise of BP in rat is not complemented by marked tachycardia as previously seen in dogs [34]. Consequently, an increase in mean arterial pressure (MAP) excites baroreceptors and causes a mutual decrease in sympathetic outflow to resistance vessels and the heart so as to restore MAP to the normal level and, consequently, originating neurogenic hypertension [6, 35].

Animal Models of Diabetes and RAS

The number of people with diabetes has been increasing in every country and the potential for the development of complications is tremendous. One of the most incapacitating of theses complications is diabetic nephropathy (DN), the major cause of chronic kidney disease (CKD) and end stage renal disease (ESRD) throughout the world. The mainstays of current therapy for DN are control of hyperglycemia and BP and inhibition of the RAS [36]. Animal models have also been largely used in diabetes research, since early studies performed pancreatomy in dogs to confirm the role of the pancreas in glucose homeostasis, culminating in the finding and purification of insulin [37, 38].

Animal Models of Hyperglycaemia

The first description of experimental diabetes goes as far as the 1880s when von Mering removed the pancreas of a dog. The animal soon developed polyuria and polydipsia and was found to have diabetes mellitus (DM) [37]. Indeed, one could think that the most direct ways of studying the effects of hyperglycaemia in an animal is to remove the pancreas, either partially or totally. Historically used in research for the convenience of size and maintenance, rats and mice are the most commonly used. Nevertheless, a key criticism of using rodents is that they may not adequately reflect the human situation justifying the use larger animals such as cats, dogs, pigs and primates [37].

The administration of chemical agents, such as alloxan and streptozotocin, is an alternative to pharmacological methods of inducing hyperglycemia, thus producing experimental diabetes [39, 40]. In the literature of RAS and induced diabetes, the vast majority of studies use streptozotocin. Streptozotocin is a powerful alkylating agent that affects glucose transport [41]. It is a nitrosourea derivative isolated from *Streptomyces achromogenes* with broad-spectrum antibiotic and anti-neoplastic activity [42]. It is postulated that diabetes can occur in rodents as a consequence of the toxic effect of a single large dose of streptozotocin in β-cells. Additionally, multiple small doses of the drug can also be used (*e.g.* 40 mg/kg on five consecutive days). In prone rodents this induces an insulinopenic diabetes in which immune damage plays a role, as in human Type 1 diabetes [37]. The streptozotocin model is widely used by groups that want to evaluate key elements of the RAS in the diabetic situation. In 2007, Ronchi *et al.*, using this model, studied the relationship of somatic and N-domain angiotensin converting enzymes from Wistar rat tissue with renal dysfunction in diabetes mellitus, suggesting an enzymatic modulation of the RAS in an attempt to protect the kidney [43].

Animal Models of Type 1 Diabetes Mellitus

Type 1 diabetes mellitus (DM1) is characterized by the destruction of pancreatic β cells, usually associated with immune-mediated damage [44]. It is common that the patient still has some remaining β cell mass before progressing to complete absence of insulin production.

Spontaneous Animal Models of Type 1Diabetes

The NOD mouse

During the study of a cataract prone colony (the JcI-ICR mouse), a diabetic mouse was identified and, after selectively breeding, the non-obese diabetic (NOD) strain was established [45]. The mice exhibit spontaneous autoimmune diabetes usually between the 14th and the 30th week of life, with variable frequency between the different colonies. In NOD mice diabetes begins with the development of insulitis around the fourth week of age, and this may or may not progress to diabetes, depending on the pattern of immune response displayed [46, 47]. It is worth noting that the environment also directly influences the development of diabetes in NOD mice, and a review of the major centers that have NOD colonies showed great diversity in the incidence of diabetes. The period of life where we usually measure the peak incidence is in the colonies in the 30th week of life [48]. In contrast to other animal models used in research, the NOD mouse seems particularly similar to human DM1 and thus many studies have been performed in the 25 years since its establishment, including studies using the NOD mice to evaluate the RAS [37]. In 2011, Colucci *et al.* published the first paper exploring the NOD mice in the context of RAS. The authors have found combined effects of increased ACE activity and expression and decreased ACE2 expression in the kidney, indicating that in NOD mice the higher ACE/ACE2 ratio in kidneys could contribute to renal injury [49].

Animal Models of Type 2 Diabetes

Type 2 diabetes is a heterogeneous group of conditions characterized by insulin resistance and reduced insulin secretion. Obesity is one of the most common triggers for insulin resistance, the first step to Type 2 diabetes (DM2). Accordingly, animal models of obesity have been used to gain insights into the human condition. Animal models of Type 2 diabetes are expected to be as complex and heterogeneous as the human condition. While some strains (ob/ob mouse and fa/fa rat) are surprisingly able to maintain normal glucose levels at the cost of a prominent and continuous compensatory β-cell response, others (db/db mouse, for instance) rapidly develop hyperglycaemia [37, 50, 51]. Multiple studies have used these animal models to investigate the RAS, many of them with focus on the kidney damage present in uncontrolled diabetes. In a 2012 study, Pichaiwong *et al.* used the ob/ob mice to develop a new model of reversible ND, BTBR ob/ob mouse [36]. It is known that RAS inhibition is the first line of treatment for DN but it is usually able to stop and/or slow its progression. With this new diabetic mouse model the authors expect to uncover new mechanisms that could reverse DN in humans as well.

Gene Targeting and Transgenic Techniques

As seen on animal models for hypertension study, the diabetes field also benefit from the development in transgenic techniques. Many animals have been created in an effort to gain perceptions into the pathogenesis of both DM1 and DM2 diabetes, mainly by manipulating insulin receptors and glucose transporters genes (IRS1 and GLUT4, for example). To overcome potential lethal manipulations, the use of conditional transgenics have been increasing in diabetes research.

CONCLUDING REMARKS

Animal models have been extremely important in the understanding of human diseases. Unfortunately, the translation of the results to man still represents the biggest challenge. To this moment no experimental model of hypertension or diabetes has proven to exactly mimic all the symptoms of the human disease. Furthermore, the results can also be influenced by variables such as duration of exposure to causal factors and dose, differences in animal species, gender as well as age of the animal at the beginning of exposure, limiting the comparison and interpretation.

CONFLICT OF INTEREST

The authors confirm that they have no conflict of interest to declare for this publication.

ACKNOWLEDGEMENTS

The authors thank CAPES (Coordenação de Aperfeiçoamento de Pessoal de nível Superior), CNPq (Conselho Nacional de Desenvolvimento Científico e

Tecnológico) and FAPESP (Fundação de Amparo a Pesquisa do Estado de São Paulo).

REFERENCES

[1] Jandeleit-Dahm K, Cooper ME. Hypertension and diabetes: role of the renin-angiotensin system. Endocrinol Metab Clin North Am 2006; 35(3): 469-490, vii. [vii.]. [http://dx.doi.org/10.1016/j.ecl.2006.06.007] [PMID: 16959581]

[2] Cooper ME, Johnston CI. Optimizing treatment of hypertension in patients with diabetes. JAMA 2000; 283(24): 3177-9. [http://dx.doi.org/10.1001/jama.283.24.3177] [PMID: 10866846]

[3] Pitt B, Williams G, Remme W, *et al.* The EPHESUS trial: eplerenone in patients with heart failure due to systolic dysfunction complicating acute myocardial infarction. Eplerenone Post-AMI Heart Failure Efficacy and Survival Study. Cardiovasc Drugs Ther 2001; 15(1): 79-87. [http://dx.doi.org/10.1023/A:1011119003788] [PMID: 11504167]

[4] Epstein M. Aldosterone receptor blockade and the role of eplerenone: evolving perspectives. Nephrol Dial Transplant 2003; 18(10): 1984-92. [http://dx.doi.org/10.1093/ndt/gfg339] [PMID: 13679471]

[5] Rothermund L, Paul M. Hypertension and the renin-angiotensin system--evidence from genetic and transgenic studies. Basic Res Cardiol 1998; 93 (Suppl. 2): 1-6. [http://dx.doi.org/10.1007/s003950050191] [PMID: 9833155]

[6] Dornas WC, Silva ME. Animal models for the study of arterial hypertension. J Biosci 2011; 36(4): 731-7. [http://dx.doi.org/10.1007/s12038-011-9097-y] [PMID: 21857120]

[7] van der Worp HB, Howells DW, Sena ES, *et al.* Can animal models of disease reliably inform human studies? PLoS Med 2010; 7(3): e1000245. [http://dx.doi.org/10.1371/journal.pmed.1000245] [PMID: 20361020]

[8] Hackam DG, Redelmeier DA. Translation of research evidence from animals to humans. JAMA 2006; 296(14): 1731-2. [http://dx.doi.org/10.1001/jama.296.14.1731] [PMID: 17032985]

[9] Burkhardt AM, Zlotnik A. Translating translational research: mouse models of human disease. Cell Mol Immunol 2013; 10(5): 373-4. [http://dx.doi.org/10.1038/cmi.2013.19] [PMID: 23934028]

[10] Okamoto K, Aoki K. Development of a strain of spontaneously hypertensive rats. Jpn Circ J 1963; 27: 282-93. [http://dx.doi.org/10.1253/jcj.27.282] [PMID: 13939773]

[11] Zicha J, Dobešová Z, Vokurková M, *et al.* Age-dependent salt hypertension in Dahl rats: fifty years of research. Physiol Res 2012; 61 (Suppl. 1): S35-87. [PMID: 22827876]

[12] Smith TL, Hutchins PM. Central hemodynamics in the developmental stage of spontaneous hypertension in the unanesthetized rat. Hypertension 1979; 1(5): 508-17.

[http://dx.doi.org/10.1161/01.HYP.1.5.508] [PMID: 541042]

[13] Engelmann GL, Vitullo JC, Gerrity RG. Morphometric analysis of cardiac hypertrophy during development, maturation, and senescence in spontaneously hypertensive rats. Circ Res 1987; 60(4): 487-94.
[http://dx.doi.org/10.1161/01.RES.60.4.487] [PMID: 2954715]

[14] Okamoto K, Yamamoto K, Morita N, *et al.* Establishment and use of the M strain of stroke-prone spontaneously hypertensive rat. J Hypertens Suppl 1986; 4(3): S21-4.
[PMID: 3465899]

[15] Trippodo NC, Frohlich ED. Similarities of genetic (spontaneous) hypertension. Man and rat. Circ Res 1981; 48(3): 309-19.
[http://dx.doi.org/10.1161/01.RES.48.3.309] [PMID: 7460205]

[16] Campese VM. Salt sensitivity in hypertension. Renal and cardiovascular implications. Hypertension 1994; 23(4): 531-50.
[http://dx.doi.org/10.1161/01.HYP.23.4.531] [PMID: 8144222]

[17] Garrett MR, Meng H, Rapp JP, Joe B. Locating a blood pressure quantitative trait locus within 117 kb on the rat genome: substitution mapping and renal expression analysis. Hypertension 2005; 45(3): 451-9.
[http://dx.doi.org/10.1161/01.HYP.0000154678.64340.7f] [PMID: 15655120]

[18] Krege JH, John SW, Langenbach LL, *et al.* Male-female differences in fertility and blood pressure in ACE-deficient mice. Nature 1995; 375(6527): 146-8.
[http://dx.doi.org/10.1038/375146a0] [PMID: 7753170]

[19] Krege JH, Kim HS, Moyer JS, *et al.* Angiotensin-converting enzyme gene mutations, blood pressures, and cardiovascular homeostasis. Hypertension 1997; 29(1 Pt 2): 150-7.
[http://dx.doi.org/10.1161/01.HYP.29.1.150] [PMID: 9039095]

[20] Cole J, Quach DL, Sundaram K, Corvol P, Capecchi MR, Bernstein KE. Mice lacking endothelial angiotensin-converting enzyme have a normal blood pressure. Circ Res 2002; 90(1): 87-92.
[http://dx.doi.org/10.1161/hh0102.102360] [PMID: 11786523]

[21] Kessler SP, Gomos JB, Scheidemantel TS, Rowe TM, Smith HL, Sen GC. The germinal isozyme of angiotensin-converting enzyme can substitute for the somatic isozyme in maintaining normal renal structure and functions. J Biol Chem 2002; 277(6): 4271-6.
[http://dx.doi.org/10.1074/jbc.M109474200] [PMID: 11723129]

[22] Kessler SP, deS Senanayake P, Scheidemantel TS, Gomos JB, Rowe TM, Sen GC. Maintenance of normal blood pressure and renal functions are independent effects of angiotensin-converting enzyme. J Biol Chem 2003; 278(23): 21105-12.
[http://dx.doi.org/10.1074/jbc.M302347200] [PMID: 12777443]

[23] Chattopadhyay S, Kessler SP, Colucci JA, Yamashita M, Senanayake Pd, Sen GC. Tissue-specific expression of transgenic secreted ACE in vasculature can restore normal kidney functions, but not blood pressure, of Ace-/- mice. PLoS One 2014; 9(1): e87484.
[http://dx.doi.org/10.1371/journal.pone.0087484] [PMID: 24475296]

[24] Mullins JJ, Peters J, Ganten D. Fulminant hypertension in transgenic rats harbouring the mouse Ren-2

gene. Nature 1990; 344(6266): 541-4.
[http://dx.doi.org/10.1038/344541a0] [PMID: 2181319]

[25] Bachmann S, Peters J, Engler E, Ganten D, Mullins J. Transgenic rats carrying the mouse renin gene--morphological characterization of a low-renin hypertension model. Kidney Int 1992; 41(1): 24-36.
[http://dx.doi.org/10.1038/ki.1992.4] [PMID: 1593860]

[26] Bader M, Ganten D. Transgenic rats: tools to study the function of the renin-angiotensin system. Clin Exp Pharmacol Physiol 1996; 23 (Suppl. 3): S81-7.
[http://dx.doi.org/10.1111/j.1440-1681.1996.tb02818.x] [PMID: 21143278]

[27] Itoh H, Mukoyama M, Pratt RE, Gibbons GH, Dzau VJ. Multiple autocrine growth factors modulate vascular smooth muscle cell growth response to angiotensin II. J Clin Invest 1993; 91(5): 2268-74.
[http://dx.doi.org/10.1172/JCI116454] [PMID: 8486785]

[28] Granger JP, Schnackenberg CG. Renal mechanisms of angiotensin II-induced hypertension. Semin Nephrol 2000; 20(5): 417-25.
[PMID: 11022893]

[29] Goldblatt H, Lynch J, Hanzal RF, Summerville WW. Studies on experimental hypertension : I. The production of persistent elevation of systolic blood pressure by means of renal ischemia. J Exp Med 1934; 59(3): 347-79.
[http://dx.doi.org/10.1084/jem.59.3.347] [PMID: 19870251]

[30] Liard JF, Cowley AW Jr, McCaa RE, McCaa CS, Guyton AC. Renin, aldosterone, body fluid volumes, and the baroreceptor reflex in the development and reversal of Goldblatt hypertension in conscious dogs. Circ Res 1974; 34(4): 549-60.
[http://dx.doi.org/10.1161/01.RES.34.4.549] [PMID: 4857066]

[31] Suzuki H, Saruta T, Ferrario CM, Brosnihan KB. Characterization of neurohormonal changes following the production of the benign and malignant phases of two-kidney, two-clip Goldblatt hypertension. Jpn Heart J 1987; 28(3): 413-26.
[http://dx.doi.org/10.1536/ihj.28.413] [PMID: 2887673]

[32] Garwitz ET, Jones AW. Aldosterone infusion into the rat and dose-dependent changes in blood pressure and arterial ionic transport. Hypertension 1982; 4(3): 374-81.
[http://dx.doi.org/10.1161/01.HYP.4.3.374] [PMID: 6279496]

[33] Doggrell SA, Brown L. Rat models of hypertension, cardiac hypertrophy and failure. Cardiovasc Res 1998; 39(1): 89-105.
[http://dx.doi.org/10.1016/S0008-6363(98)00076-5] [PMID: 9764192]

[34] Krieger EM. NEUROGENIC HYPERTENSION IN THE RAT. Circ Res 1964; 15: 511-21.
[http://dx.doi.org/10.1161/01.RES.15.6.511] [PMID: 14243890]

[35] Thrasher TN. Unloading arterial baroreceptors causes neurogenic hypertension. Am J Physiol Regul Integr Comp Physiol 2002; 282(4): R1044-53.
[http://dx.doi.org/10.1152/ajpregu.00431.2001] [PMID: 11893608]

[36] Pichaiwong W, Hudkins KL, Wietecha T, *et al.* Reversibility of structural and functional damage in a model of advanced diabetic nephropathy. J Am Soc Nephrol 2013; 24(7): 1088-102.
[http://dx.doi.org/10.1681/ASN.2012050445] [PMID: 23641056]

[37] Rees DA, Alcolado JC. Animal models of diabetes mellitus. Diabet Med 2005; 22(4): 359-70. [http://dx.doi.org/10.1111/j.1464-5491.2005.01499.x] [PMID: 15787657]

[38] Rahimi Z, Moradi M, Nasri H. A systematic review of the role of renin angiotensin aldosterone system genes in diabetes mellitus, diabetic retinopathy and diabetic neuropathy. J Res Med Sci 2014; 19(11): 1090-8.
[PMID: 25657757]

[39] Lenzen S, Panten U. Alloxan: history and mechanism of action. Diabetologia 1988; 31(6): 337-42. [http://dx.doi.org/10.1007/BF02341500] [PMID: 3046975]

[40] Junod A, Lambert AE, Stauffacher W, Renold AE. Diabetogenic action of streptozotocin: relationship of dose to metabolic response. J Clin Invest 1969; 48(11): 2129-39.
[http://dx.doi.org/10.1172/JCI106180] [PMID: 4241908]

[41] Wang Z, Gleichmann H. GLUT2 in pancreatic islets: crucial target molecule in diabetes induced with multiple low doses of streptozotocin in mice. Diabetes 1998; 47(1): 50-6.
[http://dx.doi.org/10.2337/diab.47.1.50] [PMID: 9421374]

[42] Bono VH Jr. Review of mechanism of action studies of the nitrosoureas. Cancer Treat Rep 1976; 60(6): 699-702.
[PMID: 182364]

[43] Ronchi FA, Irigoyen MC, Casarini DE. Association of somatic and N-domain angiotensin-converting enzymes from Wistar rat tissue with renal dysfunction in diabetes mellitus. J Renin Angiotensin Aldosterone Syst 2007; 8(1): 34-41.
[http://dx.doi.org/10.3317/jraas.2007.005] [PMID: 17487824]

[44] Dahlquist G. The aetiology of type 1 diabetes: an epidemiological perspective. Acta Paediatr Suppl 1998; 425: 5-10.
[http://dx.doi.org/10.1111/j.1651-2227.1998.tb01244.x] [PMID: 9822187]

[45] Makino S, Kunimoto K, Muraoka Y, Mizushima Y, Katagiri K, Tochino Y. Breeding of a non-obese, diabetic strain of mice. Jikken Dobutsu 1980; 29(1): 1-13.
[PMID: 6995140]

[46] Atkinson MA, Leiter EH. The NOD mouse model of type 1 diabetes: as good as it gets? Nat Med 1999; 5(6): 601-4.
[http://dx.doi.org/10.1038/9442] [PMID: 10371488]

[47] Delovitch TL, Singh B. The nonobese diabetic mouse as a model of autoimmune diabetes: immune dysregulation gets the NOD. Immunity 1997; 7(6): 727-38.
[http://dx.doi.org/10.1016/S1074-7613(00)80392-1] [PMID: 9430219]

[48] Pozzilli P, Signore A, Williams AJ, Beales PE. NOD mouse colonies around the world--recent facts and figures. Immunol Today 1993; 14(5): 193-6.
[http://dx.doi.org/10.1016/0167-5699(93)90160-M] [PMID: 8517916]

[49] Colucci JA, Yuri Arita D, Sousa Cunha T, *et al.* Renin-angiotensin system may trigger kidney damage in NOD mice. J Renin Angiotensin Aldosterone Syst 2011; 12(1): 15-22.
[http://dx.doi.org/10.1177/1470320310375456] [PMID: 20627940]

[50] Lee GH, Proenca R, Montez JM, *et al.* Abnormal splicing of the leptin receptor in diabetic mice. Nature 1996; 379(6566): 632-5.
[http://dx.doi.org/10.1038/379632a0] [PMID: 8628397]

[51] Phillips MS, Liu Q, Hammond HA, *et al.* Leptin receptor missense mutation in the fatty Zucker rat. Nat Genet 1996; 13(1): 18-9.
[http://dx.doi.org/10.1038/ng0596-18] [PMID: 8673096]

CHAPTER 16

Quantification of Angiotensins: Is there a Consensus in the Literature?

Zaira Palomino Jara[2], **Andréia Cristina Febba Gomes**[2], **Fernanda Barrinha Fernandes**[2], **Dale M Seth**[1], **Minolfa C. Prieto**[1], **L. Gabriel Navar**[1] and **Dulce Elena Casarini**[2,*]

[1] *Department of Physiology, Tulane University, School of medicine, New Orleans, Lousianna, USA*

[2] *Department of Medicine, Nephrology Division, Escola Paulista de Medicina, Universidade Federal de Sao Paulo, Sao Paulo, Brazil*

Abstract: The renin angiotensin system (RAS) is an essential regulator of renal and cardiovascular function. The components of this system are present in the circulation, organs, tissues and various cell types; and their syntheses in the organs are independent of the circulation. Understanding how the circulatory and organ RAS interact in the maintenance of the body function is knowledge that is not only key, but absolutely essential in helping us to unravel the implications of the RAS in a disease process. In this regard, this chapter aims to verify whether or not there is a consensus in the literature for the reported quantities and concentrations of Angiotensin I (Ang I), Angiotensin II (Ang II) and Angiotensin 1-7 (Ang1-7) in normal physiological states in mice, rats and humans. Because of the various methods for quantification of angiotensins, there is not presently a clear consensus for the absolute quantities of these peptides in plasma and the different tissues.

Keywords: Angiotensins, Angiotensin converting enzyme (ACE), Angiotensin converting enzyme 2 (ACE2), Angiotensin I, Angiotensin II, Angiotensin 1-7,

* **Corresponding author Dulce Elena Casarini:** Rua Botucatu, 740 – 2° andar, Department of Medicine/Nephrology Division, Vila Clementino – Sao Paulo/SP, Brazil, CEP 04023-900; Tel: +55 11 5904-1687; E-mail: casarini.elena@unifesp.br.

Dulce Elena Casarini, Danielle Yuri Arita, Tatiana Sousa Cunha & Juliana Almada Colucci (Eds.)

Consensus, Enzyme-linked immunosorbent assay (ELISA), Extraction of angiotensins, High performance liquid chromatography (HPLC), Liquid chromatography (LC) mass spectrometry (MS), Plasma angiotensins, Protease inhibitors, Radioimmunoassay (RIA), Tissue angiotensins.

INTRODUCTION

The renin angiotensin system (RAS) is an essential regulator of arterial blood pressure, and cardiovascular and renal functions. The first observation as a blood pressure regulator was in 1898 when Tigerstedt and Bergman discovered the rate-limiting enzyme renin [1]. The initial description of this system was related to the discovery of the circulating RAS. The circulating RAS starts with renin released from the kidney, which cleaves angiotensinogen (Agt) to form angiotensin I (Ang I). The decapeptide Ang I (Asp^{1}-$Arg^{2-}Val^{3}$-Tyr^{4}-Ile^{5}-$His^{6-}Pro^{7}$-Phe^{8}-His^{9}-Leu^{10}-COOH is converted by angiotensin converting enzyme (ACE) to form angiotensin II (Ang II: Asp^{1}-Arg^{2}-Val^{3}-Tyr^{4}-$Ile^{5-}His^{6}$-Pro^{7}-Phe^{8}-COOH) that is the first and major active angiotensin peptide (Ang). Since then, many studies have described other angiotensin peptides (Angs) and enzymes in tissues and fluids. The Angs can be biologically active or inactive, within the active peptides are: Ang III (Ang 2-8: Arg^{2}-Val^{3}-Tyr^{4}-Ile^{5}-His^{6}-Pro^{7}-Phe^{8}-COOH), Ang IV (Ang 3-8: Val^{3}-Tyr^{4}-Ile^{5}-His^{6}-Pro^{7}-Phe^{8}-COOH), Ang 1-9 (Asp^{1}-Arg^{2}-Val^{3}-Tyr^{4}-Ile^{5}-His^{6}-Pro^{7}-Phe^{8}-His^{9}-COOH), Ang 1-7 (Asp^{1}-Arg^{2}-Val^{3}-Tyr^{4}-Ile^{5}-His^{6}-Pro^{7}-COOH), Ang 3-4, Ang A and Alamandine (Ala^{1}-Arg^{2}-Val^{3}-Tyr^{4}-Ile^{5}-His^{6}-Pro^{7}-COOH). The inactive angiotensins are Ang 1-12 (Asp^{1}-Arg^{2}-Val^{3}-Tyr^{4}-Ile^{5}-His^{6}-Pro^{7}-Phe^{8}-His^{9}-Leu^{10}-Leu^{11}-Val^{12}-COOH), Ang 1-5 (Asp^{1}-Arg^{2}-Val^{3}-Tyr^{4}-Ile^{5}-COOH), Ang 1-4 (Asp^{1}-Arg^{2}-Val^{3}-Tyr^{4}-COOH), Ang 2-7 (Arg^{2}-Val^{3}-Tyr^{4}-Ile^{5}-His^{6}-Pro^{7}-COOH), Ang 3-7 (Val^{3}-Tyr^{4}-Ile^{5}-His^{6}-Pro^{7}-COOH), Ang 5-8 (Ile^{5}-His^{6}-Pro^{7}-Phe^{8}-COOH), and Ang 5-7 (Ile^{5}-His^{6}-Pro^{7}-COOH). All the Angs are formed by the action of a diverse range of enzymes such as aspartyl, serine, thiol, and metallo-proteases among other enzymes (Fig. **1**) [2 - 6].

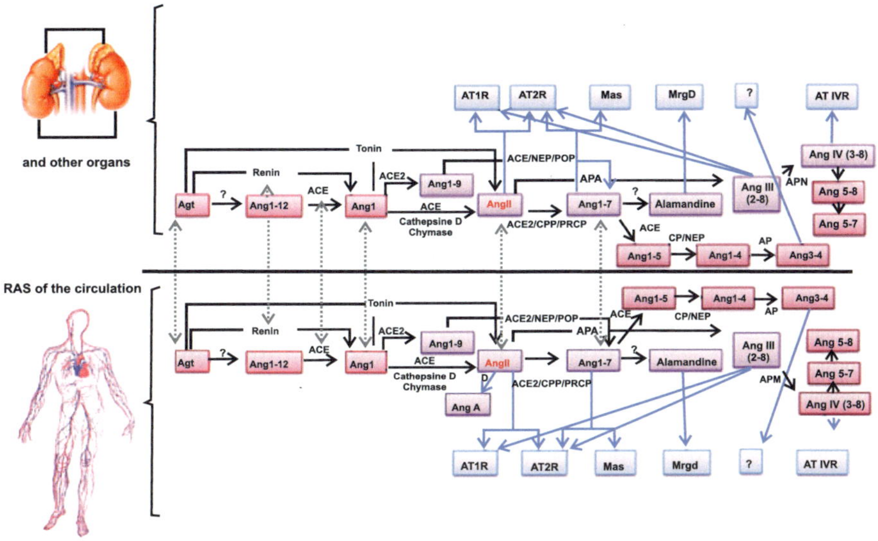

Fig. (1). Renin-angiotensin system cascade. Active peptides: Ang1-9, Ang II, Ang A, Ang1-7; Alamandine; and inactive peptides: Ang1-12, Ang I, Ang 1-5, Ang1-4, Ang 3-4, Ang5-8, Ang5-7. Protein: Agt: angiotensinogen Enzymes: renin, angiotensin I-converting enzyme (ACE), angiotensin converting enzyme 2 (ACE2) -, AP – aminopeptidase (AP), aminopeptidase A (APA), aminopeptidase N (APN), –carboxypeptidase (CP), - endopeptidase (EP), –carboxypeptidase P (CPP), prolyl carboxypeptidase (PRCP), neprilysin (NEP), prolyl oligopeptidase (PO). Receptors: AT1, AT2, Mas, MrgD, ATIVR.

Two Angs have been extensively studied, Ang II and Ang 1-7, that are present in the circulation, organs, tissues and cell types, and have endocrine, paracrine, autocrine and intracrine functions. Pathophysiologically, Ang II has been implicated in hypertension, inflammation, fibrosis, and proteinuria. On the other hand, Ang 1-7 has been shown to act as an anti-hypertensive, anti-inflammatory and anti-fibrosis peptide [7 - 12]. However, these phenotypes for Ang II and Ang 1-7 are highly generalized concepts. Further dissection of the function of Angs is necessary, so that we can better understand their pathophysiology. Indeed, Ang II acts on vascular smooth muscle cells (VSMC) causing vasoconstriction while acting on the endothelial cells to elicit vasodilation by the same angiotensin type 1 receptor (AT1R) [13]. This specific study demonstrated that what is true for one tissue may not be for others. Can Ang 1-7 behave in the same pattern as Ang II, being a vasoconstrictor and a vasodilator depending upon the cell type? The same question can be raised for the other activc Angs, which are present in the circulation, organs, tissues and cells; although their syntheses in the organs are independent of the circulating RAS. Many authors have questioned the implication that the local RAS is more important in mediating organ damage as part of disease processes. The RAS components have endocrine, paracrine, autocrine and intracrine activities, and it is not completely clear how these components interact in the disease process. Regardless, knowing the quantities of Angs in the circulation and in the tissues, in physiological and pathophysiological states, is of importance in helping us to understand the disease process of many disorders where the RAS is involved. Therefore, we can conclude that knowing the specific quantities of the Angs in various systems and in the circulation and organs is indispensable.

To further understand the behavior of RAS, more specifically of the Ang peptides, numerous studies have been performed on the development and application of methods for Angs analyses. In this chapter we present an analysis of the following methods: radioimmunoassay (RIA), high performance liquid chromatography (HPLC), HPLC followed by RIA, and the enzyme immunoassay (ELISA). These methods were used for quantification of the Ang I, Ang II, and Ang 1-7 mentioned in the Tables **1**, **2** and **3**.

Table 1. Plasma quantities of Ang I, Ang II and Ang 1-7 reported by some author since 1991 to present.

ID graph	Method	Ang I		Ang II		Ang 1-7		Specie	Author
		Quantity described	fmol/mL	Quantity described	fmol/mL	Quantity described	fmol/mL		
A	RIA	10.0 pg/mL	7.7	-	-	-	-	mouse	Senador D *et al* 2010
B	ELISA	-	-	100 pg/dL	1	-	-	rat	Zhang S *et al* 2013
C	HPLC-RIA	12.0 fmol/mL	12	10 fmol/mL	10	-	-	mouse	Xiao HD *et al* 2004
D	RIA	57.0 pg/mL	43	28 pg/mL	28	8 pg/mL	8.9	human	Mustafá HI *et al* 2011
E	RIA	75.0 pg/mL	57	-	-	-	-	rat	Carroll MA *et al* 2014
F	RIA	80.0 fmol/mL	80	30 fmol/mL	30	-	-	rat	Ferrario CM *et al* 2009
G	RIA	101.6 fmol/mL	101.6	31.2 fmol/mL	31	14.2 fmol/mL	14.2	rat	Gironacci MM *et al*, 2007
H	ELISA	-	-	35 pg/mL	35	-	-	rat	Dagan A *et al* 2010
I	?	-	-	39 pg/mL	39	-	-	rat	Granado M *et al* 2013
J	RIA	13.1 fmol/mL	13.1	42 fmol/mL	42	-	-	human	Ferrario CM *et al* 2013
K	RIA	300 pM	300	50 pM	50	125 pM	125	rat	Mori Y *et al* 2014
L	HPLC	-	-	50 fmol/mL	50	-	-	rat	Campbell *et al* 1991
M	ELISA	-	-	50.3 fmol/mL	50	932 fmol/mL	932	mouse	Wysocki J *et al* 2014
N	CE	-	-	66.9 pmol/L	66	67.9 pmol/L	67.9	human	Sim KM *et al* 2003
O	RIA	-	-	90 fmol/mL	90	-	-	rat	Ohnishi *et al* 2013
P	RIA	992 pg/mL	763	110 pg/mL	110	-	-	mouse	Cole J *et al* 2000
Q	ELISA	-	-	115 fmol/mL	115	-	-	rat	Li XC *et al* 2011
R	ELISA	-	-	150 pg/mL	150	-	-	dog	Hu J *et al* 2014
S	RIA	-	-	210 pg/mL	210	-	-	rat	Ahmed MA *et al* 2013
T	RIA	-	-	220 fmol/mL	220	-	-	rat	Walkowski A *et al* 2010
U	ELISA	-	-	249 pg/mL	249	-	-	mouse	Hara M *et al* 2002
V	RIA	1000 pg/mL	769	250 pg/mL	250	60 pg/mL	66.7	rat	Arnold AC *et al* 2011
W	?	-	-	250 pg/mL	250	600pg/mL	666.7	mouse	Peña-Silva RA *et al* 2012
Y	ELISA	-	-	1 ug/L	1000	-	-	rat	Deng J *et al* 2011
Z	RIA	-	-	100 pmol/L	100,000	-	-	dog	Imaki R *et al* 2008
AA	ELISA	-	-	0.35 ug/mL	350,000	-	-	rat	Kim JM *et al* 2012
BB	ELISA	-	-	-	-	10 ng/mL	11,111	rat	Zong W *et al* 2011

A [30]; B [28]; C [37]; D [33]; E [49]; F [38]; G [35]; H [50]; I [51]; J [52]; K [36]; L [53]; M [42]; N [44]; O [54]; P [39]; Q [40]; R [55]; S [56]; T [57]; U [58]; V [32]; W[43]; Y [59]; Z [60]; AA [29]; BB [34].

Table 2. Kidney quantities of Ang I, Ang II and Ang 1-7 reported by some author since 1991 to present.

ID graph	Method	Ang I		Ang II		Ang 1-7		Organ	Specie	Author
		Quantity described	fmol/g	Quantity described	fmol/g	Quantity described	fmol/g			
A	RIA	-	-	65 fmol/g	65	-	-	Kidney	rat	Kobori H *et al,* 2004
B	RIA	-	-	90 fmol/g	90	-	-	kidney	rat	Ohnishi K *et al,* 2013
C	ELISA	-	-	150 fmol/g	150	-	-	kidney	rat	Navar LG *et al,* 2002
D	RIA	219.8 fmol/g	219.8	158.6 fmol/g	158.6	53.1 fmol/g	53.1	kidney	rat	Gironacci MM *et al* 2007
E	ELISA	-	-	163.6 pg/g	163.6	-	-	kidney	rat	Dagan A *et al,* 2010
F	ELISA	-	-	172 pg/g	172	-	-	kidney	rat	Li XC *et al,* 2011
G	HPLC-RIA	39 fmol/g	39	200 fmol/g	200	-	-	kidney	mouse	Xiao HD *et al,* 2004
H	HPLC-RIA	40 fmol/g	40	300 fmol/g	300	-	-	kidney	rat	ONG FS *et al,* 2012
I	RIA	-	-	320 fmol/g	320	-	-	kidney	rat	Walkowska A *et al,* 2010
J	HPLC	-	-	340 fmol/g	340	-	-	kidney	rat	Campbell DJ *et al,* 1991
K	RIA	-	-	1000 pg/g	1000	-	-	kidney	rat	Ahmed MA *et al,* 2013
L	ELISA	-	-	1.5 fmol/mg	1,500	0.8 fmol/mg	800	kidney	mouse	Wysocki J *et al,* 2014
M	ELISA	-	-	10 fmol/mg	10,000	0.78 fmol/mg	780	kidney	mouse	Wysocki J *et al,* 2010
N	RIA	-	-	15 pg/mg	15,000	6 pg/mg	6,666	kidney	mouse	Senador D *et al,* 2010
O	HPLC	35 ng/g	26,923	95 ng/g	95,000	39 ng/g	43,300	kidney	rat	Ronchi FA *et al,* 2007
P	RIA	110 fmol/g	110	788 fmol/g	788	-	-	kidney	mouse	Park *et al* 2009
Q	RIA	9 fmol/mg	9,000	25 fmol/mg	25,000	14 fmol/mg	14,000	kidney	mouse	Modrall et al, 2004

A [46]; B [54]; C [11]; D [35]; E [50]; F [40]; G [41]; H[47]; I[57]; J[53]; K[56]; L 42]; M [48]; N[30]; O [45]; P [69]: Q [70]

Table 3. Hypothalamusm, heart, lung and adrenal glands quantities of Ang I, Ang II and Ang 1-7 reported by some author since 1991 to present.

ID graph	Method	Ang I		Ang II		Ang 1-7		Organ	Specie	Author
		Quantity described	fmol/g	Quantity described	fmol/g	Quantity described	fmol/g			
R	RIA	50 fmol/g	50	196.9 fmol/g	196.9	146.6	146.6	hypothalamus	rat	Gironacci MM *et al,* 2007
S	HPLC-RIA	1.1 pmol/g	1100	1.18 pmol/g	1,180	1.45 pmol/g	1450	hypothalamus	rat	Chappell MC *et al,* 1989
T	RIA	-	-	32.3 fmol/g	32.3	16.3 fmol/g	16.3	heart	rat	Gironacci MM *et al,* 2007
U	HPLC-RIA	4.2 fmol/g	4.2	48 fmol/g	48	-	-	heart	mouse	Xiao HD *et al,* 2004
V	HPLC-RIA	-	-	150 pg/mg	150,000	-	-	heart	rat	Belmadani S *et al,* 2007
X	ELISA	-	-	78.3 ng/g	78,300	-	-	lung	rat	Deng J *et al,* 2012
Z	HPLC-RIA	0.19 pmol/g	190	1.10 pmol/g	1100	0.14 pmol/g	140	Adrenal gland	rat	Chappell MC *et al,* 1989

R [35]; S[61]; T[35]; U[41]; V [62]; X[59]; Z [61]

Regardless of the measurement method, the collection is the most important step in the accurate assessment of the endogenous levels of the Angs. Appropriate precautions must be taken to arrest all enzymatic activity as the sample is collected or immediately post-harvesting using sufficient specific inhibitors. Continued enzymatic activity may lead to altered values that do not accurately reflect the endogenous levels. Accordingly, samples are either collected into a cocktail of enzyme inhibitors or immediately homogenized in methanol or other agents that instantly arrest enzymatic activity but do not degrade the peptides, followed by centrifugation [14 - 17]. The extraction of Ang peptides can be done using C18 Sep-Pak (Waters associates) columns where they are absorbed to the column to be eluted with acetonitrile [14]. The type of column matrix, elution solvent, will definitely affect the quantification of the Ang peptides. Internal standard angiotensin peptides are added to each sample to determine the recovery during the extraction process, which can routinely range from 60-90% for plasma or tissues.

Radioimmunoassay (RIA)

The radioimmunoassay has been used for Ang peptides quantification since 1967 [18]. This method uses monoclonal and polyclonal anti-Ang II, Ang I or Ang 1-7 antibodies that are able to differentiate between these peptides, but have cross-reactivity with Ang III, Ang IV and Ang V because of sequence homologies. In the literature, the cross-reactivity of anti-Ang I antiserum was described with Ang II and anti-Ang II antiserum with Ang I of 0.5%. Interestingly, authors showed 100% of cross-reactivity for anti-Ang II antiserum with Ang III [18]. Accordingly, immunoreactive Ang II includes both Ang II and Ang III. The RIA detection limit for Ang I and Ang II is about 4 pg/mL and 2 pg/mL for Ang II. Despite the non –selectivity of some antibodies for angiotensin peptides that are not able to distinguish N-terminal portion of peptides, the use of RIA allows the quantification of endogenous peptides found in the tissues or circulation [14]. The variation of plasma values obtained using RIA for Ang II described in the literature was from 28 to 100,000 fmol/mL (Table **1**).

High Performance Liquid Chromatography (Hplc) and Hplc Followed by Ria

De Silva *et al.* (1988) [14] described the association of HPLC and RIA for the determination of concentrations of Ang peptides. This analytical approach was developed because the RIA method requires antibodies of high affinity that are difficult to obtain. The HPLC system consists of pressurized pumps that control the flow of liquid through columns filled with a matrix, thereby allowing the separation of sample components. However, in order to inject a biological material into a HPLC system, the sample must be taken through an extraction process. De Silva *et al.* (1988) [14] described the extraction process using C18 Sep-Pak (Waters associates) that eliminates potential unknown substances that may interfere with the RIA. This research group tested adrenal, ovary, uterus, brain and kidney samples and they detected Ang II, Ang 2-8, Ang 3-8, Ang 4-8 in the picogram range. They found that when RIA was performed with the collected fraction of samples after HPLC separation (following C18 Sep-Pak extraction) the recovery was 93 ± 4% compared 77 ± 0.4% RIA alone. Thus, the extraction of the samples is important to provide pure samples for analysis in the RIA or HPLC [14 - 18]. In the literature the variation for tissue Ang II using HPLC-RIA was from 48 to 150,000 fmol/g (Tables **2** and **3**).

In 2002, Pelegrini-da Silva *et al.* described another analytical HPLC method for Ang quantification. They separated and detected peptides in pmol amounts as: 1 pmol Ang II (5-8); 248 pmol Phe-His-Leu; 80.6 pmol Ang II; 63.8 pmol Ang III; 83.8 pmol Ang II (3-8); 237.7 pmol Ang I (5-10); 82.5 pmol Ang I; 115.8 pmol Ang I (4-10); 121.6 pmol of human renin tridecapeptide substrate and 420 pmol of renin inhibitor (Pro-His-Pro-Phe-His-Phe-Phe-Val-Tyr-Lys) [19].

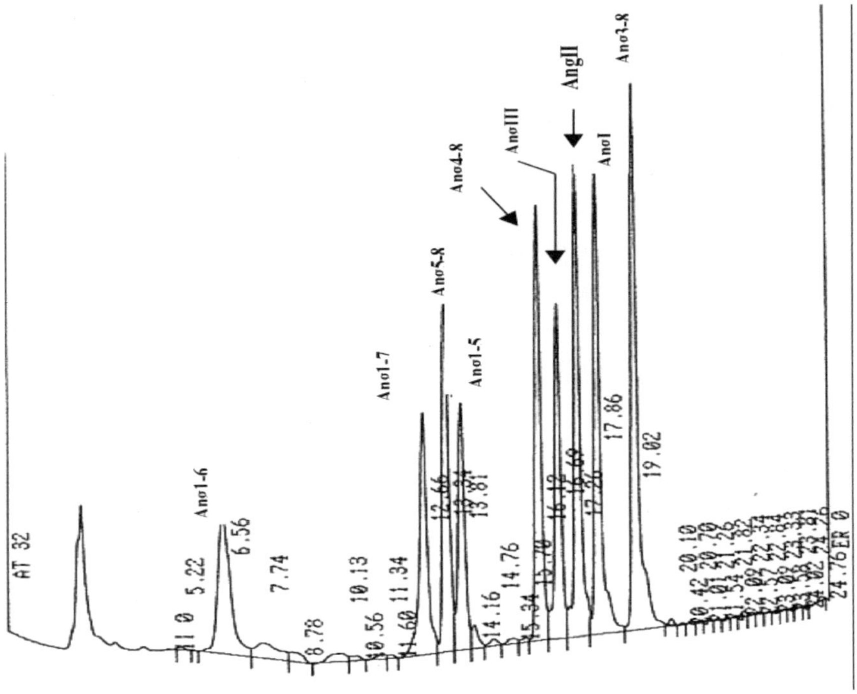

Fig. (2). Reverse-phase HPLC of angiotensin peptide standards. The effluent was monitored at 214 nm. The peptides separation was performed using an Aquapore OD 300 column, 7 mm (4.6 × 250 mm) (Applied Biosciences, USA), equilibrated with 0.1% phosphoric acid in 5% acetonitrile. The peptides were separated with a flow rate of 1.5 ml/min by isocratic elution for 5 min, followed by a linear gradient from 5 to 35% acetonitrile in 0.1% phosphoric acid during 20 min. Chromatogram of 1000 pmol of each peptide. Retention time of peptides in minutes: Ang1-6, 6.56; Ang1-7, 12.66; Ang 5-8, 13.34; Ang1-5, 13.81; Ang4-8, 15.70; AIII, 16.12; Ang II, 16.69; Ang I, 17.26 and Ang3-8, 19.02 (Casarini DE, personal data not published).

Our group also developed a HPLC method for quantification of Angs, specifically to quantify the biologically active RAS peptides of plasma, organs and different cell types cultured *in vitro* [20 - 25]. For sample collection and extraction, we use a pool of serine-, thiol-, aspartyl- and metallo protease inhibitors to avoid hydrolysis by peptidases. For the Angs separation, we used the HPLC with ultraviolet detection (214 nm). An Aquapore OD 300 column, 7 mm (4.6 x 250 mm) confers our method favorable separation of Angs. The peptides are separated by 5 minutes of isocratic elution, followed by 20 minutes of linear gradient from 5 to 35% acetonitrile in 0.1% phosphoric acid, under a flow of 1.5 ml/min. Fig. (**2**) shows the profile of the Angs separation. Identification of Ang peaks is based on the retention time, and the quantification is based on a peak area ratio. We have established standard curves for each peptide from fmol to pmol (pg to ng), and the inferior detection limit was 10 fmol. With this HPLC method, the Ang levels obtained for plasma and tissues ranges from fmol to pmol [20 - 27].

Although it has been suggested that the HPLC method based on detection with UV 214 nm does not allow the separation of all angiotensin peptides, in Fig. (**2**) we can see the chromatogram from our laboratory with all the retention times for each peptide demonstrating that they are distinct allowing complete separation thereof, and that the recovery of peptides is with high reproducibility. Based on the quality of the chromatographic profile established in our method using HPLC, we can infer that if we have a concomitant elution for example of Ang II peak and some minor fragment of angiotensin that matches between 1-2% of the total content in it, this factor does not change nor mask a physiological level found, considering that we always have a control group compared to experimental. A quality control of our method was done with the elution and collection in the same tube of Ang I, Ang II and Ang 1-7 peaks detected in each chromatogram of control and experimental groups, followed by the Edman sequencing of these peptides for confirming the existence of each of them in this eluate.

The variations found in plasma and tissues using the method of quantification of Angs by HPLC can be explained by various factors and precautions that if not correctly observed can generate erroneous values. These include: the handling of animals to avoid or minimize stress, collecting samples after anesthesia and/or decapitation, processing blood and homogenate samples in the presence of protease inhibitors, ensuring rapid centrifugation in a refrigerated centrifuge followed, recognizing differences among animal strains, and other factors.

Enzyme-Linked Immunosorbent Assay (ELISA)

This analytic approach for measuring Angs has been adopted extensively by many biotechnological companies. In this method, plates coated with antibodies detect the presence of Ang I or Ang II or Ang 1-7. Then a further specific antibody (anti-Ang I, or anti-Ang II or anti-Ang1-7) is applied over the surface so it can bind to Ang I or Ang II or Ang 1-7**.** The second antibody in general is linked to an enzyme, which reacts with a substrate causing a color change. Since the quality and reproducibility of ELISA hinges upon the availability of specific antibodies, and considering the difficulty in producing specific antibodies, potential cross-reactivity problems cannot be excluded. In the literature, Ang levels reported for plasma using ELISA quantification have a variation from 1 to 350 000 fmol/mL (Tables **1** & **2**) [28, 29].

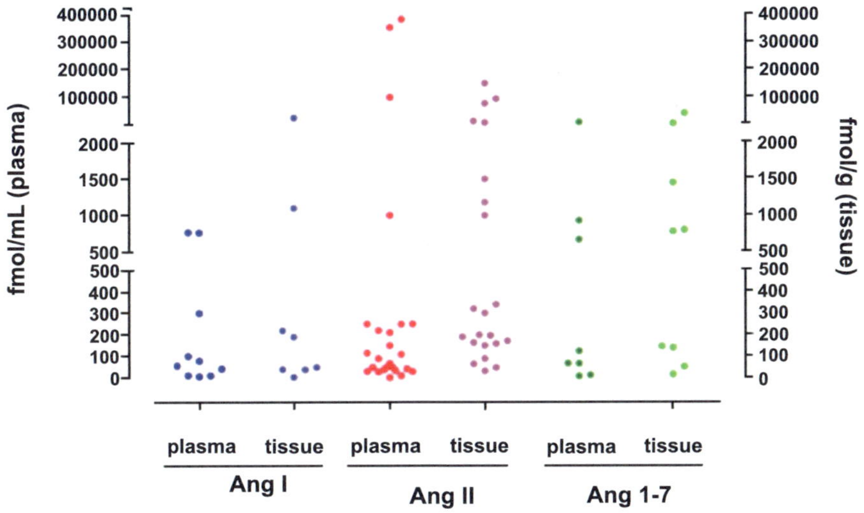

Fig. (3). Distribution of reported Ang I, Ang II and Ang 1-7 values based on data presented in Tables 1, 2 and 3. On the left "y" axis is the plasma unit (fmol/mL), and on the right "y" axis is the tissue unit (fmol/g).

Quantities of Ang I, Ang II and Ang 1-7 Reported in the Literature

Reported values of Ang I, Ang II and Ang 1-7 levels for mouse, rat, dog, and humans without physiological disorders described in the literature have been summarized. All the values were transformed to fmol/mL for the plasma, and fmol/g for tissues. The summary of plasma Ang levels are in Table **1**, the kidney in Table **2**, and the heart, hypothalamus and adrenal gland are in Table **3**. The distribution of the Angs values for both plasma and tissues are depicted in Fig. (**3**).

The summary of Table **1** indicates that:

1. In the plasma of mice, rats, and humans samples; the amount of Ang I ranged from 7.7 to 769 fmol/mL Senador D *et al.* (2010) [21, 30] = 10 pg/mL *vs* Nishiyama *et al.* (2003) [31] and Arnold AC *et al.* (2011) [32] = 1000pg/mL). The amount of Ang II ranged from 1 to 350,000 fmol/mL Zhang S *et al.* (2013) [28] = 100 pg/dL *vs* Kim JM *et al.* (2012) [29] = 1000pg/mL) and Ang1-7 ranged from 8.9 to 11,111 fmol/mL Mustafa HI *et al.* (2011) [33] = 8.9 pg/mL *vs*. Zong W *et al.* (2011) [34] = 10 ng/mL).
2. Arnold AC *et al.* (2011), Mustafá HI *et al.* (2011) Gironacci MM *et al.* (2007), measured the three Angs, and those studies reported Ang I > Ang II > Ang1-7 [32, 33, 35]. Mori Y *et al.* (2014) reported Ang I >Ang 1-7 > Ang II [36].
3. Again four studies measured only Ang I and Ang II, three of them found Ang I > Ang II [37 - 41]. One study that measured plasma Angs, reported Ang I < Ang II.
4. Three studies measured only Ang II and Ang 1-7. Two found Ang1-7 > Ang II [42, 43], the other one found equal levels of Ang1-7 and Ang II [44].

The summary of Tables **2** and **3** indicates that:

1. In tissue samples of mice and rats, the amount of Ang I ranged from 39 to 26,923 fmol/g Xiao HD *et al.* (2011) [37] = 39 fmol/g *vs* Ronchi FA *et al.* (2007) [45] = 35ng/g). The amount of Ang II ranged from 65 to 95,000 fmol/g Kobori H *et al.* (2004) [46] = 100 pg/dL, Nishiyama *et al.* (2003)[32] = 157 fmol/g *vs* Ronchi FA *et al.* (2007) [45]= 95ng/g) and Ang1-7 ranged from 53.1 to 43,300 fmol/g Gironacci MM *et al.* (2007)[35] = 53.1 fmol/g *vs* Ronchi FA *et al.* (2007) [45] = 39 ng/g).
2. Two studies measured Ang I, Ang II and Ang 1-7. One study found Ang I >

Ang > Ang1-7 [35], and the other one found Ang II > Ang 1-7 > Ang I [45].

3. Two studies only measured Ang I and Ang II, both found Ang II > Ang I [37, 47].
4. Two studies only measured Ang II and Ang 1-7, both found Ang II > Ang1-7 [30, 42, 48].
5. There is also variation described for the hypothalamus in the levels of Angs reported by Gironacci MM *et al.,* (2007) and Chappell MC *et al.,* (1989) of 50 and 1100 fmol/g for Ang I, 196.9 and 1180 fmol/g for Ang II and 146,6 to 1450 for Ang1-7, respectively [35, 61]. Specifically comparing the values obtained for hypothalamus described by Chappell MC *et al.,* (1989) using HPLC-RIA and for adrenal in the same study, the variation detected for Ang I was

The general picture of this summary indicates that there is a huge variability of Ang quantities reported using RIA, HPLC, HPLC+RIA and ELISA methods. In the last four decades a massive effort has been made to optimize the quantification of Angs, and the results are positive, with current methods, it is possible to reach inferior detection limits of fmol, which was very difficult to achieve two decades ago. Nevertheless, it seems that we still are facing some problems because there is not a consensus in the literature.

Based on the summary, quantities of Ang II in the plasma measured with RIA go from 28 to 100,000 fmol/mL and in the kidney go from 65 to 15,000 fmol/g. A very large variation is also seen in ELISA, with a range of 1 to 350,000 fmol/mL and of 150 to 10,000 fmol/g for plasma and tissue, respectively. Both assays use antibodies, and although the quality of antibodies has improved (improving the sensitivity), it seems that there are still cross-reactivity issues (lack of specificity). When comparing the HPLC, and the HPLC+RIA to the ELISA and RIA methods, we can also see the same pattern. For kidney and heart tissues the range for HPLC goes from 340 to 95,000 fmol/g and for HPLC+RIA from 48 to 150,000. Although the HPLC system has been considered having greater specificity, the variation found with this method could be related to: a) stationary phase, mobile phase, the separation method (isocratic or gradient); b) the size of the column, the size of the loop of injection, the wavelength used for detections. Other issues that may be linked to all the methods include sample handling. The method of handling blood specimens determines whether results from an accurate assay methodology represent physiological plasma levels or *in vitro* artifacts as described by Moore DJ *et al.* (1993) [63]. Many investigators recommend the use of protease inhibitors for plasma collection. For 10 mL of blood inhibitors should be used in the following concentrations: 50 μL of 0.5 M EDTA and 0.5 M captopril, trypsin inhibitor (0.15 mg/ml blood), aprotinin (2 μg/ml blood) and pepstatin A 14 (4 μg/ml blood). The majority of methods for collection of blood or preparation of tissue homogenates use pepstatin as a classical aspartyl protease inhibitor. More recently, aliskiren, a specific renin inhibitor, has been adopted. In this regard, there is a commercially available cocktail of inhibitors (Roche, Cat # 11836153001) that can be used for collection and extraction of biological samples [44]. Tissue samples also should be processed in the presence of protease inhibitors. The cocktail of inhibitors prevents both generation and degradation of the Angs prior to their measurement [64]. Finally, careful attention should be paid in order to choose an appropriate extraction/concentration (E/C) method to avoid fragmentation of the Ang peptides caused by the E/C method even in the presence of a pool of inhibitors.

Liquid Chromatography (LC) Mass Spectrometry (MS) (LC-MS/MS)

More recent methods based on mass spectrometry combined with liquid chromatography are described in the literature. They include screening for Ang metabolites using: LC-MS in MS full-scan mode [65], electrospray ionization—(tandem) mass spectrometric ESI-MS(/MS) [66], and sensitive LC-MS/MS methods in the selective reaction monitoring (SRM). Stoppacher *et al.* (2013) [67] using LCMS/MS for synthetic Ang II, Ang III, Ang IV, Ang (1-4) and Ang (4- 8) showed mass accuracy of ± 5 ppm for the specified m/z values. He separated a standard mixture containing six peptides extracted from ion current chromatograms with mass tolerance of ± 5 ppm: 552.27764 m/z (Ang 1-4; retention time 5.12 min), 4666.26106 (Ang III; retention time 24.88 min), 338.67630 m/z (Ang 4-8), 523.77453 m/z (Ang II; retention time 30.82), 3888.21051 m/z (Ang IV), and 432.89977 m/z (Ang II) [67].

Further, Ali *et al.* (2014) [68] developed LC-MS/MS method of angiotensin peptides quantification for tissues such as kidney, epididymal white adipose and fluids including urine and plasma. The results obtained for Ang 1-7 and Ang II in adipose tissue were 290 - 350 and 120-150 fmol/mg and in kidney 320 - 350 and 140 -200 fmol/mg respectively. For plasma the authors described Ang 1-7 and Ang II with 35 – 40 and 15 -20 fmol/uL and for urine 100 -105 and 45 -50 fmol/uL, respectively.

In comparing results from Ali *et al.* (2014) for kidney Ang II with the other values listed in Table **2**, the 95 fmol/mg (95,000 fmol/g) is the highest reported value. When comparing the results from the same authors for kidney Ang1-7 with 43.3 fmol/mg (43,300 fmol/g), with the others reported in Table **2** again it is the highest value. It would seem that the LC-MS/MS method is more sensitive than the existing methods for quantification of Angs [68, 70, 71]. The methods that exist today depending on their specificity often cannot recover all peptide content of biological samples, whether fluids or tissues.

The use of capillary-HPLC interfaced to an ion trap HTC from Brucker by Lortie *et al.* (2009) [71] permitted the quantification of Ang II from human plasma with high sensitivity detecting 6 fmol of Ang II. Using a nanoLC ChipCube from Agilent coupled to a XCT Ultra ion trap mass spectrometer, Schulz *et al.* (2014) [72] obtained a separation of Ang I, Ang II and Ang III, with a limit of detection per injection of 10 amole – 10 fmole.

Poglitsh *et al.* (2012) proposed the analysis of angiotensin peptide using mass spectrometry fingerprint thus introducing a new concept where the balances between the levels of the peptides are deduced from the activity of various enzymes. The limit of sensitivity of LC-MS/MS determined for human plasma in this method was 1 fmol/mL [73].

By using new forms of RAS analysis the LC-MS/MS by the system fingerprint, Poglitsh *et al.* showed new pathways not previously detected, thus opening new perspectives for the best way for the treatment of renal and cardiovascular disease. Kovarik *et al.* (2015) using this new approach described that NEP is the enzyme able to generate Ang 1-7 in kidney allografts, suggesting the possibility of new RAS therapies for transplanted patients [74].

CONCLUDING REMARKS

We must emphasize that the angiotensin peptides are regulated by a variety of different pathways in tissues, cells and fluids due to the existence of many enzymes capable of generating them. Tonin, cathepsins, prolyl endopeptidase, neprilysin, chymase, angiotensin I-converting enzyme and angiotensin converting enzyme 2 are the enzymes responsible for forming angiotensin peptides. From angiotensinogen, tonin and cathepsin are able to produce AngII directly in tissues and also in circulation [75, 76].

The values for the RAS peptides range widely despite the efforts of many authors to establish consensus values for plasma and tissues; thus, it is difficult to determine the true level. Because of the ranges observed, it is important to consider not only the different methods reported in the literature, but also to critically evaluate the methods for sample collection and extraction, animal manipulation and other parameters that can affect the measured concentrations. RIA or HPLC-RIA have been considered as the best methods to quantitate angs, but when comparing them to LC-MS / MS, commonly held belief may not be valid considering the cross-reactivities of the antibodies for Ang II with Ang I and Ang 1-7 that exist, and thus may overestimate the concentrations. Although LC-MS / MS has high specificity and sensitivity in the quantification process, that is a result of identification of mass/charge peptide ratio, the values reported for the angs concentration have generally been much higher than those obtained from RIA or HPLC-RIA, and have raised questions about the validity of these values. The importance of the intracellular RAS system is gaining increased recognition and the use of highly sensitive techniques such as LC-MS/MS for angiotensin quantification is critical. Studies during the last 2 decades have described the compartmentalization of intrarenal Ang II. These studies showed high concentrations of Ang II in the proximal tubular fluid, in interstitial fluid and also in the intracellular compartments, showing that the intrarenal regulation of angiotensin peptides is important to maintaining renal homeostasis [77 - 81].

Considering all the aforementioned, it seems that the accuracy of Angs measurement has clearly increased; however, we cannot yet be certain about the absolute quantities of a specific Ang in a physiological state or in a disease state.

Nevertheless, the quantity of Angs described in pathophysiological states should be taken as a relative quantity compared to the control. By doing that, we can avoid the bias caused by the lack of either sensitivity or specificity that may be linked to the existing methods. The physiological profile of a study should not differ as a consequence of different methods despite differences in the absolute values.

Despite the massive use of RIA, HPLC-RIA, HPLC methods, the LC-MS/MS analysis will increase our ability for peptide quantification, directing us to novel discoveries related to the RAS which will contribute to the treatment of renal and cardiovascular diseases.

CONFLICT OF INTEREST

The authors confirm that they have no conflict of interest to declare for this publication.

ACKNOWLEDGEMENTS

We would like to thank CAPES Coordenação de Aperfeiçoamento de Pessoal de nível Superior, CNPq Conselho Nacional de Desenvolvimento Científico e Tecnológico and FAPESP Fundação de Amparo a Pesquisa do Estado de São Paulo.

REFERENCES

[1] Tigerstedt R, Bergman PG, Kreislauf N. Skand Arch Physiol 1898; 8: 223-71. [http://dx.doi.org/10.1111/j.1748-1716.1898.tb00272.x]

[2] Santos RA, Simoes e Silva AC, Maric C, *et al.* Angiotensin-(1-7) is an endogenous ligand for the G protein-coupled receptor Mas. Proc Natl Acad Sci USA 2003; 100(14): 8258-63. [http://dx.doi.org/10.1073/pnas.1432869100] [PMID: 12829792]

[3] Carey RM. Newly discovered components and actions of the renin-angiotensin system. Hypertension 2013; 62(5): 818-22. [http://dx.doi.org/10.1161/HYPERTENSIONAHA.113.01111] [PMID: 24082058]

[4] Carey RM, Siragy HM. Newly recognized components of the renin-angiotensin system: potential roles in cardiovascular and renal regulation. Endocr Rev 2003; 24(3): 261-71. [http://dx.doi.org/10.1210/er.2003-0001] [PMID: 12788798]

[5] Hall JE. Historical perspective of the renin-angiotensin system. Mol Biotechnol 2003; 24(1): 27-39. [http://dx.doi.org/10.1385/MB:24:1:27] [PMID: 12721494]

[6] Villela DC, Passos-Silva DG, Santos RA. Alamandine: a new member of the angiotensin family. Curr Opin Nephrol Hypertens 2014; 23(2): 130-4.
[http://dx.doi.org/10.1097/01.mnh.0000441052.44406.92] [PMID: 24389733]

[7] Ferrario CM, Chappell MC, Tallant EA, Brosnihan KB, Diz DI. Counterregulatory actions of angiotensin-(1-7). Hypertension 1997; 30(3 Pt 2): 535-41.
[http://dx.doi.org/10.1161/01.HYP.30.3.535] [PMID: 9322978]

[8] Guyton AC. Blood pressure control--special role of the kidneys and body fluids. Science 1991; 252(5014): 1813-6.
[http://dx.doi.org/10.1126/science.2063193] [PMID: 2063193]

[9] Itoh H, Mukoyama M, Pratt RE, Gibbons GH, Dzau VJ. Multiple autocrine growth factors modulate vascular smooth muscle cell growth response to angiotensin II. J Clin Invest 1993; 91(5): 2268-74.
[http://dx.doi.org/10.1172/JCI116454] [PMID: 8486785]

[10] Meng W, Busija DW. Comparative effects of angiotensin-(1-7) and angiotensin II on piglet pial arterioles. Stroke 1993; 24(12): 2041-4.
[http://dx.doi.org/10.1161/01.STR.24.12.2041] [PMID: 8248986]

[11] Navar LG, Harrison-Bernard LM, Nishiyama A, Kobori H. Regulation of intrarenal angiotensin II in hypertension. Hypertension 2002; 39(2 Pt 2): 316-22.
[http://dx.doi.org/10.1161/hy0202.103821] [PMID: 11882566]

[12] Tao X, Fan J, Kao G, *et al.* Angiotensin-(1-7) attenuates angiotensin II-induced signalling associated with activation of a tyrosine phosphatase in Sprague-Dawley rats cardiac fibroblasts. Biol Cell 2014; 106(6): 182-92.
[http://dx.doi.org/10.1111/boc.201400015] [PMID: 24641355]

[13] Ramchandran R, Takezako T, Saad Y, *et al.* Angiotensinergic stimulation of vascular endothelium in mice causes hypotension, bradycardia, and attenuated angiotensin response. Proc Natl Acad Sci USA 2006; 103(50): 19087-92.
[http://dx.doi.org/10.1073/pnas.0602715103] [PMID: 17148616]

[14] De Silva PE, Husain A, Smeby RR, Khairallah PA. Measurement of immunoreactive angiotensin peptides in rat tissues: some pitfalls in angiotensin II analysis. Anal Biochem 1988; 174(1): 80-7.
[http://dx.doi.org/10.1016/0003-2697(88)90521-0] [PMID: 2851278]

[15] Campbell DJ, Lawrence AC, Towrie A, Kladis A, Valentijn AJ. Differential regulation of angiotensin peptide levels in plasma and kidney of the rat. Hypertension 1991; 18(6): 763-73.
[http://dx.doi.org/10.1161/01.HYP.18.6.763] [PMID: 1660448]

[16] Chappell MC, Brosnihan KB, Welches WR, Ferrario CM. Characterization by high performance liquid chromatography of angiotensin peptides in the plasma and cerebrospinal fluid of the dog. Peptides 1987; 8(5): 939-42.
[http://dx.doi.org/10.1016/0196-9781(87)90084-2] [PMID: 3432137]

[17] Nagata S, Hatakeyama K, Asami M, *et al.* Big angiotensin-25: a novel glycosylated angiotensin-related peptide isolated from human urine. Biochem Biophys Res Commun 2013; 441(4): 757-62.
[http://dx.doi.org/10.1016/j.bbrc.2013.10.124] [PMID: 24211583]

[18] Haber E, Koerner T, Page LB, Kliman B, Purnode A. Application of a radioimmunoassay for

angiotensin I to the physiologic measurements of plasma renin activity in normal human subjects. J Clin Endocrinol Metab 1969; 29(10): 1349-55.
[http://dx.doi.org/10.1210/jcem-29-10-1349] [PMID: 4311082]

[19] Pelegrini-da-Silva A, Prado WA, Juliano MA, Wilk S, Martins AR. High-performance liquid chromatographic separation of renin-angiotensin system peptides and most of their metabolic fragments. J Chromatogr B Analyt Technol Biomed Life Sci 2002; 780(2): 301-7.
[http://dx.doi.org/10.1016/S1570-0232(02)00542-1] [PMID: 12401356]

[20] Graciano ML, Cavaglieri RdeC, Dellê H, *et al.* Intrarenal Renin-Angiotensin system is upregulated in experimental model of progressive renal disease induced by chronic inhibition of nitric oxide synthesis. J Am Soc Nephrol 2004; 15(7): 1805-15.
[http://dx.doi.org/10.1097/01.ASN.0000131528.00773.A9] [PMID: 15213268]

[21] Hilzendeger AM, Morais RL, Todiras M, *et al.* Leptin regulates ACE activity in mice. J Mol Med 2010; 88(9): 899-907.
[http://dx.doi.org/10.1007/s00109-010-0649-7] [PMID: 20614101]

[22] Prieto-Carrasquero MC, Botros FT, Pagan J, *et al.* Collecting duct renin is upregulated in both kidneys of 2-kidney, 1-clip goldblatt hypertensive rats. Am J Physiol Renal Physiol 2008; 295(4): F904-11.
[PMID: 18632790]

[23] Prieto MC, González-Villalobos RA, Botros FT, *et al.* Reciprocal changes in renal ACE/ANG II and ACE2/ANG 1-7 are associated with enhanced collecting duct renin in Goldblatt hypertensive rats. Am J Physiol Renal Physiol 2011; 300(3): F749-55.
[http://dx.doi.org/10.1152/ajprenal.00383.2009] [PMID: 21209009]

[24] Dias AT, Rodrigues BP, Porto ML, *et al.* Sildenafil ameliorates oxidative stress and DNA damage in the stenotic kidneys in mice with renovascular hypertension. J Transl Med 2014; 12: 35.
[http://dx.doi.org/10.1186/1479-5876-12-35] [PMID: 24502628]

[25] Hagihara GN, Lobato NS, Filgueira FP, *et al.* Upregulation of ERK1/2-eNOS *via* AT2 receptors decreases the contractile response to angiotensin II in resistance mesenteric arteries from obese rats. PLoS One 2014; 9(8): e106029.
[http://dx.doi.org/10.1371/journal.pone.0106029] [PMID: 25170617]

[26] Silva SD Jr, Zampieri TT, Ruggeri A, *et al.* Downregulation of the vascular renin-angiotensin system by aerobic training - focus on the balance between vasoconstrictor and vasodilator axes -. Circ J 2015; 79(6): 1372-80.
[http://dx.doi.org/10.1253/circj.CJ-14-1179] [PMID: 25808225]

[27] Almeida WS, Maciel TT, Di Marco GS, Casarini DE, Campos AH, Schor N. Escherichia coli lipopolysaccharide inhibits renin activity in human mesangial cells. Kidney Int 2006; 69(6): 974-80.
[http://dx.doi.org/10.1038/sj.ki.5000134] [PMID: 16528246]

[28] Zhang S, Li Y, Li H, Zheng X, Chen X. Renal-protective effect of nicousamide on hypertensive nephropathy in spontaneously hypertensive rats. Biomed Rep 2013; 1(1): 34-40.
[PMID: 24648890]

[29] Kim JM, Heo HS, Ha YM, *et al.* Mechanism of Ang II involvement in activation of NF-κB through phosphorylation of p65 during aging. Age (Dordr) 2012; 34(1): 11-25.
[http://dx.doi.org/10.1007/s11357-011-9207-7] [PMID: 21318332]

[30] Senador D, Key M, Brosnihan KB, Irigoyen MC, Elased KM, Morris M. Cardiovascular interactions between losartan and fructose in mice. J Cardiovasc Pharmacol Ther 2010; 15(1): 68-77. [http://dx.doi.org/10.1177/1074248409351409] [PMID: 19995939]

[31] Nishiyama A, Seth DM, Navar LG. Renal interstitial fluid angiotensin I and angiotensin II concentrations during local angiotensin-converting enzyme inhibition. J Am Soc Nephrol 2002; 13(9): 2207-12. [http://dx.doi.org/10.1097/01.ASN.0000026610.48842.CB] [PMID: 12191964]

[32] Arnold AC, Shaltout HA, Gilliam-Davis S, Kock ND, Diz DI. Autonomic control of the heart is altered in Sprague-Dawley rats with spontaneous hydronephrosis. Am J Physiol Heart Circ Physiol 2011; 300(6): H2206-13. [http://dx.doi.org/10.1152/ajpheart.01263.2010] [PMID: 21460193]

[33] Mustafa HI, Garland EM, Biaggioni I, *et al.* Abnormalities of angiotensin regulation in postural tachycardia syndrome. Heart Rhythm 2011; 8(3): 422-8. [http://dx.doi.org/10.1016/j.hrthm.2010.11.009] [PMID: 21266211]

[34] Zong WN, Yang XH, Chen XM, *et al.* Regulation of angiotensin-(1-7) and angiotensin II type 1 receptor by telmisartan and losartan in adriamycin-induced rat heart failure. Acta Pharmacol Sin 2011; 32(11): 1345-50. [http://dx.doi.org/10.1038/aps.2011.96] [PMID: 21963897]

[35] Gironacci MM, Brosnihan KB, Ferrario CM, *et al.* Increased hypothalamic angiotensin-(1-7) levels in rats with aortic coarctation-induced hypertension. Peptides 2007; 28(8): 1580-5. [http://dx.doi.org/10.1016/j.peptides.2007.06.016] [PMID: 17646033]

[36] Mori Y, Aritomi S, Niinuma K, *et al.* Additive effects of cilnidipine, an L-/N-type calcium channel blocker, and an angiotensin II receptor blocker on reducing cardiorenal damage in Otsuka Long-Evans Tokushima Fatty rats with type 2 diabetes mellitus. Drug Des Devel Ther 2014; 8: 799-810. [PMID: 24970998]

[37] Xiao M, Wang Y, Zhu Z, *et al.* Influence of the 5′-proximal elements of the 5′-untranslated region of classical swine fever virus on translation and replication. J Gen Virol 2011; 92(Pt 5): 1087-96. [http://dx.doi.org/10.1099/vir.0.027870-0] [PMID: 21307229]

[38] Ferrario CM, Varagic J, Habibi J, *et al.* Differential regulation of angiotensin-(1-12) in plasma and cardiac tissue in response to bilateral nephrectomy. Am J Physiol Heart Circ Physiol 2009; 296(4): H1184-92. [http://dx.doi.org/10.1152/ajpheart.01114.2008] [PMID: 19218503]

[39] Cole J, Ertoy D, Lin H, *et al.* Lack of angiotensin II-facilitated erythropoiesis causes anemia in angiotensin-converting enzyme-deficient mice. J Clin Invest 2000; 106(11): 1391-8. [http://dx.doi.org/10.1172/JCI10557] [PMID: 11104792]

[40] Li XC, Cook JL, Rubera I, Tauc M, Zhang F, Zhuo JL. Intrarenal transfer of an intracellular fluorescent fusion of angiotensin II selectively in proximal tubules increases blood pressure in rats and mice. Am J Physiol Renal Physiol 2011; 300(5): F1076-88. [http://dx.doi.org/10.1152/ajprenal.00329.2010] [PMID: 21307128]

[41] Xiao HD, Fuchs S, Campbell DJ, *et al.* Mice with cardiac-restricted angiotensin-converting enzyme

(ACE) have atrial enlargement, cardiac arrhythmia, and sudden death. Am J Pathol 2004; 165(3): 1019-32.
[http://dx.doi.org/10.1016/S0002-9440(10)63363-9] [PMID: 15331425]

[42] Wysocki J, Ortiz-Melo DI, Mattocks NK, *et al.* ACE2 deficiency increases NADPH-mediated oxidative stress in the kidney. Physiol Rep 2014; 2(3): e00264.
[http://dx.doi.org/10.1002/phy2.264] [PMID: 24760518]

[43] Peña Silva RA, Chu Y, Miller JD, *et al.* Impact of ACE2 deficiency and oxidative stress on cerebrovascular function with aging. Stroke 2012; 43(12): 3358-63.
[http://dx.doi.org/10.1161/STROKEAHA.112.667063] [PMID: 23160880]

[44] Sim MK, Qui XS. Angiotensins in plasma of hypertensive rats and human. Regul Pept 2003; 111(1-3): 179-82.
[http://dx.doi.org/10.1016/S0167-0115(02)00289-6] [PMID: 12609766]

[45] Ronchi FA, Irigoyen MC, Casarini DE. Association of somatic and N-domain angiotensin-converting enzymes from Wistar rat tissue with renal dysfunction in diabetes mellitus. J Renin Angiotensin Aldosterone Syst 2007; 8(1): 34-41.
[http://dx.doi.org/10.3317/jraas.2007.005] [PMID: 17487824]

[46] Kobori H, Prieto-Carrasquero MC, Ozawa Y, Navar LG. AT1 receptor mediated augmentation of intrarenal angiotensinogen in angiotensin II-dependent hypertension. Hypertension 2004; 43(5): 1126-32.
[http://dx.doi.org/10.1161/01.HYP.0000122875.91100.28] [PMID: 15037565]

[47] Ong FS, Lin CX, Campbell DJ, *et al.* Increased angiotensin II-induced hypertension and inflammatory cytokines in mice lacking angiotensin-converting enzyme N domain activity. Hypertension 2012; 59(2): 283-90.
[http://dx.doi.org/10.1161/HYPERTENSIONAHA.111.180844] [PMID: 22203735]

[48] Wysocki J, Ye M, Rodriguez E, *et al.* Targeting the degradation of angiotensin II with recombinant angiotensin-converting enzyme 2: prevention of angiotensin II-dependent hypertension. Hypertension 2010; 55(1): 90-8.
[http://dx.doi.org/10.1161/HYPERTENSIONAHA.109.138420] [PMID: 19948988]

[49] Carroll MA, *et al.* Azilsartan Is Associated With Increased Circulating Angiotensin-(1-7) Levels and Reduced Renovascular 20-HETE Levels. Am J Hypertens 2015; 8(5): 664-71.
[http://dx.doi.org/10.1093/ajh/hpu201] [PMID: 25384409]

[50] Dagan A, Gattineni J, Habib S, Baum M. Effect of prenatal dexamethasone on postnatal serum and urinary angiotensin II levels. Am J Hypertens 2010; 23(4): 420-4.
[http://dx.doi.org/10.1038/ajh.2009.274] [PMID: 20075846]

[51] Granado M, Fernández N, Monge L, *et al.* Long-term effects of early overnutrition in the heart of male adult rats: role of the renin-angiotensin system. PLoS One 2014; 8(6): e65172.
[http://dx.doi.org/10.1371/journal.pone.0065172] [PMID: 23755190]

[52] Ferrario CM, Jessup JA, Smith RD. Hemodynamic and hormonal patterns of untreated essential hypertension in men and women. Ther Adv Cardiovasc Dis 2013; 7(6): 293-305.
[http://dx.doi.org/10.1177/1753944713513221] [PMID: 24280597]

[53] Campbell DJ, Lawrence AC, Towrie A, Kladis A, Valentijn AJ. Differential regulation of angiotensin peptide levels in plasma and kidney of the rat. Hypertension 1991; 18(6): 763-73. [http://dx.doi.org/10.1161/01.HYP.18.6.763] [PMID: 1660448]

[54] Ohnishi K, Murase M, Nakano D, *et al.* Angiotensin-converting enzyme inhibitor does not suppress renal angiotensin II levels in angiotensin I-infused rats. J Pharmacol Sci 2013; 122(2): 103-8. [http://dx.doi.org/10.1254/jphs.13045FP] [PMID: 23698111]

[55] Hu W, Zhao QY, Yu SB, *et al.* Renal sympathetic denervation inhibits the development of left ventricular mechanical dyssynchrony during the progression of heart failure in dogs. Cardiovasc Ultrasound 2014; 12: 47. [http://dx.doi.org/10.1186/1476-7120-12-47] [PMID: 25416926]

[56] Ahmed MA. Effect of angiotensin II type 1 receptor blocker on renal function, arterial blood pressure and parathyroid hormone related protein over expression in cadmium induced nephrotoxicity in adult male rats. Int J Physiol Pathophysiol Pharmacol 2013; 5(2): 109-19. [PMID: 23750309]

[57] Walkowska A, Skaroupková P, Husková Z, *et al.* Intrarenal cytochrome P-450 metabolites of arachidonic acid in the regulation of the nonclipped kidney function in two-kidney, one-clip Goldblatt hypertensive rats. J Hypertens 2010; 28(3): 582-93. [http://dx.doi.org/10.1097/HJH.0b013e328334dfd4] [PMID: 19940786]

[58] Hara M, Ono K, Hwang MW, *et al.* Evidence for a role of mast cells in the evolution to congestive heart failure. J Exp Med 2002; 195(3): 375-81. [http://dx.doi.org/10.1084/jem.20002036] [PMID: 11828013]

[59] Deng J, Wang DX, Deng W. [Effect of angiotensin II on expression of alveolar epithelial sodium channel in rat]. Zhongguo Wei Zhong Bing Ji Jiu Yi Xue 2011; 23(9): 551-4. [http://dx.doi.org/10.3760/cma. j.issn.1003-0603.2011.09.009] [PMID: 21944177]

[60] Imaki R, Niwano S, Niwano H, *et al.* Neutral endopeptidase inhibitor suppresses the early phase of atrial electrical remodeling in a canine rapid atrial pacing model. Indian Pacing Electrophysiol J 2008; 8(2): 102-13. [PMID: 18379655]

[61] Chappell MC, Brosnihan KB, Diz DI, Ferrario CM. Identification of angiotensin-(1-7) in rat brain. Evidence for differential processing of angiotensin peptides. J Biol Chem 1989; 264(28): 16518-23. [PMID: 2777795]

[62] Belmadani S, Bernal J, Wei CC, *et al.* A thrombospondin-1 antagonist of transforming growth factor-beta activation blocks cardiomyopathy in rats with diabetes and elevated angiotensin II. Am J Pathol 2007; 171(3): 777-89. [http://dx.doi.org/10.2353/ajpath.2007.070056] [PMID: 17640965]

[63] Moore DJ, Perrino PJ, Klerer CP, Robertson P. High-performance liquid chromatographic assay for two rifamycin-derived hypocholesterolemic agents in liver and biological fluids. J Chromatogr A 1993; 612(2): 310-4. [http://dx.doi.org/10.1016/0378-4347(93)80178-7] [PMID: 8468390]

[64] Braithwaite JE, Yandle TG, Nicholls MG, Lewis LK. Interference by o-phenanthroline in the

radioimmunoassay of angiotensin II in small volume blood samples. Clin Biochem 2012; 45(1-2): 168-70.
[http://dx.doi.org/10.1016/j.clinbiochem.2011.10.008] [PMID: 22040809]

[65] Bujak-Gizycka B, Madej J, Wołkow PP, *et al.* Measurement of angiotensin metabolites in organ bath and cell culture experiments by liquid chromatography - electrospray ionization - mass spectrometry (LC-ESI-MS). J Physiol Pharmacol 2007; 58(3): 529-40.
[PMID: 17928648]

[66] Wang X, Sha Y, Hou X, Li R. Electrospray ionization tandem mass spectrometric analysis of fragmentation patterns of dithiocarbamate derivatives. Rapid Commun Mass Spectrom 2006; 20(4): 719-22.
[http://dx.doi.org/10.1002/rcm.2344] [PMID: 16444799]

[67] Stoppacher N, Josephs RD, Daireaux A, Choteau T, Westwood SW, Wielgosz RI. Impurity identification and determination for the peptide hormone angiotensin I by liquid chromatography-hig--resolution tandem mass spectrometry and the metrological impact on value assignments by amino acid analysis. Anal Bioanal Chem 2013; 405(25): 8039-51.
[http://dx.doi.org/10.1007/s00216-013-6953-7] [PMID: 23708692]

[68] Ali Q, Wu Y, Nag S, Hussain T. Estimation of angiotensin peptides in biological samples by LC/MS method. Anal Methods 2014; 6(1): 215-22.
[http://dx.doi.org/10.1039/C3AY41305E] [PMID: 24489613]

[69] Park S, Bivona BJ, Kobori H, *et al.* Major role for ACE-independent intrarenal ANG II formation in type II diabetes. Am J Physiol Renal Physiol 2010; 298(1): F37-48.
[http://dx.doi.org/10.1152/ajprenal.00519.2009] [PMID: 19846569]

[70] Modrall JG, Sadjadi J, Brosnihan KB, *et al.* Depletion of tissue angiotensin-converting enzyme differentially influences the intrarenal and urinary expression of angiotensin peptides. Hypertension 2004; 43(4): 849-53.
[http://dx.doi.org/10.1161/01.HYP.0000121462.27393.f6] [PMID: 14981053]

[71] Lortie M, Bark S, Blantz R, Hook V. Detecting low-abundance vasoactive peptides in plasma: progress toward absolute quantitation using nano liquid chromatography-mass spectrometry. Anal Biochem 2009; 394(2): 164-70.
[http://dx.doi.org/10.1016/j.ab.2009.07.021] [PMID: 19615967]

[72] Schulz A, Jankowski J, Zidek W, Jankowski V. Absolute quantification of endogenous angiotensin II levels in human plasma using ESI-LC-MS/MS. Clin Proteomics 2014; 11(1): 37.
[http://dx.doi.org/10.1186/1559-0275-11-37] [PMID: 25505856]

[73] Poglitsch M, Domenig O, Schwager C, *et al.* Recombinant expression and characterization of human and murine ACE2: Species-specific activation of the alternative renin-angiotensin-system. Journal of Hypertension 2012; 2012(Article ID 428950): 8.
[http://dx.doi.org/10.1155/2012/428950]

[74] Kovarik JJ, Kaltenecker CC, Domenig O, *et al.* 8d.03: evidence for an ace-independent tissue-specific ras regulation after kidney transplantation. J Hypertens 2015; 33 (Suppl. 1): e113-4.
[http://dx.doi.org/10.1097/01.hjh.0000467657.23414.54] [PMID: 26102690]

[75] Belova LA. Angiotensin II-generating enzymes. Biochemistry (Mosc) 2000; 65(12): 1337-45.

[http://dx.doi.org/10.1023/A:1002848402911] [PMID: 11173502]

[76] Kobori H, Nangaku M, Navar LG, Nishiyama A. The intrarenal renin-angiotensin system: from physiology to the pathobiology of hypertension and kidney disease. Pharmacol Rev 2007; 59(3): 251-87.
[http://dx.doi.org/10.1124/pr.59.3.3] [PMID: 17878513]

[77] Navar LG, Imig JD, Zou L, Wang CT. Intrarenal production of angiotensin II. Semin Nephrol 1997; 17(5): 412-22.
[PMID: 9316209]

[78] Navar LG, Harrison-Bernard LM, Imig JD, Wang CT, Cervenka L, Mitchell KD. Intrarenal angiotensin II generation and renal effects of AT1 receptor blockade. J Am Soc Nephrol 1999; 10 (Suppl. 12): S266-72.
[PMID: 10201881]

[79] Navar LG, Nishiyama A. Intrarenal formation of angiotensin II. Contrib Nephrol 2001; (135): 1-15.
[http://dx.doi.org/10.1159/000060154] [PMID: 11705276]

[80] Navar LG. The intrarenal renin-angiotensin system in hypertension. Kidney Int 2004; 65(4): 1522-32.
[http://dx.doi.org/10.1111/j.1523-1755.2004.00539.x] [PMID: 15086502]

[81] Zhuo JL, Imig JD, Hammond TG, Orengo S, Benes E, Navar LG. Ang II accumulation in rat renal endosomes during Ang II-induced hypertension: role of AT(1) receptor. Hypertension 2002; 39(1): 116-21.
[http://dx.doi.org/10.1161/hy0102.100780] [PMID: 11799089]

SUBJECT INDEX

A

B

C

G

H

I

J

K

L

M

R

Made in the USA
Las Vegas, NV
03 November 2026

57424117R00231